AF685892

# Heal Yourself the European Way

Betsy Morscher

Parker Publishing Company, Inc.

West Nyack, New York

© 1980 by

Betsy Morscher

All rights reserved. No part of this book may be reproduced in any form or by any means, without permission in writing from the publisher.

*This book is a reference work based on research by the author. The opinions expressed herein are not necessarily those of or endorsed by the publisher. The directions stated in this book are in no way to be considered as a substitute for consultation with a duly licensed doctor.*

**Library of Congress Cataloging in Publication Data**

Morscher, Betsy
Heal yourself the European way.

Includes index.
1. Health. 2. Therapeutics, Physiological.
3. Health resorts, watering-places, etc.—Europe.
I. Title.
RA776.5.M64 613 80-13653
ISBN 0-13-384404-8

Printed in the United States of America

*Heal Yourself the European Way is dedicated to Harriet Stern, M.D. who helped me begin to heal myself and to Dagmar Liechti-von Brasch, M.D. who believed in me and my destiny.*

*A special thanks to my children, Monica, Maria, Vincent; to Boobie; to the Sisters at Queen of Peace Oratory and Marycrest Convent; to the staff at Beth Joseph Synagogue; to Nancy O'Brien and Lucy Arnold; to Agnes and Grif Griffiths; and to all those anonymous people who urged me onward by saying that I couldn't do it.*

# Medical Doctor's Comment

During the past several years, numerous books and articles have awakened the American public to the issue of responsibility for one's own health. Doctors Friedman and Rosenman wrote about "Type-A" behavior and cardiac disease; Norman Shealy, M.D. has written a great deal about holistic treatment approaches; Dr. Cooper started an "aerobic" revolution; Adelle Davis and Dr. Cheraskin increased public awareness of proper nutrition, and so on. Recently, Norman Cousins (*Anatomy of An Illness*) described his creative approach for dealing with a near-fatal degenerative disease. The evolving theme underlines an increasing awareness that the individual has a crucial role to play in both the prevention and amelioration of illness.

It is not necessary to feel like a helpless victim, overwhelmed with life's afflictions. The days of passive patienthood appear to be numbered, while newer methods are presented for active participation in one's health and well-being. Most of us have experienced the phenomena of getting a common cold or some other illness at a time when our resistance was low. We are continually surrounded and bombarded by the seeds of disease throughout our lives. Yet, our own immunity and inner strength prevents most illnesses from gaining a foothold. It takes a vulnerable host to permit illness to flourish. There is even some recent evidence that major diseases such as cancer, arthritis, hypertension and others are related to lifestyle and host susceptibility. If so, there is a glimmer of hope in the contention itself. It would imply that these individuals can shed the role of demoralizing helplessness and assert an active, more vital role in regaining their health.

Traditional medicine has focused for too long on only two facets of a three-faceted health paradigm. There have been brilliant advances in the discovery and reduction of illness-producing agents. Secondly, we have made unparalleled drug discoveries. However, we have drifted in a rather neglectful manner from the vital role of host resistance. It's not merely the bug or the medicine that's crucial, but also the defensive strength of the individual. This developing field truly offers a panorama of opportunities. Yet, the concept is difficult for many. It requires courage and persistence to shift from a life-long illusion that health is a temporary condition of chance, while illness is "for the doctor to handle." Yet again, while the price of responsibility is high, there is the reward of feeling more control over one's life.

*Heal Yourself the European Way* will be welcomed into the ever-expanding holistic health literature. It delightfully underscores the cornerstone theme that sound health is an individual endeavor, not available from a doctor's prescription pad. As the word "heal" implies, one must be total in one's approach (the words "heal," "health," "whole," "holy," "total" are all derived from the same word root.) Betsy Morscher takes you on an enriching odyssey into the European world of holistic wellness. She provides a witty and vibrant account of her experiences in Europe's major health spas, as well as her abundant knowledge of wellness and stress management methods.

In reading this book, I couldn't help wondering where we have been for the past 2500 years. The European health spas seem to have recaptured the essence of the Temples of Asclapias in ancient Greece, where "whole-person" healing had its inception. In those bygone Temples, an ailing citizen was provided with a serene environment in the country, massage, soothing music, water therapy, relaxation techniques, nutritional guidance and a spiritual counselor to aid with dream interpretation. Although reminiscent of the past, Betsy's book has moved eons ahead, providing a veritable treasure-house of valuable information. It is written clearly, and free of either professional or aquarian jargon. Any serious reader can immediately apply any one of numerous and imaginative health concepts.

What makes this book even more enjoyable to read is the knowledge that Betsy Morscher lives what she writes. It is no rarity for her to whip out a jump rope from her purse and get in a few minutes of intense exercise while waiting for a bus. Or, she might surprise a coffee group by pulling out one of a variety of herbal tea bags she keeps handy for such occasions. I was particularly impressed with her chapter on creating a home spa. All of the author's accumulated knowledge of nutrition, family relationships, exercise, yoga, and stress management is skillfully synthesized into a humorous and factual assortment of practical "how to do what each day" ideas. One can even learn along the way that "relief is spelled p-a-p-a-y-a."

*Joel F. Miller, M.D., P.C.*

# A Word from the Author

"Why take a twenty-thousand mile odyssey to all those glorified watering holes of Europe?" asked a friend of mine. "Prevention of illness," was my response. A few years ago I discovered that the basic difference between the European and American approach to medicine is: in Europe, healthful measures are built into the life style to ward off future illness. In the United States the method is curative in nature. The idea "if you've got an illness, we've got an antibiotic," has not always worked. Americans with minimal health insurance, or those who desire to assume responsibility for their own health care, question this "after the fact" attitude.

Rising American hospital expenses, which escalate daily, rivaling the National debt, made me believe that health care alternatives had to be available.

As one who feels no compunction to subsidize the American health industry, I trekked to Europe to discover my personal health choices.

In early summer, 1977, I arrived in Germany for the first phase of my new health orientation in Bads, spas and kliniks on the other side of the Atlantic. Fasting at the Buchinger Sanitorium in Bad Pyrmont was just the beginning. My sojourn took me throughout northern, southern and eastern Europe. Each experience added another stepping stone in my personal path to a healthier life and the avoidance of illness.

When I returned to the United States, I made radical changes in my life style. Rather than run through the Austrian woods at dawn, I jogged in a local park. At midday I napped, as is the custom in Europe. I gave out different programs to my friends to see if these European regimes were adaptable to the American way of life. Home treatments mentioned in this book have been personally tried.

The most impressive part of my European adventure was the genuine concern and care that was evidenced by medical doctors in the spas and kliniks. They saw the patient as a human being with a problem, not "an appendix, gall bladder or bed number." Their dedication undoubtedly contributed to the well-being of their patients.

I learned that health results from harmony of living . . . the body, mind and spirit working together to bring about healing or the prevention of illness. This is the basis of the home program that I have initiated in this book. *Heal Yourself the European Way* will show you how to use natural, do-it-yourself health programs in the home and to alleviate common ailments and to enjoy youthful vitality.

The European health secrets are now yours. Turn the pages—see for yourself how you can cope with stress, tap hidden sources of dynamic energy and experience more zest in your life.

The foods mentioned in my book can be obtained at any nearby supermarket or health food store. The programs are not a substitute for medical treatment, merely a supplement. Anyone seriously ill should consult a medical doctor rather than attempt self healing.

Arthur Schopenhauer, the German philosopher, represented a profound truth when he said: *Health Is All . . . Without Health, All Is Nothing!*

Betsy Morscher

# PREFACE

*As you begin a self-healing journey in the quest of health,*
*your own Holy Grail, you may bring with you and share*
*with others on life's path . . .*
*a bit more truth,*
*and more justice*
*with a bit more love,*
*than there would have been;*
*and a solemn thank you for the gift of life and vitality.*

*To you my readers, I wish the best of health . . .*
*and L'Chaim . . . "To Life" . . . yours and mine.*

# Contents

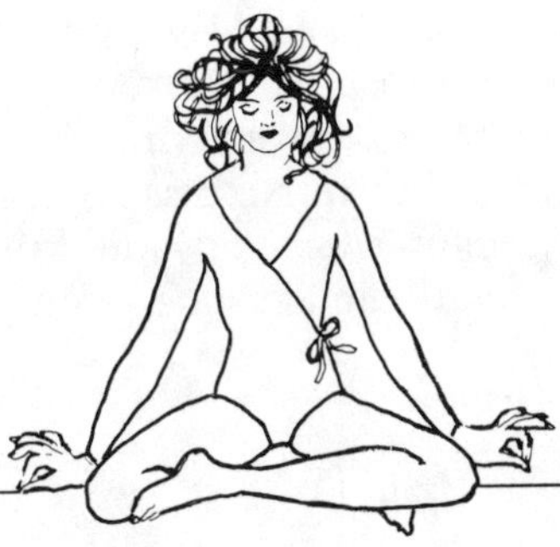

# 1

# Live Longer the European Way

*Fear less, hope more*
*Eat less, chew more*
*Whine less, breathe more*
*Hate less, love more*
*And all good things are yours . . .*
*Swedish proverb*

Imagine yourself strolling down a verdant path. Everywhere you look lush foliage welcomes you, emanating fragrances in pollution-free air. You meander down a cure path and hear the strains of a symphony in the distance as you pass picturesque scenery and classic statuary. Become aware of the nurturing atmosphere. Every sense seems stimulated with positivism and health. Is this the Garden of Paradise? No, it's a European spa where millions trek annually to take a "Kur," the German word for cure.

In the distance people are dining on freshly picked fruits and vegetables, basking on herbal baths or resting. An octogenarian is vigorously walking up a rugged path that goes through the Black Forest. This is part of the terrain cure. That attractive woman who is participating in the gymnastics program by the laurel bush has been coming here every year since her cancer was arrested.

Beyond her is a tall gentleman who used to be confined to a wheelchair, who now walks five miles a day with a cane, despite his advanced years. See the young girl smiling? When she came here she was crippled with rheumatoid arthritis. That disease is now just a memory for her. Now she vigorously skates, dances and lives an active life. What about those droves of people who seem so relaxed as they stroll along? They are spa regulars who come to prevent illness.

*Prevention!* That's the magical word to health success here. It is served with smiles and understanding at many spas, Bads and kliniks throughout Europe. While our American medicine is concentrating on disease, the emphasis here is on health.

## MUSIC AIDS IN TREATMENT

Music in the background is coming from the Kur park orchestra that is a regular part of the setting. Often a medical doctor will write out a prescription for a patient to listen to Strauss waltzes as part of his treatment, just as his American medical counterpart would write a prescription for penicillin.

Music therapy is a regular feature of some spas and Bads. Certain sounds and tonal qualities affect a particular body organ or person in various ways. Medieval Baroque and Renaissance music are calming, orderly, meditative and lend themselves to the healing climate. Chopin waltzes, triumphant marches and entrancing symphonies offer a sense of healing joy. Bach's musical style is emotionally inspiring and reportedly schizophrenic children and adults recover more quickly if exposed to his works. By being in touch with how you are affected, you can profit from the healing principles of music.

Kur doctors emphasize that your health depends upon the quality of your daily life. They attempt to assist you in finding a life style for you that will encourage wellness. You are asked if you are interested in your work, in your relationships, in the world out there and the world within you. The belief is that interest plus vitality equals wellness. That is, a healthy life is a dance between the extremes of newness and tradition.

## WHAT HAPPENS AT A SPA?

Health seekers who have experienced failure with conventional medical approaches may rejoice in "spa-ing." In these healing settings you can let nature and harmless, drugless naturopathic methods give you a new lease on life.

The spa therapy of naturopathy is based on finding the cause of the illness, eliminating it and having the body heal itself. Remedies used include fasting, hydrotherapy, fresh air, sunshine, pleasant surroundings, exercise, rest and recreation, and most importantly, proper nutrition that emphasizes fresh fruits, vegetables and grains.

Working with a medical advisor, the patient learns how to regain his health and protect himself from a relapse after he has left the spa, Bad or clinic. Every aspect of the person, not merely the medical one, must be brought into focus.

In places like Switzerland's renowned Bircher-Benner Klinic, a total environment which regulates one's way of life under medical supervision, helps a person to develop his own vital forces for recovery. An atmosphere of security and confidence helps the person to find courage and to gain personal power and energy.

Dr. Liechti von Brasch, medical director of the Bircher-Benner Klinik in Zurich, said, "Until a person establishes a code of life and brings his system into balance by understanding the rhythm and harmony, he will continue to be ill."

## NATURE USED TO CURE

The basis of the European cures that have been successful for centuries consists of the natural remedies of the earth, climate and landscape as applied in spa therapy. Waters, herbs and fresh fruits and vegetables are some of the natural resources that are taken unchanged from nature, and used therapeutically. They, in turn, touch off natural reactions in the human body.

## THE ENVIRONMENT SETS THE STAGE FOR HEALING

The cure environment is just as critical as the "kur" itself. Most spas are nestled in verdant areas where the air is charged with invigorating qualities of ozone, the climate is pleasant, the vistas are outstanding and serenity prevails.

Magnificent old-world architecture and its accompanying elegant ambiance are coupled with modernistic klinik facilities that hug a mountain site, seashore or center of a village. Those that are called *Bads*, the German word for "bath," are built around mineral springs whose healing waters are used to relax, rejuvenate and ease aches and pains while cleansing the system.

Since early Romans restored their battle-scarred bodies in hot mineral springs, Europeans have traveled to various watering hamlets. The natural qualities of the waters act favorably upon affected organs. Many Kur directors—professionals who oversee the Bads functions, say chemical reactions in mineral baths create antibody formations, enhancing circulation in the adrenal glands and the muscles. Roman physiologists say that the skin absorbs water just as the intestines do, which aids in the prevention of disease.

In the 1500s when the ancient physician Paracelsus advised, "Go on your journey to a watering place when the days are getting longer," he used intuition to discover the healing powers of the springs and moors rather than relying on scientific arguments. Today science has furnished proof of the healing power of the mineral springs. The character of each mineral spring is determined by its ion content. Magnesium, sodium and calcium sulphate are only some of the compounds that are used and applied in internal and external hydrotherapies (mineral baths).

## NATURE HEALS IN NATUROPATHIC THERAPIES

Many spas and Bads base their therapies on the philosophy of naturopathy. This belief declares that much acute disease is nature's way of eliminating waste matter in the tissues of the body. Within the organism itself lies the essential healing force for overcoming disease. The body can build up its own resistence to disease if given a chance. In this relaxing spa setting the body begins to use its curative powers to heal and strengthen itself against further illness. No drugs or surgery are used; as opposed to the American approach which removes the symptoms surgically or with synthetic drugs—without dealing with the basic cause of the disease.

## NATUROPATHIC MEDICINE

Since the time of Hippocrates, naturopathy has developed into a blend of scientific knowledge and an instinctive reliance on nature. Medical doctors who practice homeopathy in Europe, which many do in spas and kliniks, seek to understand the body/mind relationship and work in harmony with the natural laws to create balance. In a sense, naturopathy is an attempt to combine the scientific with the intuitive. People become in tune with their own bodily signals and share these with the doctor. The modern medicine that the doctors use in this treatment is drugless, but it has plenty of humanity and spirit. They use such treatments as water therapy, foods, rest, massage, exercise, reflexology and botanical herbs.

One of the primary phenomenon that occurs with this treatment is a "Law of Cure," which means that as the body becomes better nourished and internally cleansed, the symptoms of old illnesses begin to reappear in reverse chronological order. For example, if a 45-year-old person has arthritis as his chief illness, but has a history of poor digestion, migraines, constipation, headaches and stomach problems, he might experience some of these problems in the course of his healing. Although he may generally feel better in the course of his healing, he may go through periods of "healing crises" for short periods of time. The Naturopathic doctor can distinguish "healing crisis symptoms" from the same symptoms within a current disease process.

Naturopathic treatment, unlike traditional medicine, requires that a person take a very active role in his own healing process. Patience, fortitude and a willingness to overcome past destructive health habits are part of the requirements for co-working in self healing.

## WHAT IS THE FIRST STEP OF THE HEALING PROCESS?

Cleanse the body! Some people need a building and repairing process because their systems are depleted. A person who is frail and overburdened with stress may not be able to endure additional trauma at this time. Yet, a cleansing process may make a relatively well-nourished person feel better and increase his emotional stamina. *The better-nourished person will be able to cooperate with the healing process. His healthier body will be able to discharge toxins more efficiently.*

Education or re-education in the proper nutrition is essential to sustain the body with new vitality. Not only is it a matter of knowing that eating raw fruits and vegetables, grains and herb teas is important, but so are where and how to shop for food, how to prepare it, as well as when and how to eat certain foods.

## BUILDING UNDERSTANDING ABOUT FOOD AND EMOTIONS

A person must regain and give himself power over his own body and permit himself to be healthy. If he felt "married to an ulcer" he must understand he may have chosen it in response to a life situation.

I once felt destined to an early demise from cancer. After all, both my parents and 12 family members had succumbed to this dreaded disease at an early age; why not me? I presumed that the digestive problems, occassional insomnia and weight fluctuations I experienced over the years were pre-cancer symptoms. Finally, when I experienced the full spa treatment and assumed the responsibility for my own health, I realized that I did not have to become ill. I began making healthy choices to encourage my body to self heal. After I had turned my own state of health around to an optimal level, I felt that I should share that information with others, thus this book.

## FINDING SPIRITUAL NOURISHMENT

Ask yourself what gives your life meaning. Find a spiritual mentor to help you along the way. I'm not advocating "guru-hopping," but I do suggest that you choose a spiritual leader and discipline that enables you to live more fully. I first began my spiritual self healing when I realized that I was strolling down the wrong path. I was learning how to die prematurely. It was only until I could honestly admit that fact to myself and take the appropriate action to change that I began to live spiritually, psychically and emotionally. I owe a debt of gratitude to Dr. Viktor Frankl, the renowned Viennese psychiatrist who, during World War II, spent years in concentration camps before evolving his philosophy of Logotherapy. One summer day when I was interviewing him for a radio program, he stopped, looked me right in the eye with his steady gaze and said, "What really does give your life meaning? If you were to die tomorrow, would it have been worth it? Have you really lived? Would you have any regrets?" Those questions created a long, pregnant pause in my life. It took years before I could begin to answer them. But when I did, I knew that I was not only heading down the road to health but I was jogging at a good clip.

## WHAT IS HOMEOPATHY?

This system, like naturopathy, is geared toward treating the person and not the disease. Homeopathy is based on the premise that a remedy can cure a disease if it produces symptoms similar to those of the disease in a healthy organism.

A homeopathic doctor is not concerned with killing bacteria, as many American medical doctors feel, but with bringing the whole human organism into a state where it is impossible for bacteria to thrive. For the homeopathic doctor, a patient is ill if he feels sick. For the allopathic doctor, a patient is ill only if his doctor can see it in the laboratory via a tumor or pathological tissue change. The homeopathic doctor honors the patient's bodily observations and helps him cure his functional disorders before they have a chance to become pathological tissue.

## A PERSON IS TREATED—NOT JUST A BODY PART

As mentioned before, this whole approach to health is centered in the person not—an organ of the body. Many people go to spas to prevent future illness, while others go to restore health. Whether the motivation is preventive or curative, they know that they will be respected as people who want to take responsibility for their health and have the medical doctors function as auxiliary support.

"Joie do vie," joy of living, as the French say, occurs when a daily rhythm involves a balance between tension and relaxation, work and rest, physical and mental activities, and a reasonable diet. European "spa-ers" know that health is dependent upon the quality of life as well as the body, mind and spirit working together.

This concept is not new. Awareness of the connection between the health of the body and the mind has been around since the early Greek and Roman civilizations, when spas had their genesis. The Latin saying: "Mens sana in corpore sano," means "A healthy mind in a healthy body." Our ancestors knew that physical and mental health were clearly related.

Somewhere in our most recent past, we moderns in America have lost this awareness of the synthesis between body and mind. In American medicine there is fragmentation: "He is a heart problem," "She is a psychosomatic." There seems to be a division between mental problems and physical illness.

Not so in Europe. Ganzheit therapy, or "total" therapy, refers to the body, mind and spirit working together to heal, to prevent illness. This concept of integrative health has full, vibrant well-being as its objective, rather than symptom removal and crisis intervention. Ganzheit in a process of centering, integrating, balancing and finding harmony in your daily life. This approach to health is based on a love of life rather than a fear of death.

## WHAT IS HEALTH?

Wherever I traveled, I asked this question and received assorted responses. Here are some of the concepts: "Positive health is a state of maximum preparedness the person can have to accomplish his life goals and withstand the constant exposure and adaption to stress." Another said: "Health is the delicate balance . . . a state of equilibrium in every period of life between physical, mental, spiritual function." And yet others said . . . "Health is aliveness and vitality." My favorite definition is from Dr. Max Bircher-Benner, who said . . . "Health is life and wisdom." He further stated: "The deeper you sense life, the more life approaches wisdom and health. If I could grasp life in its deepest sense, I would know that it is the same as wisdom and the same as health. I need not become sick nor remain sick. I can recover as soon as I understand life."

Maladaptive life styles, frayed nerves, junk food eating patterns and improper rest are all targets in the spa treatments.

## YOU HAVE THE ANSWERS TO YOUR HEALTH

The belief is widely held in European spas that we each possess an inner wisdom that knows how to heal any disease in our systems, as well as to maintain our energy at an optimal level.

Learning to listen to your inner wisdom, you can tell the nature of your imbalance. Is the headache set off by too many stimulants, such as coffee? If you've been working too hard or have some unresolved emotional problem, colds and minor accidents often occur. Such symptoms are not only signs of imbalance in your body. Low energy, irritability or restlessness may all indicate that something is not right.

Many Kur directors state that as you tune-in more and more to that inner direction, you will see the importance of responding to positive feelings as well as understanding the negative ones.

The movement towards health involves experimenting with your life style, listening to the feedback and attempting to do those things you want to do that bring joy and achievement to your life.

"Tune into the realization of your own uniqueness" is a phrase that resounds in many a curist's ear.

## WE HAVE FORGOTTEN HOW TO LIVE

Many first-time spa-goers find that in our rush towards the 21st century, we spend 90 percent of our waking hours doing what we like to do least. Health is dependent upon the quality of life. In our 20th century rat race we get caught up with go, run, do. We acquire quantities of possessions, but what about the quality, the meaningfulness of life? Learning how to live, to really enjoy what we do with our allotted time on earth is a question of health. Interest in living can often prevent overdrinking, overeating and the developing of self-destructive habits that destroy health.

## CONTRAST WITH AMERICAN VALUES

While Europeans emphasize preventive measures in their approach to medicine, Americans stress curative means. Our research in the areas of cancer, arthritis and heart diseases have been directed toward drugs that will cure or control the disease. European research has been directed toward finding the causative factors of disease and developing means of preventing it.

Europeans consider nutritious food as the basis of many healing remedies. In the United States, nutrition as a contributing factor in health or illness has been virtually ignored, even though the 1977 U.S. Senate Hearings before the Committee of Nutrition and Human Needs pointed out the relation of diet to diseases.

Is it an accident that very few American medical schools offer classes in nutrition? Have you received valid nutritional information from your medical doctor? Is it economically profitable in the United States for doctors not to know about nutrition? Sickness: big business . . . Health: no business?

Nutrition is the most acute factor affecting health. Yet a recent Department of Agriculture survey indicated that only half the American public is eating a nutritionally adequate diet. This means that the other half are malnourished. Strange, that in a country that has the most abundant food supply in the world, one-half of the population is malnourished!

In the United States we have a love affair with meat; yet such excessive animal protein is responsible for many degenerative diseases.

The mortality rate in the United States is higher than in most civilized countries. In life expectancy among nations, the United States ranks 22nd for men and 10th for women. Despite billions of dollars spent here on health care each year, there are still over 86 million chronically ill people.

*Look at the countries with the highest life expectancies:*

| | Men | Women | Average |
|---|---|---|---|
| 1. Sweden, Europe | 71.8 | 76.5 | 74.2 |
| 2. The Netherlands, Europe | 71.0 | 76.4 | 73.7 |
| 3. Iceland, North Atlantic | 70.8 | 76.2 | 73.5 |
| 4. Norway, Europe | 71.0 | 76.0 | 73.5 |
| 5. Denmark, Europe | 70.6 | 75.4 | 73.0 |
| 6. Ryukyu Islands, West Pacific | | | |
| 7. Canada, North America | | | |
| 8. France, Europe | 68.0 | 75.5 | 71.7 |
| 9. Japan, Asia | | | |
| 10. United Kingdom, Europe | 68.5 | 74.7 | 71.6 |

More alarming is the fact that the situation worsens each year. Today the major medical problems in the United States are chronic, debilitating illnesses rather than infectious diseases. There seems to be an almost epidemic increase in heart problems, cancer, arthritis, allergies and multiple sclerosis, to mention just a few. Why? "The average person does not know the kinds of foods that are necessary for good health and vigor," reports a spokesperson for the Secretary of Agriculture. Ignorance of proper nutrition coupled with highly chemical foods containing preservatives, additives and pesticides can only result in deteriorated health, hence, illness. The urban air we breathe and the chemically over-treated water we drink are hardly contributing to good health.

In many European countries, legislative efforts have been made to protect the public from poisonous pesticides and food additives. In France, chemical additives are not permitted in bread, nor is bleach used in flour. In Germany there are strict laws regulating additives in food, while Spain and Israel have legally reduced the chemical treatment of fruit.

Where are our values? If an American shows interest in eating right and preserving his health, he is labeled a "health nut." In Europe such a person is considered enlightened and wise.

## GOVERNMENTS AND INDUSTRY ENCOURAGE PREVENTIVE HEALTH MEASURES

This attitude is also reflected in government policy. Many health insurance plans in Europe, notably in Sweden, Germany, France, and Italy provide for spa treatment. For example, a worker in a factory might go to the resident doctor and complain of headaches, arthritis or whatever. In Germany, the doctor today would suggest one of 250 approved spas or Bads in the Federal Republic of Germany. The worker would then go to the prescribed Bad for approximately three or four weeks, depending upon the course of treatment. The health insurance organization would underwrite the treatment costs, traveling expenses and a number of additional social benefits. Despite the obvious costs involved for such a program, the ultimate cost is radically less than American health care programs that are curative in nature.

Industries in Europe are concerned with preventing stress and heart attacks in their executives. They spend a considerable amount of money on establishig cardiac reconditioning centers around the country or sending their executives to such programs as the Anti-Stress regimen in Baden-Baden. In these centers, businessmen learn life style changes that enable them to cope with present and future pressures and to prevent heart disease, high blood pressure and the other executive illnesses.

## FOOD AND HEALTH

As mentioned earlier, food is a grave consideration for quality health. The American media bombards us with fast-food commercials that sell better drinking glasses rather than nutrition. Our life style of hurry, eat-on-the-run, contributes to fast-food stress mania. Have you tried that old-time favorite . . . Southern fried chicken? One bite makes you believe that the War between the States is still going on . . . Sugar and white flour remain as American as apple pie; yet the effect is about as beneficial as drinking sump water.

An encouraging sign of health emerging in America is the adoption of the European concept of holistic health. The philosophy of holistic medicine encourages a person to reeducate himself concerning nutrition, exercise and taking responsibility for his own physical and psychological well being.

Many American life styles are filled with self-destructive habits such as smoking, excessive alcohol, lack of exercise and poor eating and resting habits. Often people seek assistance in altering their life habits in crisis situations when preventive measures are no longer appropriate.

One pragmatic reason for adopting a holistic approach could be money. Some experts predict that within fifteen years American hospital costs will be $700 a day. Medical costs are rising at such a phenomenal rate that the day may arrive when only the wealthy can afford hospitalization. The future status symbol may be "going to the hospital." Society editors may be assigned to report that "Mrs. Van der Laan of Palm Beach and Paris wore a Halston hospital gown for her gall bladder operation."

A person using preventive health measures has the opportunity to utilize time and energy that he would normally spend combating illness in living as fully as possible.

What can you do for your own health care? The answer is . . . adequate diet, rest, exercise, and most importantly, a philosophy of life that encourages you to use your creative resources. In Europe, one often hears that the body, mind, and soul work together for health. Dr. Otto Buchinger, at the world renowned Buchinger Sanitorium in Bad Pyrmont, Germany, has stated, "that when a spiritual life is not in harmony with the body, then illness soon sets in. When you lose contact with your inner being you soon become a series of mirrors, reflecting what 'society' wants you to be, not necessarily what is right for you. It is important to know what you really want from life and to pursue it."

## EXERCISE FOR FITNESS

Exercise is vital for maintaining health. Fortunately in America we are rediscovering the joys of the body. Only a decade ago we were sedentary people whose big weekend activity was getting up for a can of beer during the half time of a TV football game. Now, fitness is in vogue. Legions of joggers take to the streets, parks, and indoor gyms. Marathons are very popular for promoting commercial products as well as exercise. Biking, tennis, hiking, swimming, skiing, racquet-ball are all gaining in popularity. What about including walking in our life style? Perhaps our labyriths of freeways do not encourage a pedestrian stroll. Walking through an American city's park can often be an invitation for mugging or rape.

However, as the fuel crisis increases, we will have to find viable ways to walk or skate to our respective destinations. Walking is so therapeutic and relaxing that it is a shame to miss it.

Exercise is also important as a means of detoxifying the body. Constructive movement, whether it be calisthenics, running, or walking, loosens the debris that is accumulating in the tissues. Circulation is improved, muscles are developed and their elasticity is maintained. Dr. Ken Cooper of Aerobics fame, believes that people who exercise regularly will not have problems with irregularity. He has said: "I never saw a jogger who had an elimination problem."

Exercise, coupled with sound nutrition and relaxation, can be a real energy boost. In the course of hard exercise the heart and lungs have to work harder to get blood and oxygen to the cells for improved functioning. As the body becomes stronger from regular work-outs, stamina will increase.

In many European cities, there are specified paths in the woods, parks and throughout the city that are designed for strollers. In Northern Germany a frequent sight is octogenarians strolling hand in hand at sunset through the Kur paths. In parts of Switzerland, Germany, and Austria, people arise early to run or walk through the woods before going off to work. While I was in Zurich, I found the woods conveniently located about seven minutes from the city. It was possible for local business people to run or walk through the verdant paths of foliage then, within a few minutes, to be enroute to their places of business.

Another feature of health maintenance in many European cities is that at midday, shops close for an afternoon rest. I have had the experience of having a business meeting or interviewing doctors at noon when they will politely say, "It's time for my rest," and off they go.

The custom of visiting in sidewalk cafes over tea contributes to a less hurried pace of life. Early evenings find people taking walks through the woods, strolling on the Banhofstrasse promenade, through a Kur park or meandering down a city street.

## CONTRASTING AMERICAN VS. EUROPEAN SPA ATTITUDES TOWARDS HEALING

You don't have to be ill . . . unless you want to be. Some Americans assume that sickness is their inalienable right, along with voting and bearing arms. Just because your place of employment offers a health care plan such as Blue Cross/Blue Shield, there is no reason for you to take advantage of it unless you have an affinity for illness. You could be a whole lot healthier and still take your sick leave.

Many Europeans think that is it not necessary to be ill. Preventive health measures are built into the life style. The process is self healing and on going, which contrasts with our American approach of instantism in health care.

When ill, how often do we rush to a physician for a shot to get over an ailment, and go back to our regular pace within 24 hours? When we become sick again, we rush to our medical magician and expect an instant healing from his arsenal of pills, potions, needles and knives. The dependency that is created when we abdicate our responsibility for preventive health care is as devastating for the doctor as it is for the patient. We can say that doctors in America harbor dehumanized attitudes, yet we are poor physicians to ourselves. When we lead debilitating life styles that create unneeded stress, eat junk food, smoke incessantly, hold anger and resentments in our daily lives, we are being a foe to ourselves. When we multiply the number of people who journey daily to an overworked doctor and expect him to perform miracles, we can begin to understand the problem.

In 1975, the Canadian government under Dr. Thomas Boudreau, Assistant Deputy Minister of Health, made the statement that: "The health status of each person is related to life style, environment, both physical and social and human biology. Biomedical research will not provide the primary answers to these problems. The problems reflect life style and involve changes in our way of thinking as well as living."

## ATTITUDES AND LIFE STYLES IN EUROPE

"Life can be enjoyed when one has good health and knows about a balance in living," says one elderly Bad regular. Undereating, a concept alien to Americans, is considered a viable health measure. Many spas substitute exercise for excess eating. Scheduled runs or walks before a meal help burn excess calories as well as condition the body.

Those who adhere to the undereating principle are definitely healthier than those of us who prefer such Ben Franklinisms as "waste not, want not." How often have we begun digging our graves with our forks at restaurants where we can eat all we want for $5.99? How many cases of homicide and suicide occur over a dinner table? Deteriorated health and bulges in the wrong places are by-products of our great American eating patterns!

In European spas, defeating patterns of living are altered with behavior modification, just as in America. However, Europeans have the advantage of societal reinforcement.

That we have to take more responsibility for our health is not being emphasized in some medical circles. In September 1979, at the 55th annual Colorado Hospital Association convention in Vail, Dr. Donald Ardell of Mill Valley, California, author, lecturer and fitness consultant said: "Wellness is no longer something a few California hippies are talking about, it must become an integral part of the hospital program." He went on to say: "Hospitals are the place for wellness because that is where sick people go. They can be caught at a "teachable moment" when they are ready for a cure or a change of life style." Ardell further stated that wellness doesn't require one to be a fantastic jogger or a health food nut but should include a proper diet, physical fitness and a style of living that emphasizes the positive and spurns the negative. Let people know there are alternatives to Valium.

Life style changes are easier to make when we see other people exercising regularly, eating natural foods and adopting a more natural approach to living. "Balance" is a word used repeatedly to emphasize the basis of a total health plan.

Life was meant to be simple: we make it complex. Many times we are our own worst enemy. We overschedule our time doing unimportant things that deplete our energies. We overeat and overtax our bodies. We forfeit needed rest by our late night vigilance with an innane TV show and wonder why we are fatigued and all strung out. Sound familiar?

Well, my friends, we got trouble, "right here in River City" as the song goes. We need to think . . . reevaluate our lives and see which side we are fighting on. Are we promoting health or illness? That is the question.

## SELF-POISONING

Autointoxication is self-poisoning. It occurs when we overeat, overdrink, underexercise and overstress our bodies. Consider the average person walking down the street . . . chances are he is at least half sick. Often people say, "but there is nothing wrong with me now . . . I can continue to smoke my two packs of cigarettes, it hasn't hurt me yet. I can overeat rich foods that are difficult to digest, such as those with white flour, sugar and excess salt. I can continue to overstress my body by lack of exercise and inadequate rest."

## TWILIGHT ZONE OF ILL HEALTH

Many people who "appear" to have good health have built-in or incubating diseases. People can be unaware that they are ill. Dr. Bircher-Benner has indicated that often a disease is hidden by the effective regulatory mechanisms of the body. However, when confronted with acute stress, or when an advanced phase of the disease occurs, bodily compensations become insufficient and obvious disease occurs.

According to Dr. Karl Menninger, of the Menninger Institute in Topeka, Kansas, "only about 0.7 percent of the population could pass as really healthy in mind and spirit. The rest are struggling through life burdened with nervous obsessions and other prejudicial complexes." The promotion of optimal health throughout life is an important factor in the prevention of chronic illness.

It's like the familiar story of a man who fell out of a twenty story window. As he passed the second story window, he remarked, "Well, I'm all right so far!" So it is with living dangerously on wrong food and living habits. All right so far . . . but how long will it last?

Have you ever thought that you might be toxic? Toxic? That's like poison. Yes, that's exactly what many of us are. In fact, a recent medical report indicates that the majority of people are. "Constipation is either a chronic or acute disease in many people." Dr. William Hunter of London's Royal Society of Medicine, states: "Almost every chronic disease known is directly or indirectly due to the influence of bacterial poison absorbed from the intestine. The colon is a veritable Pandora's box . . . let it stagnate and it will distill the poisons of decay, fermentation and putrefaction into the blood. Depression and irritability, weakness and foul breath are the by-products."

In short, every organ of the body is poisoned. We age prematurely, look and feel old. The joints are stiff and painful; neuritis, dull eyes and a sluggish brain all overtake us. The pleasure of living is gone.

All this information indicates the importance of bowel regularity. In America, we are more inclined to discuss our sex life than our bowel habits. Europeans differ in this regard. They will freely say that they had a colonic, a water treatment to irrigate the colon. This glorified enema allows water to circulate in and out of the colon simultaneously. Its purpose is to improve flexibility, and clean out the pockets that ordinary laxatives and purgatives miss.

That is one way to begin the waste removal. Many of the exclusive health spas in Europe feature detoxification programs that help cleanse the body and make you feel healthy and youthful.

## HOW TO DETOXIFY YOUR BODY AS EUROPEANS DO

Diet and exercise mark the beginnings of this all natural treatment. Raw fruits and vegetables coupled with natural juices are a good way to remove impurities from the body. Some Scandinavian spas have a once-a-week cleansing program. For three days, fresh fruit and vegetable juices are consumed exclusively. Nothing else is eaten or drunk. After these days of elimination, one feels youthful and alert. I particularly like an Austrian program in which distilled water, lemons and honey are consumed.

*Austrian Detoxification*

*To two quarts of distilled water, squeeze 3 fresh lemons and 3 limes. Add 2 tablespoons of raw honey or maple syrup. The sweetener is used to keep the blood sugar level up. Shake the mixture and drink it through the course of the day or days. This should be consumed alone, no food is allowed. The lemons and limes are particuarly good for flushing out wastes in the kidney and liver. One or more days on this liquid regimen and one's energy level skyrockets as the body rids itself of accumulated wastes.*

I frequently try this when I anticipate a day of stress. On these supposed "trying days" I am able to function in a more positive way and view crisis as an opportunity.

Eating generous amounts of raw vegetables and fruits aids in the elimination process on a continual basis. Chew the food thoroughly and eat slowly. Whole grains, seeds and nuts are also nutritious foods. Fresh foods are more nutritious than canned or frozen products. During detoxification times, avoid alcoholic beverages. They generate body heat and upset your metabolism. This can interfere with your detoxification program.

## STAYING WELL AND STRENGTHENING YOUR HEALTH AS EUROPEANS DO

### How To Detoxify the Body

The five main organs that involve detoxification and removal of wastes from the system are the colon, lungs, liver, kidneys and skin.

### Cleaning the Colon

Its important to detoxify the body. When waste products accumulate, they overburden the system causing either disease or death from toxemia. To begin this process, Glauber salts are usually taken as a cathartic in Europe. However, one tablespoon of Epsom Salts dissolved in a half glass of distilled water works just as well. Repeat every 30 minutes until three doses are consumed. After your purging, drink alkalizing punch every 2 hours . . .

## Alkalizing Punch

Using all fresh fruits, juice 6 lemons, 12 oranges and 6 grapefruits. Place in a gallon jar and fill with distilled water. It is important to drink water in addition to the alkaline punch. Without sufficient fluids, the toxins become concentrated and are not eliminated in a natural way.

In some Mediterranean spas, this treatment is used once a week for removal of impurities from the body. In Austria, this regime is usually continued for two days once-a-week and followed by one day of fresh fruits and vegetables.

You may experience such uncomfortable symptoms as nausea, headache, cramps and dizziness. This signals success, indicating that your body is cleansing itself of poisons that have accumulated for years and are suddenly released from your system. After the toxins are eliminated from the system, you feel youthful and alert.

It is necessary to take either enemas or colonics to further facilitate waste removal. You can look in the yellow pages of your phone book for a chiropractor who offers colonic treatments. Should you prefer your own treatment, give yourself a daily enema made of coffee. The caffeine is beneficial in stimulating the liver to aid in elimination. Coffee is effective only in this way, not in the conventional methods of consumption.

## Cleansing the Kidneys

The kidneys filter 4000 quarts of blood daily to maintain the acid/alkaline balance and eliminate wastes. Vitamin C is especially suggested to help in this organ's function. To aid the kidney, drink plenty of fluids plus the juice of one lemon in a cup of hot water once a day mid-morning or mid-afternoon.

## Lungs Cleaning

Life is dependent upon an adequate exchange of gases in the lungs. Most significant is the removal of carbonic acid and the flow of oxygen in the blood. Deep breathing, as yoga breaths, helps the cleansing action. (Refer to Chapter 7 for more detailed information.)

Mucus producing foods such as white bread, refined flour, and sweet milk products should be avoided for a period of time if a person has asthma or a breathing problem.

## Can Your Skin Breathe?

Elimination via the skin can occur either when sweating or bathing. In an air-polluted city, skin pores often become clogged. Two purgative baths follow. For further bath information refer to Chapters 3 and 4.

### *Epsom Salts Bath Purgative*

Fill a bathtub with lukewarm water and two cups of Epsom Salts. As you recline in your own spa, gradually lower the temperature by adding cool water. The salts are beneficial in eradicating accumulated wastes from the skin. After your bath, cool your body by rubbing with witch hazel. Put on a loose cotton robe and lie down with your feet elevated. This treatment is so good it is worth repeating. Try it again later on in the day.

### *Apple Cider Vinegar Bath*

One time a week rub the skin from head to toe with a mixture of olive oil and castor oil in equal parts. Soak in a hot bathtub of water to which one cup of apple cider vinegar has been added. This aids in the acid/alkaline balance of the skin. Relax for 15 minutes and allow the oil to penetrate the skin.

After bathing, wear clothes that allow your body to breathe. Select natural fabrics such as cotton, silk and wool. These materials allow your body to "breathe" and thereby eliminate toxic wastes through the pores of the skin. Synthetic fabrics tend to seal in body excretions and may cause toxic substances to accumulate. This is particularly true of some brands of pantyhose which induce vaginal infections.

Air baths are very popular in many Swiss spas. You can try the same thing at home by sunbathing in the nude or, a modified version, by wearing loose cotton clothing.

These detoxifying methods are an inexpensive way to rid your body of unneeded wastes and allow it to self heal.

### *Detoxifying Your Feet*

This treatment is a popular one in Bavaria. Soak your feet in warm, soapy water. Then place them in a basin of cold water. Repeat three times and conclude with a cold water soak. Since nerve endings are in the feet, you will feel invigorated throughout your body as a result. Pat your feet dry and apply a generous amount of chilled witch hazel to the entire foot and ankle area. This is a terrific aid for walking more comfortably . . . that, coupled with good fitting shoes and adequate posture.

## PRODUCING A HEALING CRISIS WITHIN THE BODY

A diet of raw fruits and vegetables always brings on a healing crisis. Fresh fruits and vegetables, green herbs and nuts all provide the impetus for self healing. Detoxification reduces the surplus of acidity plus accumulated metabolic wastes that impair the system. During this time, critical days occur: in chronic conditions it may appear that the condition has worsened. In other words, you will feel temporarily worse before becoming better. Symptoms such as mood changes, perspiration, and flatulence will be apparent. This is because a cleansing diet of raw vegetables and fruits will dissolve huge amounts of accumulated debris and throw them into the bloodstream for removal. The organs of elimination—kidneys, liver, lungs and skin—will be overloaded. This healing crisis is temporary, and unpleasant symptoms of excessive elimination, such as skin eruptions, catarrhal discharge and fever will subside. Within several days you will experience improvement as your body cleanses itself and becomes stronger.

In extremely toxic conditions, as in severe arthritis, repeated short fasts are advised. This is done to prevent too rapid elimination from overt toxicity.

### Personal Account of a Healing Crisis

The fourth day of dining on raw foods seemed to be the beginning of my healing crisis. Initially, I experienced a tremendous surge of energy. However, I later learned that such a sign is ominous. It means that the body is ready to detoxify. During my crisis I cried profusely for no apparent reason, was unable to sleep at night and thought of various experiences from my past that I had forgotten over the years. I later learned that as the body begins self healing it retraces, step-by-step in reverse order, the diseases or conditions experienced throughout life. This passed after several days and I then encountered more energy than I had experienced in years. I learned that in times of healing, the body eliminates the debris first. Body tissues that have been built from poor food and bad living habits are dispelled from the body. The next stage is transitional, which is where a crisis occurs. The third stage involves building new tissues as a result of self healing.

## ONE-DAY REPRIEVE

To give your body a twenty-four hour reprieve, try fasting and resting for one day. Begin the day by taking a vegetable laxative or one tablespoon of olive oil mixed with one tablespoon of lemon juice. This is one of the best ways to detoxify the body.

Plan on spending the entire day in bed. Complete rest, physical and psychological, is necessary to aid in the process. During this day, drink only liquids. The menu for your elimination day consists of;

Chamomile tea with a teaspoon of honey.

Fresh juice at noon.

Clear broth and no salt in the evening.

During the course of the day you can drink as much water as you need.

At the end of the day take an enema to assist the debris removal.

A detoxification day in bed is a great boon to weight-loss also. In many of the European fasting spas, people lose between one and two-and-a-half pounds a day. While fasting in Bad Prymont, I was able to lose two and a half pounds a day while confined to bed. In the Bircher-Benner klinik, I lost two pounds a day with a similar regimen.

Rest cannot be underestimated as a part of the reprieve from stress: one day can do wonders for restoring the psyche and body. I first became aware of this benefit when I spent Shabbat with an Orthodox Israeli family in Jerusalem. A day with no work, no noise, and pure rest was so revitalizing that I was able to accomplish twice as much the following day as I ever did before. I have learned that this is the best deposit to make in one's energy bank account.

## GIVE YOURSELF ONE DAY A WEEK

When God created the world, he rested on the seventh day. The observant Moslems have Friday. Orthodox Jews have Saturday (or Shabbat, in Hebrew). The Christians in a bygone era strictly observed Sunday. If, for no other reason, it's a tremendous health boon.

Why not take a day solely for yourself? Plan such quiet activities as reading, taking long walks, doing Yoga, enjoying music or starting a creative project. Spend some time on innovative day dreaming, become aware of the silence around you, listen . . . open up your senses. What do you feel? Are there aromas around you that were not evident before . . . the smell of herbs and spices, plants, air by the ocean, freshly baked bread? Touch people, fabrics, yourself. How does it feel? Do you notice the difference in textures and touches? Spend a day not talking. You will be amazed at the extra energy you will have the following day. Give your senses a holiday. Declare a moritorium on the hustle and bustle of daily routine.

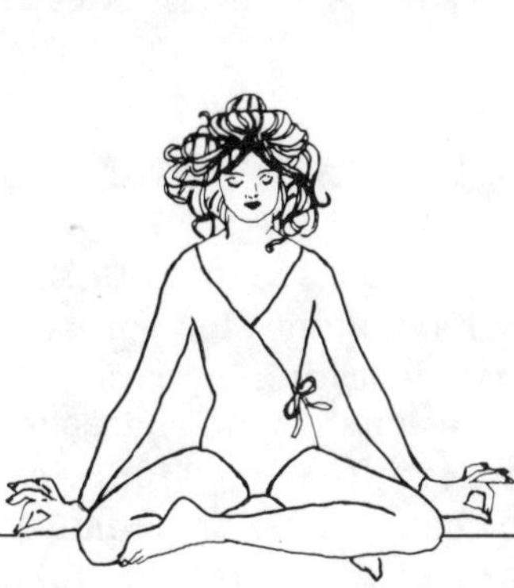

# 2

# Europe's Best Health Secret Is Ours

*"Man eats too much, lives on 1/4 of all he is eating and the remaining 3/4ths serves as a livelihood for doctors."*

Europeans often practice some form of fasting: omitting all forms of eating for a period of time. This can be the most freeing ritual of purifying the body. Having fasted in various spas, Bads and kliniks throughout Europe, I can attest to its effectiveness. It is easier than dieting, which involves a constant interaction with food. Often I feel like an alcoholic tending bar as I prepare a low calorie meal while fattening foods are beckoning me like a choir of Loreleis. Not so with fasting: it is a reprieve from thinking about food, and seems to stimulate other activity, alertness, euphoria, and aliveness.

After the second or third day of fasting, there are pleasure and exhilaration associated with a mental lightness, and a clarity of thinking and perception. I have found that while fasting I am able to function more creatively, music sounds more resonant, colors are brighter and feelings are more intense. (Maybe it's a cheap high!)

When fasting you are in good company with Moses, Pythagoras, Plato, Mohammed, Abraham and Jesus, who spent forty days fasting in the desert. I've often wondered if He did it according to the spa program . . . one week of nutritional build-up following the fast? To the remark of St. Clement, a frequent faster, who said "Fasting is better than prayers," I say a hardy Amen!

## FASTING AND RELIGION FOR SPIRITUAL AWARNESS

Fasting has played a vital role in the Jewish, Oriental, Christian, and Moslem religions. Reason? Foregoing food offers a time of rest and renaissance for mind, body and spirit. Periodic fasting increases visual and mental perceptions; and awareness of aesthetics are sharpened.

Super yogis and eastern philosophers fast for energy four-times-a year, according to the seasons, in order to change the blood. Many yogi fasters report that when fasting they become very centered and know how to use their energy better. Fasting, like yoga, is an opportunity to alter the consciousness. When internal cleansing occurs during fasting, the mind changes as the oxygen level varies. Euphoria results as a feeling of lightness, spirituality and cleansing.

While in Jerusalem at the end of Ramadan, the Moslem fasting period, I was invited to celebrate with Arabs in the Old City. Many of the Moslem adherents said that they felt more alive and festive after abstaining from food. "Foods taste better, senses are heightened," are some of the comments made after fasting.

The Christian observance of Lent is a forty-day-period of self-discipline, reminiscent of the time Jesus spent in the desert. Yom Kippur, the Jewish fast-day of Atonement, is devoted to redemption and meditation. Despite the absence of food and water from sundown to sundown, there is a presence of hope and a time for new beginnings. I have observed Orthodox Jews outside the synagogue mending torn relationships for the start of the new year. Just as Yom Kippur commemorates an opportunity to begin again, so, too, is a secular fast a time for physical, psychic and spiritual renewal.

## BENEFITS OF FASTING

- Improved health
- Reduced tension
- Sense of physical and mental well-being
- Time and money saved
- New vitality and buoyancy
- Younger looks
- Enhanced sleep
- Heightened spiritual awareness

The advantages of fasting are far reaching. Preventive fasting is ideally suited for cleansing the whole body. "It does not damage nerves or vital organs but a majority of acute and chronic ailments can be improved or even cured," says Dr. Otto Buchinger, who is considered to be the world's leading fasting authority.

Fasting can mean victory for anyone fighting the perennial battle-of-the-bulge. I have interviewed many Europeans who were former victims of obesity, but viewing their present svelte figures, it is hard to imagine that they had experienced a weight problem. To guard against future gains, they annually fast to prevent added avoirdupois.

## NEW ENERGY WITH FASTING

A therapeutic fast is known in Europe to be the best way to build up the physical stamina in order to resist illness and revitalize the functions of all the vital organs. It is amazing how intensely energy is increased after abstaining from food. At the conclusion of my initial European fast, I was able to travel many miles from spa to Bad to klinik without experiencing the usual traveler's fatigue. After a day of complete spa treatment I would write until the wee hours of the morning while other curists slept. Prior to fasting, I seldom had that kind of endurance. The loss of weight coupled with rejuvenation of the endocrine glands creates a feeling as well as appearance of youth. After my second European fast, I felt like a seventeen-year-old. I had so much energy that I would half skip and half run when I went into the cities. What a sense of aliveness!

## CHRONIC DISEASES SUBSIDE WITH FASTING

Fasting is an effective means of healing various diseases. According to Professor Parade of the University of Innsbruck, cancer, diabetes, appendicitis, serious forms of rheumatism, skin and intestinal diseases decreased impressively during World War II and post-war period. Between 1939–1949 a dramatic reduction of diseases occurred in Germany which has been attributed to the compulsory diet reduction of that time. According to an old Roman sage: "The first illness was due to eating and the first treatment has been fasting."

While fasting, the body will rid itself of accumulated wastes such as tumors, dead cells, abcesses, damaged tissues and fat deposits. When disease takes hold of the body, it is usually due to the weakened defense mechanisms and impaired functions of the vital organs. The metabolic rate slows down and the lung, kidneys, skin, and colon lose their eliminative efficiency.

Self-digestion or "autolysis" is the process by which your body will burn and digest its own unnecessary tissues. Years of dining on highly seasoned foods, pastries, heavy starches, and abundant proteins create an acid condition in the blood. As a raw juice regimen is begun, the living matter of the fresh fruit and vegetable juices will dispel the old dying and decayed cells. During this time the eliminative organs, the lungs, liver, kidney, and skin, work overtime to relieve the body of accumulated wastes and toxins. As the old cells and diseased tissues are eliminated, the building up of new and healthy cells is stimulated and increased. If given the opportunity, the body has a marvelous ability to self heal. Nature's internal physician brings about a harmony within mind and spirit.

## WHAT SYMPTOMS TO EXPECT WHEN YOU FAST

Positive signs that the body is working in your behalf are evidenced by perspiration, skin eruptions, offensive breath, mucus discharges, coated tongue, chilliness, and concentrated urine. Don't be discouraged by your momentary odor. Actually, it's the sweet smell of success, signaling that your body is in the act of purification for healing. As the body self-digests internal debris, you are on the road to new health. Consider that you have voluntarily placed yourself in a temporary state of sickness to prevent long-term illness. The current inconvenience will be well worth your effort.

## WHAT TO DO ABOUT THE OFFENSIVE TASTE IN YOUR MOUTH

- Take sips of natural lemon juice
- Chew on natural chlorophyll herbs like parsley, chives, thyme, or chervil
- Brush the tongue with a toothbrush coated with baking soda

This corrects the mouth odor in a simple and inexpensive way.

If wastes are not removed from the body, they are then deposited in arteries and small capillaries, constricting and hindering the flow of blood.

## AFTER-EFFECTS OF FASTING

A fast gives the digestive system a holiday: the assimilative and protective organs of the body get a physiological rest. After fasting, food is digested more completely because nutrients are more readily assimilated into the system, the body experiences a time of balancing, the nervous system is improved, plus mental abilities are more acute. Glandular chemistry and hormone secretions are stimulated while the tissues' mineral balance is normalized. Is it any wonder that people feel rejuvenated after fasting?

## WHO SHOULD NOT FAST?

According to Dr. Otto Buchinger, who has supervised over 80,000 fasts, there are those conditions in which a person may fast, those in which a person must fast, and certain conditions in which therapeutic fasting is to be avoided. Among persons who should not fast, he cites specifically: cases of mental imbalance, climacteric psychosis, hysteria, tuberculosis, cancer, bleeding ulcers, kidney or liver disease and advanced diabetes. Cases of diphtheria or scarlet fever should be recovered for at least one year before any effort is made to fast.

Dr. Buchinger says that some conditions of susceptibility to disease smolder in readiness but are still not always recognizable. With these diseases, one may fast and often should. Chronic fatigue is a sign that the body is toxic and needs a fast. The preventive fast is important for following the rhythm of nature. Thus a preventive fast should be undertaken every year in the spring, as a "spring-cleaning" to remove accumulated impurities.

The conditions in which a person should therapeutically fast are: (1) metabolic disorders, like obesity, chronic underweight, rheumatism, sciatica, and diabetes in the initial stages; (2) diseases of the heart, circulation, and blood vessels, such as angina pectoris, high or low blood pressure, and congestion of the blood stream. This type of fasting would involve medical supervision.

## FASTING AND SLIMNESS

In Europe fasting has been used to successfully combat obesity. Studies indicate that up to 40 percent of chronically obese people can and do maintain the lower weight they reach after prolonged, supervised fasting. It's interesting to note that in Europe, people pursue the same fad diets as we do in the United States. The hard boiled egg, brown rice, high protein, and low carbohydrate diets have all been tried on both sides of the Atlantic with about the same results.

For all those involved in calorie counting, it is reassuring to know that even when you do not eat or receive any kind of nourishment, the body still uses up fuel. At complete rest, the body of an average person will use up about 1300 calories per day. Light or moderate exercise will bring the calorie requirement up to 2000 to 2500 per day, depending upon the weight and size of the body. That is why fasting enables a quick reduction in weight.

During a fast, there is a weight-loss of one or two pounds per day; it is no wonder that Dr. Buchinger calls fasting the "zero diet." It provides a needed reprieve from counting calories, fad diets and a love affair with the kitchen. For the legions who daily weigh in at weight-loss clinics, fasting is a viable alternative to three square meals a day and a distended stomach.

Another "plus" of fasting is constant feedback. Daily you can see yourself changing for the better. While fasting at the Buchinger Sanitorium, I was amazed that after the third day of fasting, I noticed that extra pounds on my hips and stomach were dramatically disappearing. They were not the only thing to go: wrinkles, aging lines, and fatigue were vanishing as well. As a result of such feedback, I felt a sense of determination to continue. New self-confidence also builds as thinness approaches.

## FEARS AND FASTING

Dr. Allan Cott, author of *Fasting, the Ultimate Diet,* suggests that fear of starvation need not be a deterrent to fasting. Abstaining from food is the best healing measure of nature. "The body tolerates a fast far better than a feast." Fear-inspired overeating can become a deeply ingrained life-long compulsion, beginning in infancy and continuing to an early grave.

Dr. Cott suggests that a one day fast is a good beginning for those who have not previously fasted. He stresses that it is important to realize that fasting and starvation are not the same. Fasting is a positive, elective action that produces equally positive results, whereas starvation is an imposition of fate. Involuntary wasting away due to the unavailability of food or inadequate amounts of food is a definite contrast to fasting.

## WHAT HAPPENS DURING A FAST?

Fasting activates the body's own healing powers. Any defect, disturbance or damage to tissues has an opportunity for self-regeneration during this time.

In a fast that exceeds three days, the body will burn and digest its own tissues via autolysis or self-digestion. Wisely, it will decompose only those tissues which are diseased, damaged, or of lesser importance to the body such as tumors, abscesses, and fat deposits. These are utilized first, while vital organs and essential tissues are spared.

Lungs, liver, kidneys and skin cleanse and eliminate accumulated metabolic wastes and toxins. The previously mentioned symptoms: offensive breath, dark urine, skin eruptions, and perspiration all give evidence of this action. Since the digestive and protective organs of the body have received a physiological rest, after fasting, digestion and utilization of food are greatly improved, making assimilation of all the important nutrients more effective.

## PERSONAL ACCOUNTS OF FASTING SUCCESSES

Many people sing the praises of fasting. The following are typical comments:

> *"Having spent many wakeful nights with insomnia, I was relieved to discover that after three days of fasting I slept soundly and have had many restful nights since." Hans K., Karlsruthe, Germany.*

> *"I look twenty years younger after fasting for one month." Eric B., Bad Hofgastein, Austria.*

> *"My arthritis seemed to miraculously disappear about the tenth day of fasting at the sanitorium. It has been three years since I experienced any arthritic symptoms. Now I fast annually as a preventive measure." Evelyn W., Hanover, Germany.*

> *"Migraine headaches have been my constant companion. They are no longer . . . thanks to my annual fasting regime." Daren A., Strasburg, France.*

> *"For many years I had an overweight problem, fifteen kilo to be exact. Ten years ago I fasted for the first time and lost the added avoirdupois. Each year I return to the Buchinger Sanitorium and fast to make sure I don't gain back the weight. Despite my 78 years, I am still able to work a 40-hour week." Paris, France.*

> *"Rheumatism was incapacitating. I had to stop work because of it. My doctor suggested that I go to the Buchinger Sanitorium and fast. Twenty-one days of fasting and one week of nutritional build-up was the answer. I have not experienced rheumatoid symptoms since. However, I do fast each year and maintain a diet of raw fruits and vegetables." Jerome L., Vals, Switzerland.*

> *"When my body is cleansed by a fast, I feel more in touch with myself and seem to have an extra sensory perception. I feel younger. I like myself more." Hannah G., Hamlin, Germany.*

> *"Energy, more than I've had in years. That's what I got from fasting." Monica K., Newark, New Jersey.*

### New Stamina and Still Going

Helene is a healthy, youthful looking woman who works a 60-hour week in an import-export business. If one were to guess her age judging by her appearance, the guess might be 50. The truth is, she is 78! Helene was not always blessed with good health. Nineteen years ago she was plagued with insomnia, overweight, and depression. She decided to try fasting as an approach to her problems, and at the end of a three-week fast with a week of nutritional build-up, she felt so improved that she decided to make it an annual ritual. When I met her at Buchinger's Sanitorium it was her nineteenth year of fasting.

### Fatigue and Weight Lost with Fasting

Henrick was always tired. No energy . . . no motivation . . . but lots of weight. In fact, Henrick was obese. He had tried every conceivable diet: low calorie, grapefruit, banana, high protein, but nothing worked. He could lose weight for a brief period of time but he always regained it. His doctor suggested that he try fasting under supervision, so he began at the Bircher-Benner Klinik. Although it took several fasts before he reached his desired weight, after seven years he has maintained a normal weight for his height. Henrick reports that he feels more alive than he ever felt before, and has more energy, concentration, and vitality than he ever dreamed possible.

## BEGINNING A FAST

It is necessary to begin with a purge. Before any disease can be overcome, the waste accumulations in the system must first be cleansed from the system.

At Buchinger Sanitorium a bowel cleanse consists of Glauber Salts and a quart of warm water on the first morning of fasting. The taste is not the most delicious, so it is followed with a glass of fruit juice. There is no doubt that the Glauber salts are effective, since the body feels like a volcano erupting as repeated evacuations cleanse the system.

### Types of Cleansers for Your Bowel Catharsis

1. *Epsom Salts.* Dissolve one tablespoon of Epsom Salts in half a glass of distilled water, which is the best to use. Add to this the juice of two lemons, and drink. Twenty minutes later take half a glass full of carrot and celery juice or orange juice.

2. *Castor Oil.* In some European kliniks two tablespoons of castor oil are given in a glass of water. Here again, add the juice of a lemon to cut the taste.

3. *Herb Lax.* A milder form of bowel cleansing is that of taking a prepared laxative made of herbs. This can be purchased at any health food store, and you may find it necessary to repeat the dosage several

times a day. The usual amount taken is one teaspoon with water every two hours until the evacuation is completed.

4. *Enemas.* When fasting for several days, it is advisable to take daily enemas or colonics which cleanse the intestines and rid the body of toxins that have been loosened from the various cells of the body. If these poisons are not removed from the system, they are re-absorbed into the bloodstream. Enemas can be made of warm water into which the juice of one lemon has been squeezed. Some Swiss kliniks use chamomile tea rather than plain water, since they feel that the tea offers a more complete cleansing. Coffee enemas to stimulate the kidneys are used in German kliniks.

5. *Colonics.* Another cleansing possibility is a colonic. This flushing of water throughout the entire colon is usually performed at a klinik in Europe. In the United States, it is possible to have a colonic at a chiropractor's office where special equipment is available or in a holistic clinic. The usual cost is about $12.00. This cathartic system is indeed successful, and there is no doubt that one has been purged after it; you do feel cleansed.

## WATER FASTING VS. JUICE FASTING

When I asked Dr. Otto Buchinger about the advantages of water fasting—eating or drinking nothing but water—he replied that he does not advocate drinking water alone. He says that our bodies are loaded with many toxins. Foods often are contaminated with additives and preservatives, and these cumulative poisons are stored in the fat-tissues of the body. During fasting, the body begins to feed on its own tissues, and fat is broken down and digested, releasing harmful amounts of DDT into the bloodstream. If a person is fasting on water alone, symptoms of DDT poisoning often occur. However, when one drinks raw fruit or vegetable juice during a fast, DDT is released into the bloodstream more slowly due to the neutralization of the toxins by the juice. Poisons are also more safely excreted by the body because of the vitamin and mineral content of the juices.

## WHY RAW JUICES?

Raw fruit and vegetable juices as well as freshly-made vegetable broth are rich in vitamins, minerals, enzymes and trace elements, which help normalize bodily processes and speed up toxin removal. Such juices are easily assimilated directly into the bloodstream without putting a strain on the digestive organs.

Fresh fruits and vegetables are more potent than any medicine. Fruits are the cleansers of the human system. Vegetables are the regenerators of the building blocks of the body, yet neither have the toxic effect of drugs. Scientists relate that many diseases are the result of a diet deficient in trace-vitamins and organic minerals. Anemia, pellagra, rickets, malnutrition, overweight, underweight and even the common cold can be traced to a lack of these life-sustaining elements of health.

### Vegetable Broths

In many kliniks, a vegetable broth is made of half-inch pieces of vegetables of the season like carrots, potatoes, and celery, which are cooked for 30 minutes in water. After straining, the vegetables are thrown away and the remaining liquid, a highly alkaline, mineral-packed broth, is retained.

### Herb Teas

Herb medicines are one of the oldest remedies known. In all kliniks that I visited, the particular favorites were rose hips which are rich in Vitamin C, peppermint, Chamomile, Linden, and Golden Seal.

## CHOOSING YOUR JUICE

When beginning your juice-fast, you have many choices as to the types of juice to try. You can stick with one, such as orange or apple, or try a variety. Personally, I prefer trying different fruits and vegetable juices. In the European kliniks a variety is often the rule unless there are specific health conditions that indicate a certain juice, such as carrot.

A pint or more of fresh, raw, fruit or vegetable juice taken on an empty stomach will be absorbed by the bloodstream and glands within 15 minutes.

*Carrot.* Carrots are an excellent source of Vitamin A, the healing vitamin. Carrot juice is the most popular of all the vegetable juices. At the world-renowned Ringburg Cancer Klinik, carrot juice is a standard for treatment. Containing practically the full range of vitamins and minerals needed by the body, it is used for treatment of hay fever, asthma, lung trouble, eye problems; and for beautifying the hair and skin. Carrot juice is the total juice for restoring pep and energy.

*Carrot and Celery.* In addition to the benefits of carrot juice, celery offers a calming effect on the nerves. The juice seems able to dissolve calcium deposits which occur in the system in cases of arthritis, high blood pressure and hardening of the arteries. The high alkaline content of this juice is valuable for correcting inflammation of the urinary tract and for conditions of rheumatism, and neuritis. It is a great complement to carrot juice.

*Carrot and Cucumber.* Known as a beauty aid when applied to the skin, cucumber juice is equally effective when taken internally. It is high in silicon and fluorine, which is essential to the health of the skin, hair and fingernails. Its rich sodium content is also valuable in dissolving calcium deposits in high blood pressure, hardening of the arteries, and gall and kidney stones. Cucumber is also effective as a diuretic, with a taste that is compatible with the carrot juice.

*Apple.* Eve knew what she was doing when she offered Adam an apple. This fruit is a good cleanser of the digestive tract, gall bladder and liver and, being mildly laxative, aids a sluggish pancreas. The cleansing action of apple juice can cause gas distress, so it is not advisable to drink it before going to bed. The silicon content of this juice is recommended for improved hair, skin, and fingernails.

*Beet Juice.* Reportedly beet juice is very effective for poor circulation and vitality, while being a good blood cleanser as well as a builder of new cells. In some European kliniks it is given in cases of low blood pressure, suppressed menstruation and heart trouble. It is not recommended when diabetes is present, due to its natural sugar content.

*Grape Juice.* The grape cure is famous throughout Europe. Although the grape is low in vitamins, it is a very effective cleanser of the body. Grape juice is used in cases of anemia, low blood pressure, overweight and skin problems, but should not be used in cases of inflammation of the digestive tract or diabetes.

*Lemon Juice.* Lemons are a good source of vitamins C and B. It has long been used for treatment of flu and cases of colds. It is also recommended for rheumatic conditions, liver, and bladder problems, pyorrhea, scurvy, and as a beauty aid. Lemon juice is a strong antiseptic and can be used on wounds where no other antiseptic is available. It is fairly stressful to the system and should not be used where there is inflammation of the digestive tract.

*Orange Juice.* Possibly one of the most popular of all the fruit juices in European fasting programs, orange juice is a great source of vitamin C, as well as A and B. Calcium and phosphorus are also found in this juice.

*Tomato Juice.* Tomato juice is a good source of vitamins A, B, C, G, and iodine, which is useful for thyroid and glandular troubles. It is useful in blood cleansing, improving the skin, treating pyorrhea, liver and gall bladder problems.

*Pineapple Juice.* Raw pineapple juice is one of the most delicious of the fruit juices. It contains a digestive enzyme that aids in the digestion of foods, and is a good body cleanser useful in treatment of gum conditions.

*Parsley Juice.* Parsley is one of the richest sources of vitamins A, C, B, some E, and iron. Known as an aid to the optic nerves, it is suggested for improving the skin, mucous membranes, treating anemia, liver, and gall bladder problems and menstrual difficulties. Parsley is a powerful juice and should not be taken alone. Drink about one-half glass with carrot, celery, or cucumber juice.

*Cabbage Juice.* Cabbage owes its fame to its vitamin U, the anti-ulcer factor. Used in cases of stomach and duodenal ulcers, it is a good source of vitamins A, B, and C. It is not very palatable, but the flavor is improved by the addition of celery or celery juice. Cabbage juice contains an abundance of practically all the minerals making it valuable for almost any condition of ill health.

## CALORIE CONTENT OF JUICES

Below is a run-down of the calorie content of the juices for those who are conscious of calorie consumption. Using a pint as the standard amount, the juices contain the following amounts of calories:

| | | | |
|---|---|---|---|
| apple juice | 250 | lemon juice | 210 |
| beet juice | 220 | orange juice | 265 |
| carrot juice | 217 | parsley juice | 283 |
| celery juice | 89 | pineapple juice | 207 |
| cucumber juice | 84 | tomato juice | 112 |
| grape juice | 462 | | |

Novelist Upton Sinclair has said this about fasting: "I have found a perfect health, a new state of existence, a feeling of purity and happiness, something unknown to humans." Fasting, that perfect state that Sinclair refers to, can be experienced in several ways. For the ultimate fast, try a four-week experience at a sanitorium or klinik. If that is not possible, try any of the following: go off for a weekend and fast with a trusted friend, or try it for one day at home.

## HOW TO BEGIN A FAST AT HOME

On the day prior to fasting, have a "fruit day." On this day, eat only fruit, preferably in season, like apples, pears, oranges, figs, and prunes. The fruit flushes out quantities of fluids retained by the body and begins removing excess toxins from the system. The three meals of fruit can be eaten in any combination, e.g., oranges and grapefruits, with figs or bananas and apples sliced with currants. Usually not more than two pounds of fruit should be consumed during this day, and thirst should be quenched between meals exclusively with water.

A one-day fast can be done either at work or at home. If a person elects to stay at home, then try to stay in bed. This period of rest allows the body to cleanse itself more completely than if involved in work activity. Even one or two days of fasting can have an amazing effect upon one's energy level.

## FASTING FOR ONE DAY OR LONGER

Freshly made juice is the best to use. If you have a juicer or blender you can make your own but be sure to drink the juice within ten minutes after preparation. When the juice is allowed to stand longer, it loses its enzymes and some of its effectiveness.

Should you have neither time nor juicer you can buy bottled apple juice. This is very convenient for taking to the office, and you can also take along herb tea bags or herb tea in a thermos.

| | |
|---|---|
| What to do: | Get up and take a brisk walk. |
| Time of arising: | Herb tea such as Chamomile, Rose Hip or Fenugreek with one teaspoon of honey. |
| Midday: | Fresh juice or vegetable broth. Rest for 20-30 minutes. |
| Mid-afternoon: | Juice or herb tea such as Lemon Grass or Alfalfa Mint with honey. Walk again for 10 minutes. |
| Dinner time: | Fresh juice. |

During the course of the day you can consume as much water as you desire. Distilled, artesian well or mineral water is better than tap water. Water from the faucet often is loaded with debris. While your body is attempting to rid itself of wastes, it does not need contributions from another source.

## ONE-WEEK FAST OR LONGER

Dr. Buchinger suggests the following nourishment:

| | |
|---|---|
| Breakfast: | Herb tea: rose hips, chamomile, golden seal or peppermint, with one teaspoon of honey or milk sugar. |
| Lunch: | Fresh juice: orange, tomato, or fruit in season. |
| Mid-afternoon: | Tea and one teaspoon of honey. |
| Supper: | Vegetable broth or juice. |

- Throughout the day, drink about two quarts of water, either spring water or artesian well water.
- Exercise, preferably first thing in the morning and again in the evening: this stimulates the supply of oxygen through deep breathing and increases the flow of nutritive matter to the cells.

- Do not take any medications.
- Avoid coffee, black tea and non-caloric soft drinks.
- Keep warm. Lack of warmth impedes the process of elimination.
- Get plenty of fresh air.
- Rest, especially midday, but sleep isn't necessary.
- Do not smoke or consume alcohol.
- Sunbathe, if possible, for 20 minutes in the early morning and late afternoon when temperature is not at its highest.
- Shower or bathe frequently but avoid hot baths or saunas. Alternate hot and cold baths lower energy levels.
- Exercise—with long walks in fresh air.
- Be careful of sudden movements; lowered blood pressure can make you dizzy.
- Take an enema every second day.

NOTE: For added weight loss, spend a day fasting in bed.

## WEEKEND FASTING ADVENTURE

Go off for a weekend with a trusted friend to a different environment; to mountains, woods, or seaside. The change of scenery and being apart from the everyday influences that prevent fasting will encourage you to get into your self healing. Plan the last meal on either Thursday or Friday evening. Fast completely on Saturday and Sunday on herb teas, fresh juices and water.

What to do? Take leisurely walks through the woods, by the sea or in the mountains. If you are retreating in an urban area, walk around the block, through the park or in a scenic area. The visual effect of appreciating beautiful surroundings contributes to your emotional well-being. While fasting the senses are more heightened, the flowers are more fragrant, the sky seems bluer and your feelings about your environment more intense.

Rest, preferably outside, if the weather permits, and leisurely watch the clouds roll by. Sleep is not necessary, but the body does need a period of relaxation so that it can begin its internal cleansing to make a more vitalized you. Take along some light reading that would enhance your spirits, and enjoy your mini-vacation. Start a diary. Write down your thoughts, feelings, impressions, and get acquainted with yourself. This could be the beginning of a new and trusted relationship with your best friend . . . you! Note the sensations that you experience when fasting . . . euphoric, light-headed, spiritual. (This could mark the beginnings of *your* book on fasting.)

A weekend fasting adventure could be the beginning of your personal renaissance. You can use this time apart from your usual life style to discover new aspects of your personality and interests. The only limitations are self-imposed . . . let your creativity reign. At the end of your weekend adventure, your new found energy, lightness and sense of well-being can help you to return home with a new perspective on life.

## HOW TO BREAK THE FAST

This is the critical issue: many people can fast, but the real test is in breaking it. The beneficial effects of a fast can be totally undone if the fast is broken incorrectly. As Dr. Otto Buchinger says: "Even a fool can fast, but only a wise man knows when to break the fast properly and build up properly after a fast."

The rules of breaking a fast are:

(1) Eat slowly, chewing each mouthful thoroughly.

(2) Avoid overeating; you don't have a license to splurge.

(3) Allow several days of gradual transition to a normal diet.

Some European clinics use fresh juice, but I have found that Dr. Buchinger's idea of using a fresh apple is better. There is no rush of hunger after a fresh apple as there can be with liquids. Slowly chewing the apple has a relaxing effect and promotes the peristaltic movement of digestion. If false teeth prevent thorough chewing, the apple can be grated. No liquids should be consumed with the apple, but drink water throughout the day. Eat an apple for breakfast and lunch, while the evening meal can consist of plain potato soup or a vegetable broth.

The food eaten following a fast can be as follows:

*First Day—Building-Up Day*

Breakfast: Muesli (cereals, cereal germ—see recipes at end of book) and three apples between meals. Herb tea at conclusion of meal.

Lunch: Fresh salad, mashed potatoes with parsley, fresh carrots.

Dinner: Fresh fruit salad (e.g., apples, bananas, oranges), ⅓ of an ounce of butter, crisp bread and rose hip tea.

*Second Day—Building-Up Day*

Breakfast: Prunes or figs soaked in water, granola, one cup of milk, 12 hazel nuts. Three apples for snacks between meals.

| | |
|---|---|
| Lunch: | Salad, carrots cooked lightly in butter, unpolished rice, bowl of junket as a sweet. |
| Afternoon: | Butter, crisp bread, herb tea. |
| Evening: | Mixed salad, cheese, rose hip or lemon tea. |

In the building-up days following a fast, you discover that your energy increases daily. As you grow stronger, there is a renewed joy in living resulting from the cleansing process that has occurred within. Often there is a feeling that "less is more." Fasting has a way of injecting a new positiveness as it changes your weight and possibly your way of life.

## AN INNER SOURCE OF HELP

A period of fasting often stimulates dreams, which can be powerful soothsayers providing direction in our daily lives, and an inner source of information and strength that can offer new insights about our lives. As one who has been keeping a dream journal for many years, I believe that the best book on dreams is the one that you write yourself.

Throughout history, people have regarded dreams reverently and sensed a meaningful relation between the inner world of their dreams and the outer world of waking life. Hippocrates, the ancient Greek physician, practiced dream therapy and encouraged his ritual of dream incubation. This ritual began in Egypt and was extensively practiced for more than a thousand years in ancient Greece.

Ancient dream incubation involved a pilgrimage to a sacred temple in which one went to sleep in hopes of having a curative or prophetic dream.

When I was at the Acropolis in Athens, I tried having a cat-nap and dreamed of the flowing waters of the Aegean Sea. For two years thereafter I continued to dream of waters. At the same time I thought "I'm either all wet or water is symbolic of energy and life." Later, I became very interested in water as a healing force. The two chapters in this book give testimony to this interest.

EXERCISE: Think of a place that has had special impact in your life, go there and take a nap. People have been doing that in Sunday sermons, during a symphony, or in a garden for centuries. I wonder if there has been any research done on the subject?

When you are sleeping with someone you love, flukey as it sounds, have pen and paper beside your bed and see what you dream about.

As you keep a dream diary or journal, note the kinds of dreams that you have in certain locations, or seasons of the year, with specific people, or when its raining, snowing, etc.

## Keeping a Dream Diary

Pen and paper at your bedside are prerequisites. Certainly you can't interpret your nocturnal adventures the same way that a professional would, but that doesn't preclude the possibility of gathering clues from them anyway. You can train yourself to remember more by writing dreams down immediately upon awakening. The data that you gather will help you understand more about your dealings in everyday situations.

1. Before you go to sleep, tell yourself that you are going to remember your dreams and write them down promptly, even though the time is 2 a.m. Record your dreams, no matter how fragmentary, fearful or unimportant they may be.
2. As you begin scribing your dreams, get an overall picture of them first, e.g., setting, people involved and colors. Then fill in the details, like size of objects, facial expressions, or time of day.
3. Realize that no dream is nonsense. When you view them over a period of time you will be able to gather more knowledge about yourself and recall your dreams in greater depth.
4. Pay attention to the emotions expressed in the dreams, e.g., the fear or frustration you express when running down a dark alley with no light at the end.
5. Note your feelings upon awakening. Often if a dream has great psychic impact: you may be perspiring and your heart palpitating.
6. Accept your feelings about your dreams. Be aware of their message then take appropriate action.
7. Nightmares are urgent signals from your inner-self to take action. (It was via a dream that I decided to go to Europe and begin to self heal upon learning that I needed curative help.)
8. Nightmares can help you resolve inner conflict. Write them down and then share them with a trusted friend to reduce anxiety.

## HOW BETTINA R. CHANGED HER LIFE

Bettina R., age 30, was a compulsive eater. Her marketing job for a large corporation was extremely stressful, so whenever she felt she could not cope with the situation, she would reach into her desk drawer and pull out some type of sweets to nibble on until she got through the momentary crisis. The more job pressure, the more she ate. Finally she decided to go to a Bad and try juice fasting. On the third night of her fast she had a vivid dream in which she was sitting at her desk being strangled by a marketing report and candy wrappers. Two days later she had a similar dream. In a week, her dream centered on being in a small room that was filled with marketing reports and food piled to the ceiling. She was backed in a corner and could not move, and awakened from her dream perspiring. In two weeks, she returned home and resumed her stressful job. After the first day on the job she went to bed exhausted. That night she dreamed that she was being buried in a coffin of food and the company's annual report was on top of her. Again she awakened with perspiration but this time she made a decision. She would quit her job and work in a less stressful free-lance public relations position. Without the overt tension, Bettina was able to control her eating. She continued to record her dreams, and had solved the missing link in her life. She no longer experienced the marketing and candy-wrapper nightmares.

## PROVIDING MYSTERIOUS DATA THAT HELPS US BEGIN HEALING

Dreams remind us of missing links in our waking life. These signals tell us what we need to change or clear up. When we ignore them, they recur until they come to the forefront of our conscious mind, when we must take the necessary action, as with Bettina. Jung, the renowned Swiss analyst has said that: "To be concerned with dreams is a form of self-realization."

The first time that I went to the spas in Europe I met Marjorie Freer, a journal facilitator for Dr. Ira Progoff's Intensive Journal workshops. Although I had taken these workshops in the States, I found the experience particularly helpful in a spa setting. While fasting I discovered that my dreams were intensified, and I would write four or five pages a night. Fellow fasters were having similar experiences, so we began sharing our scribed dreams and writing dream enlargements. That is, we would take a specific dream, think about it while in a relaxed state after doing autogenic training, and then let our imaginations go. Result? We acquired important data to help us resolve some areas of conflict within our lives. One woman, Eloise M., was very angry that her husband had died three years before and left her alone. On a conscious level she was feeling constantly depressed, had digestive problems and was withdrawing from people. After a series of vivid-red dreams about her husband, Eloise realized that she had been holding in much anger that had been internalized in depression and health problems. She began to actively talk about the situation with some of her friends, write dream enlargements and was eventually able to say a final goodbye to her husband in a dream. She confided that the dream was white, which is a healing color. When Eloise checked out of the spa she was an avid dream correspondent, without digestive problems or depression.

## HOW TO DISCOVER HIDDEN DATA ABOUT YOURSELF

During fasting, the brain rises to heights of efficiency particularly in the area of recall and insight. It is said that we never forget any facts that we have ever encountered. When ideas seem forgotten, they are merely mislaid. Somewhere in the inner consciousness of the subconscious mind these facts are still recorded, and on certain occasions when something happens to suggest them, they will rise again into consciousness.

While fasting when the bloodstream is well cleared of debris, all these forgotten or mislaid facts are again uncovered and ready for instant use. This seems to indicate that all we need to uncover mislaid facts is to clean up our act, so to speak, and have a more hygenic mind and body via fasting. At this point dreams can be an effective healing tool.

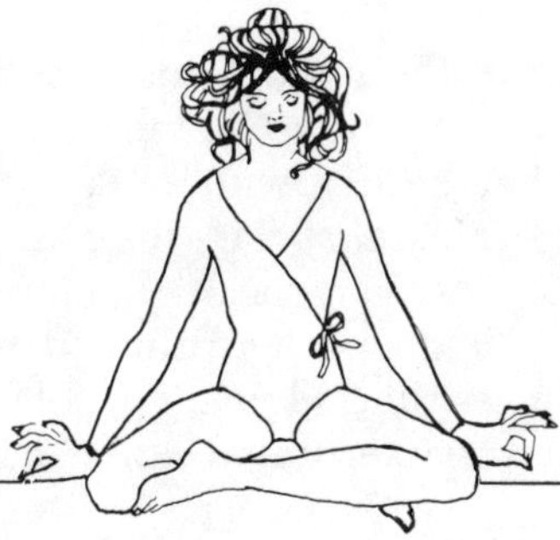

# 3

# Water Therapy

*Go to a watering place when your days are getting longer.*

*Paracleus*

## HOW CONTINENTAL WATER THERAPIES WILL WASH AWAY YOUR ILLS

Water, that magical cleanser of disease, tension and dirt; quencher of thirst; purifier of bodies; and relaxant, is one of the best healing sources in our natural medicine chest. Europeans appreciate the healing powers of water.

Nature provides us with water healing every time we emerge from a hot bath, and step into a cool environment. First the heat of the bath increases surface circulation, dilates pores and encourages sweating. Next, the cold air stimulates internal circulation while contracting surface blood vessels and pores. The two used either one right after the other, or on different parts of the body at the same time, will greatly increase circulation throughout the whole body.

This means that cells receive more nutrition and have their waste-matter collected sooner and more efficiently. The organs that deal with waste-removal, namely, the kidneys, bowels, skin and lungs become better fed and able to function.

## HOW YOU CAN WASH AWAY YOUR ILLS

Water therapy has been appreciated throughout history. The prophet Elisha experienced healing waters at the River Jordan as noted in II Kings, 2:22. Cleopatra enhanced her beauty with milk baths. Caraculla and the Roman legions found mineral-springs helpful for many purposes: battle-fatigue, rheumatism, orgies, relaxation, church-guardianship and riot-control as well as hygiene. It's rumored that Charlemagne held court from a large tub where he had floating tables in order that his backgammon game would not be interrupted while he had "le bain," the French bath.

Greeks were the original people to find relief by using water therapy. They built resplendent temples with baths, and various gods and sea nymphs served as protectors of these elegant watering holes.

Romans, who usually did things bigger and better than their Greek counterparts, built luxurious temples near mineral-springs. When Rome's Tiber became too polluted for public bathing due to urban expansion, an alternative had to be found. Wealthy Romans built lavatrinae, which were early bathrooms. Eventually public baths were built, and when the Emperor Constantine came to power, there were 360 baths and 11 thermae. It has been estimated that the city's water, which was brought in by huge aqueducts, totalled 200,000,000 gallons a day, which is approximately how much modern Romans use.

The emperors, particularly Caraculla, built opulent baths, such as Caraculla's own, which accommodated 16,000. Rich Patricians, as well as poor Plebians, bathed together. Perhaps these early Roman watering-holes were a means of riot-control. After a dousing of hot, tepid, and then cold water, the Plebians were probably too relaxed to rise up against Caesar. The public baths were a sight to behold. The old Pennsylvania station in New York was a replica of the Roman baths of Caraculla.

Cold water treatments were favored by early Greeks. The Spartans proclaimed bathing in cold waters as holy, which is why we probably still call a ruggedly health life "Spartan." Even Pythagoras, the teacher of geometric theorems, insisted his pupils take cold baths to strengthen body and spirit.

In the 19th century, water therapy, or balneology, was recognized for its curative powers by the European medical world. Vincent Priessnitz, an Austrian, first introduced the water cure to European doctors. His cold water applications were aimed at stimulating and encouraging sluggish vital organs to eliminate wastes more effectively.

## How Anais G. Overcame Menstrual Irregularities

Anais G., age 32, chose St. Moritz as the setting for her cure for menstrual irregularities. The Engadine in St. Moritz offers cut peat and alpine herbs for bathing. Each day she took either a mineral bath or herb bath that caused a slow yielding of over-heating. Blood circulation was strongly intensified as were her supradrenal glands and ovarian activities. The cure effectively helped Anais strengthen her own circulation and bodily functions.

A hydrotherapist tells me you can get the same results by:

*Taking a Ginger Bath*

Add 1 cup ground ginger to bathwater. Get in and sit for 20 minutes while you perspire. When you get out, dry off and lie under an electric blanket, turned up high. Perspiration and improved circulation will result.

A later pioneer of hydrotherapy was Father Sebastian Kneipp, a Bavarian monk. The name of Kneipp has become the German noun for water cure. Like most water treatment, his purports to stimulate the body's own defense against disease. Father Kneipp had cured himself of consumption by bathing in the Danube's cold water. He believed that fresh cool "living" water improved circulation in the feet, legs and internal organs thereby speeding up the healing process.

Like Priessnitz, he believed strongly in using cool water. However, he also used alternating hot and cold water treatments that ended with cool water, which was sun-exposed and drawn from a spring or river. Father Kneipp is better known for some of his treatments such as walking barefoot in the snow, alternating hot and cold pools, walking barefoot in the grass, and sulphur baths.

## ADVANTAGES OF COLD WATER BATHING

Cold water almost sounds like a panacea when you consider the many advantages of its use. Here are some of its benefits:

- It improves circulation and increases muscle tone.
- It aids metabolism and improves digestion.
- It influences the central nervous system, the brain and all vital organs of the body.
- It enhances glandular functioning, particularly the adrenals and hormonal production.

- It assists in preventing premature aging.
- It builds up resistance against colds and infections.
- It promotes beauty and keeps you younger longer.

## FATHER KNEIPP'S RULES FOR COLD WATER TREATMENT:

1. Cold water treatment must not be used by anyone who feels chilled.
2. A cold plunge bath should not last more than four or five minutes, including dressing and undressing.
3. After any application, the body, with the exception of the face and hands, must not be dried. The body should at once be covered, while wet, with dry clothing to protect it from the outside air.

## WHY DRYING IS TABOO

Drying involves rubbing which can not be done evenly over every part of the body, and it leads to an unequal distribution of heat over the skin. The simpler plan of not drying quickly produces a regular, uniform and natural heat. Like throwing water on a fire, the body's own warmth promptly utilizes the water adhering to its outer surface to generate an intense heat.

## WHAT TO DO AFTER A COLD WATER TREATMENT

After each application of water it is necessary to walk around briskly. This is done until every part of the body is completely dry and has regained normal warmth. Walk quickly at first and slow down as the body heat returns. Those who warm up quickly and perspire should walk slowly at first and take a longer walk. Then, lie down and rest for 20 minutes.

## FATHER KNEIPP'S THEORY

His theory is akin to the naturopathic or homeopathic approaches presently acceptable in most European Bads or kliniks. The theory includes:

1. A water cure in which water of different temperatures is applied in various ways to stimulate the body;

2. Phytotherapy, the usage of plants or parts of plants to heal;
3. Kinesotherapy which includes active motion, walking, hikes, sports, as well as passive-motion massage;
4. Dietetics, a change of diet to organic food, which eliminates toxins, such as tobacco, coffee, black tea and high caloric substances and substitutes organic foods;
5. An "Order of Life" therapy to restore natural life rhythm and psychic harmony, as a prerequisite for health, efficiency and joy of life.

## WHY LIVING WATER?

The living water that Father Kneipp considered so curative is sun-drenched from fast-flowing streams and lakes. Its replenished water is better for health and healing because the sunlight enriches water, which absorbs solar energy. This energy influences the growth and reproduction of beneficial micro-organisms, which exercise a destructive influence on disease causing organisms that pollute water.

The great physician Hippocrates believed in the healing power of living waters. The Greeks cured themselves by drinking running water from temple fountains that was given maximum exposure to sunlight.

## WHAT CAN YOU DO FOR COLD WATER TREATMENT?

One of the best ways to start the day is with a cold shower. It is invigorating, improves circulation and is guaranteed to lift you from lethargy.

As you take your cold shower, consider the notables throughout history who have done likewise. Paracelsus, a cold-water advocate, and the controversial revolutionary physician of the 15th Century, was so impressed with balneological treatment that he wrote about it in *Bader-Buchlein, The Little Book of the Baths.*

## HEADACHE RELIEF WITH COLD WATER

Cold water is used to treat many common and uncommon maladies. The Faecher douche is a popular treatment in Europe. "Faecher douche" is a German word meaning "fan spray or shower." It consists of spraying the soles of the feet with cold water. This can be done outdoors with a garden-hose, or in the bathtub if you have a portable spray attachment. (A hand spray can be purchased at a hardware store for less than five dollars.)

Apply cold water by spraying the soles of the feet for one minute only. This draws the excess blood from the brain and relieves the cranial congestion. Follow this treatment by massaging your neck and shoulders with your fingertips, then rest in bed for about 20 minutes.

When I first was told of this treatment, I was skeptical of its benefits. However, I tried it when fatigued and suffering from an enormous headache from political hassles in an East-European country. As the cold water hit the soles of my feet, I began to feel relaxed. My headache soon dissipated.

## HOW TO REV UP YOUR SEX-LIFE WITH WATER

Potential lovers take note. When the Faecher douche, fan spray, is applied to the lower back and tailbone, sex-life is revitalized.

A cold sitz bath also has an invigorating and stimulating effect on the libido. Fill your bathtub two-thirds of the way with cold water. The temperature should be about 50–65°. Granted, the cold water is a

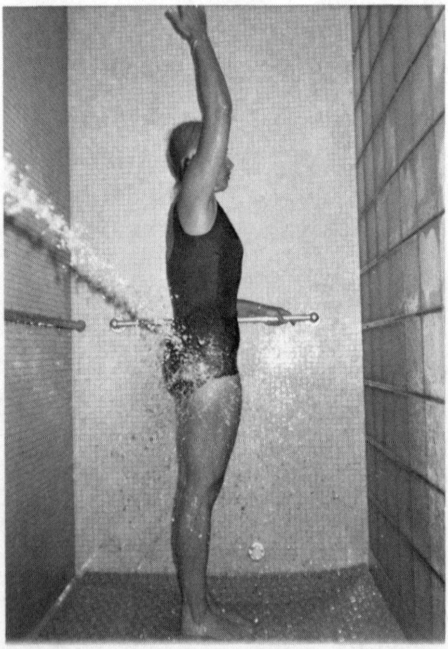

**Photo 3-1.** Faecher douche for improved circulation.

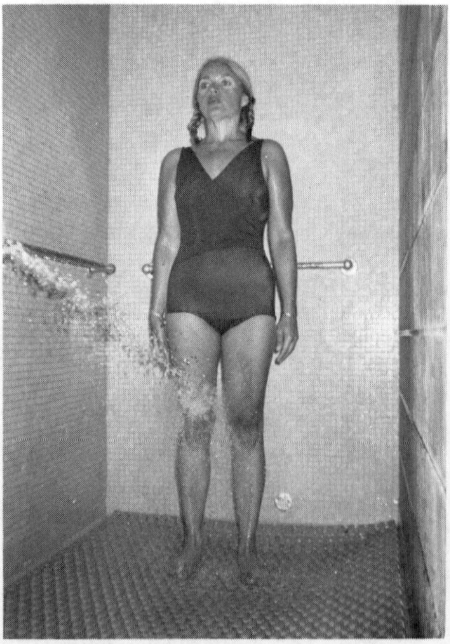

**Photo 3-2.** Faecher douche for circulation and vitality.

shocker, but the three to five minutes that you spend in the tub will be beneficial. The cold sitz bath is popularly called a "youth bath" because of its rejuvenating effect of increasing blood circulation to the vital centers.

## HOW TO "TURN ON" FOR LOW ENERGY DAYS, OR WHAT TO DO THE MORNING AFTER THE NIGHT BEFORE

Upon leisurely rising, get up and exercise for fifteen minutes. This can include jogging, either in place or outdoors, skipping rope, practicing yoga, taking a brisk walk, or doing calesthenics or isometrics. Refer to Chapter 8 for complete exercises.

Exercise until your body feels warmed up. Brush your body with a stiff-bristled brush, beginning at the soles of your feet and progressing up the body, with the exception of the breasts and face.

Take an alternate warm and cold shower, concluding with water as cold as you can endure.

Dry with a corse towel, until you feel warm. This simple routine will build up your resistance to infection, improve circulation to important organs and glands, and prevent premature aging.

If this cold water treatment does not send you off to work skipping and singing, try it again the next day and see what happens.

## WATER TREATMENT FOR OVERWEIGHT

In Europe, the word "overweight" is rarely used. Obesity is the exact term. Even one kilo overweight, which is approximately 2.2 pounds, puts one in the obesity category. The standard water treatment for obesity is the underwater massage. As a veteran of several such treatments, I can attest to their effectiveness. An oversized bathtub, complete with underwater jets, is the locale for this high-pressure treatment. As one reclines in this mammoth tub, the jets of water pulsate every pore of the body, or so it seems. To help this action along, a hydrotherapist, with a quasi-firehose starts at the bottom of the feet and hoses up to the shoulders. After a quick turnover from stomach to back, the procedure is complete. An overweight person might feel he has earned a piece of high-calorie Black Forest Torte after that treatment, but willpower sets in and he goes without.

## HOW TO FIGHT FAT WITH COLD WATER

Cold water therapy is a good supplement to weight control. As cold water hits the body, it produces a warming reaction that increases

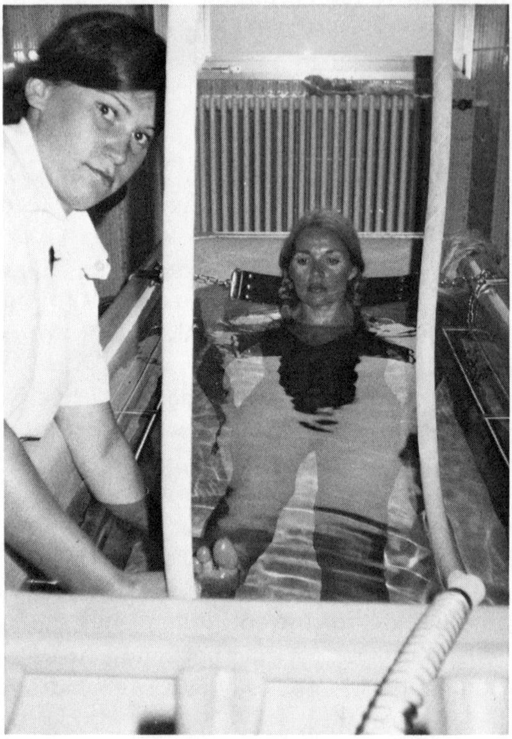

**Photo 3-3.** Underwater massage for the overweight.

the metabolism and reenergizes the body process for health. As the system's energy-glands begin to function, the fat is consumed. While digestion and absorption are also improved.

Recline in a tub half-filled with cold water at 50–75° for approximately five minutes. Then stand up and take a quick, cold shower. Don the now familiar woolen shroud blanket and head for the sack. Rest 20 minutes and dream that the mirror shows less of you. Take a cold-water treatment three-times-a-week for a period of one month to see results.

This should also be done as part of an exercise program and food-reduction plan.

## CONSTIPATION AND WHAT TO DO ABOUT IT

There are several water treatments that are used for constipation. A cold sitz bath is used in the morning and evening, with an alternating hot-and-cold sitz bath, epsom salts, and full baths taken twice weekly as an adjunct to this program. Abdominal massage, biking, hill-climbing or walking up flights of steps, plus swimming are the forms of exercise that are suggested to reduce constipation. This problem usually accompanies a weight problem and is treated accordingly. Water and fruit-juice fast for three to five days followed by two weeks of raw, grated vegetables and fresh fruits. This diet aids both the overweight and the constipated.

## COLD HIP SITZ BATH

Allow two inches of warm water, about 95°, to flow into the bathtub. Sit in it and turn on the cold water, permitting it to run until mid-stomach level. Get up and rub down with a coarse Turkish towel, followed immediately by a massage. (Refer to Chapter 4 for the "how to" of Dry Brush Massage.)

## ALTERNATE HOT AND COLD SITZ BATH

Half-fill the tub with hot water, at about 110°. Sit in the water for five minutes, then refill the tub with cold water, at 50°. Alternative this water treatment twice ending with cool water. Follow this with a cold-friction-rub on the stomach, by taking a wrung-out washcloth that is dipped in cold water and rub it over the abdominal area. This invigorates the stomach organs and their functions and helps to eliminate toxic wastes.

## EPSOM SALTS BATH FOR TOXIN REMOVAL

Epsom salts in warm bath water help rid the system of poisonous wastes. As the Epsom salts are absorbed through the skin, toxins are neutralized in the bloodstream and tissues. This treatment also softens the skin:

Add one pound of Epsom salts to one inch of water in the bathtub. Mix well, sit in the tub, and slowly add water. While the tub is filling up, begin rubbing yourself all over with a salt-water-saturated, soft towel. When the water is up another inch, add another pound of Epsom salts, and continue rubbing. When sweat breaks out on your forehead, quit! The treatment is ended. Stand up and take a quick shower. Rub down with a dry, coarse towel. Treatment time is approximately fifteen minutes.

Note: Rheumatism, sciatica, arthritis, lumbago, neuritis and colds also respond well to Epsom salts baths.

## TREATMENT FOR DIARRHEA

Cold showers and fasting are the prescribed treatment for diarrhea. The fasting program lasts for three days and consists of mineral water and fresh juices followed by a potato diet. The potato is steamed or boiled with the skin on and served with no salt. The first time I saw those small spuds staring up at me from their Dresden platter, I could not believe this was the meal of the day. After two days, the potatoes, along with the water and juice therapy, worked. A potato diet is also effective to rid the system of excessive uric acid caused by overconsumption of meats, black tea and coffee. At the Bircher-Benner Klinik in Zurich, potatoes are used as a diurectic in their fasting program. Try eating three small potatoes at each meal for one day and see if you don't shed a pound or two.

### Cold Sponge Bath for Diarrhea

While standing in the tub, rub the skin quickly with either a loofah sponge or a coarse terry cloth soaked in cold water. Begin at the feet and progress up to the shoulders, repeating every three hours. This stimulates the body and helps get rid of toxic waste.

## WHAT TO DO FOR LOW BLOOD PRESSURE

Low blood pressure is my companion. After my first Bad treatment for this condition, I felt the two of us had parted company. The cold water was so effective and dramatic, that if my blood pressure had been on the stock market it would have been a good buy.

### Home Treatment for Low Blood Pressure

Take a cold shower for one minute. Turn off the faucet, then turn it on again for another minute. When finished, wrap yourself in a woolen blanket and retire for twenty minutes.

The chief hydrotherapist in Bad Hofgastein, Austria informs me that cold showers of short duration are used to stimulate the blood vessels under the skin. They act reflexively on all organs of the stomach and chest. Due to this stimulation, the metabolic function is stepped up and blood pressure increases. Use the cold shower for only one minute to raise your blood pressure. Short cold treatments stimulate. Prolonged cold therapy sedates. The body's warming process causes you to become drowsy.

## HIGH BLOOD PRESSURE

High blood pressure is the illness of the overworked, overstressed, middle-aged businessman. In many of the Bads, high blood pressure is a frequent problem. In Austria, prolonged, one-hour neutral baths are given. The Kneipps foot and leg bath are also part of the treatment.

You can give yourself water therapy at home for high blood pressure:

*Neutral Bath.* Each day, take a bath in 95° water. Keep a cold washcloth as a compress on your head during the entire one hour bath. After leaving the tub, wrap yourself in a warm woolen blanket and rest for at least 20 minutes.

*Kneipps Foot and Leg Bath.* If you are agile, stand in a bathtub full of warm water. Take a hand hose and spray up and down the spine with cold water. If you prefer, sit on the edge of the bathtub with your feet in buckets of hot water, simultaneously spraying your extremities with a hose. Ten minutes is ample time for this treatment. Again, encase yourself in a wool blanket and recline for 20 minutes.

## COLD SALTWATER TREATMENT FOR YOUNGER SKIN

Sea saltwater has the best curative power of all the neutral living waters. Do you remember the invigorating feeling you had when you spent a vacation by the ocean or sea? In Germany, many of the Bads and spas are located along the North Sea or Baltic coast to take advantage of the healing effects of the seaside saltwater. Marinotherapy is the term that describes these water "kurs". Many of the spas build seawater swimming pools to make use of the saltwater during cooler months. They realize that sea water is rich in beneficial minerals which are absorbed through the skin and also through the inhaled mineral-rich air of the seaside. Such conditions as allergies, eczema and varied skin problems, abnormalities of blood pressure, circulation and dry skin respond very well to the saltwater treatments.

For health's sake, spend your next holiday or vacation by the sea. If that is impossible, then bring the sea to your bathtub.

## HOW TO BRING THE SEA TO YOUR BATHTUB

In addition to providing the usual benefits of cold water bathing, saltwater and its accompanying minerals will recharge your system and create a more youthful appearance for your skin. As the salt is absorbed through the skin, it attracts more water via a magnetic action, which creates a moisturization in the skin. As moisture is retained by the skin, and the tissues are lubricated, fine lines of dryness disappear, as do flaky and rough patches. What you need:

At a health-food store or pharmacy, purchase:

*Seasalt,* or use the following ingredients:

3½ lbs. of common table salt

½ lb. of magnesium chloride

½ lb. of Epsom salts

Dissolve four and a half pounds of seasalt mixture in a tub half full of cool water.

Immerse yourself and envision yourself basking in the Baltic Mediterranean, Caribbean, or any of your favorite beaches.

Turn up your stereo or radio with mood music in another room, or sing to yourself to create atmosphere in your own seaside bathtub resort. Rub yourself briskly with the seasalt and enjoy your saltwater adventure.

Dry and warm yourself with coarse Turkish towels, which are more effective for retaining body warmth. Then, start your day with a smile.

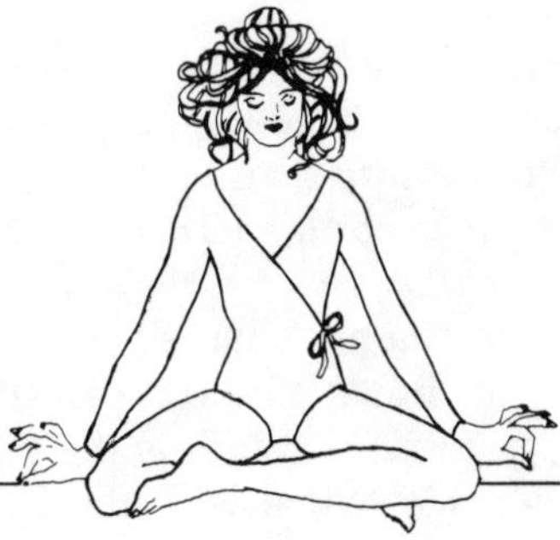

4

# At the German Bad You Discover How to Feel Good

*"Water Works Wonders."*
*Sebastian Kneipp*

The Germans call it *Bad,* others say "spa," but whatever your ailment, Western Germany has a Bad for you. Health spas total over 240 mineral, mud, marine, Kneipp and climatic treatment centers. Bad Pyrmont, Bad Nauheim, Weisbaden, Badenweiler, and Bad Wiessee are some of the names that come to mind. Each Bad offers natural mineral springs that are unique to its location. Natural hot, bubbling mineral, saltwater, carbonated and brine baths are some of the options.

During a water treatment the body absorbs these minerals. European medical people do not state that the water itself is healing, but rather that the mineral water helps the body to self heal. In most Bads, the essence of the treatment is hydrotherapy. Bathing, drinking, internal irrigation and vapor inhalation are some of the curative methods. Like the early Romans, present day spa-goers can also enjoy sensuous baths made from fruit, minerals, milk, honey, hot and cold water and flower extracts.

## BADEN-BADEN

As one of the best known remnants of the Roman migrations, Baden-Baden offers the dualism of therapeutic baths and elegant social spa. Nestled near Germany's Black Forest and less than an hour from Strasbourg, France, it is the ultimate, with the world's best anti-stress program.

What makes it special? Elegance is in the air charged with invigorating quantities of ozone. As you stroll down the Kur path that meanders along the romantic River Ooos, you will be treading the same paths where Brahms, Dostoevski, Napoleon III, Kaiser Wilhelm I and Marlene Dietrich once walked. There you can see Europe's most lavish Casino, where solid gold chips are still used on gala nights.

Nearby is the most fabulous hotel, the Brenner's Park Hotel. The guest-register reads like the world's Who's Who. Located on tree-lined Lichtentaler Allee, it is elegance personified, with exquisite furnishings, very personal service, gourmet foods that can't be compared. Further down the path is the Friedrichbad, which is located over thermal springs. This communal bath with its regal columns, marble tiles and painted murals was built over the ruins of Aquae Aureliae, the Roman baths, some 200 years ago. It was here amid sodium-chloride springs that I was baptized in the Bad treatments and discovered their by-product, supreme relaxation.

## IRISH-ROMAN BATH FOR STIMULATION AND IMPROVED CIRCULATION

When I spoke with the Kur director on the Augustplatz, I was told that the principle of water therapy is that of balancing stimulation with relaxation. Alternating hot and cold water provides a shock to the system improving circulation and vitality. During a thermal bath, the active elements of the water actually penetrate into the skin and body. Taken over a period of time, these hot saline waters have demonstrated curative effects on neurological, respiratory, cardiovascular, rheumatic and psychic ills. That sounds like a large order, but to understand it fully, I will give you a bath-by-bath account of the proceedings in Irish-Roman communal baths.

## MY COMMUNAL BATH EXPERIENCE

An Irish-Roman Bath? The term sounded incongruous to me as I walked up an expansive staircase in the Friedichsbad. I was led into a small cabin to disrobe, grab a towel and head for my first treatment. Looking like a latter-day vestal virgin in sheets, I entered a pink-tiled, dry heat chamber and studied the mosaic water birds and lilies that adorned the walls while basking in its warmth. After fifteen minutes of hot steam, I was shown into a smaller, hotter space for ten minutes of more of the same. Just as I was about to relax, a hardy Amazon attendant summoned me to an adjoining massage room to strip.

I was about to experience a massage to end all massages. After a liberal sudsing with generous amounts of lathered soap with a brush that felt like steel wool, I was vigorously massaged, and I mean vigorously, from the soles of my feet to my neck. Improved circulation, dead skin removal and rejuvenated skin-tone are some of the benefits of this treatment. As the indelicate brush was rotated from one extremity to another, my skin became the rosiest hue it had ever been.

After this cathartic brush-off, I gingerly made my way to another steam room where the ceiling perspired and so did I. While reclining on a white marble slab, I studied the Roman graffiti on the walls, and wondered who wrote it.

A succession of warm thermal baths followed. Feeling like a Roman Centurion going from kalidorium to frigidorium, I floated, reclined and basked in the waters, imagining I would soon be sought by Caesar for an orgy or, at least, a Roman banquet.

The piece de resistance was a quick plunge in frigid waters. Although I was in that glacial basin for only one minute, it seemed like an interminable length of time. At last an attendant shrouded me in a sheet and wool blanket and escorted me into a faintly lit, domed, sleep rotunda. Here I was laid to rest in a semi-circle of sleeping curists. I felt as energetic as Caesar did when he uttered "Et tu, Brute" in another rotunda, and immediately sank into a deep sleep. The rest was so profound that when I awakened I was convinced that I had died and was awaiting processing at heaven's gates.

## BATHING AS A HEALTH MEASURE

Do you really know how important bathing and proper skin care are to your health? That was a question asked of me by a Kur director in Bad Hofgastein before I took the plunge in Austria's healing waters. He went on to tell me that the skin is not generally thought of as a vital organ as are the heart, liver or lungs. Yet science tells us that if our skin fails to function for even a few hours, all the internal organs can break down. the nervous system can become paralyzed and the kidneys, liver and heart poisoned. In severe scalding or third degree burns, when two-thirds of the skin is destroyed, death shortly follows as a result of the reflex destruction of the internal organs.

## WHAT THE SKIN DOES FOR YOU

The word "pore" comes from the Greek *poros* meaning passage. The millions of pores in your skin are important gateways for eliminating waste products from your body in the form of perspiration from tiny sweat-glands. About one quart of moisture is excreted during a 24 hour period. The sudorific glands secrete and discharge a thin oil which lubricates your skin and hair as well as acting as a protective device against invading bacteria.

Your skin also functions in aiding the regulation of body temperature and prevention of the escape of necessary body heat to a considerable extent. When your body becomes overheated through strenuous exercises, such as aerobics or carrying a grand piano up three flights of stairs, external heat escapes through your skin. As an organ of respiration and absorption, your skin takes in oxygen and exhales poisons and gases.

The most important function of your skin is the elimination of impurities. In fact, it works overtime casting off more wastes than your lungs, bowels and kidneys combined. Since your skin plays such a vital role in eliminating toxins, the importance of bathing cannot be overestimated. Unless you take frequent baths, wastes accumulated on the skin can be reabsorbed, causing your system to become toxic and ill.

As an illustration of what can happen, recall that with the advent of the Dark Ages, the public baths, which were so popular in Roman times, were abandoned. In the opinion of Michelet, the noted historian, this loss was responsible for the terrible plagues and pestilence of that period. Maybe the moral of the story is to bathe relatively often or wear a clove of garlic around your neck as the survivors of the Plagues did!

## CLEANLINESS IS NEXT TO GODLINESS . . . OR IS IT?

The ancients recognized the value of bathing, not only for hygiene, but as a religious ritual. Mohammed instructed his people to bathe before each of the five daily prayers, and Moses commanded his fellow Israelites to be scrupulously clean.

Bathing was incorporated into the Jewish religion with the advent of the Micvah. Baptism, a spiritual cleansing, is widely practiced among Christians, both in the Baptist submersion variety and the Catholic symbolic sprinkling from a font. North American Indians used vapor baths for treatment of illness and had sweat lodges, or holy places where they contemplated their own spirituality and warded off evil spirits.

I can readily understand why the skin, along with the kidneys, liver and colon, is one of the greatest organs of elimination. As a veteran of having my epidermis rubbed, hosed, pounded and squeezed, all for the sake of health, I have come to believe that it has removed as much accumulated metabolic waste as possible.

## DRY BATHING

Dry skin brushing is one of the most effective of all baths. The French use the dry brush massage as a means of invigoration in the morning and as a sleep conducive at night.

It is also a good means of eliminating dead skin, and no soap can wash the skin as clean as the new skin you have under the old. Your body makes new skin every 24 hours. With dry skin brushing, the top layer is removed, which helps to eliminate uric acid crystals, catarrh and various acids in the body. The skin should eliminate about two pounds of waste daily.

*Materials needed:* Use any one of the following:

Dry vegetable-bristle massage brush with a long handle, a loofah sponge or mitt, a horsehair mitt or brush, or a bathbrush, other than nylon.

*Procedure:* First thing in the morning begin rubbing gently at the soles of the feet. Progress up the legs, torso, chest, arms and neck. Be sure to rub gently so that only the top layer of dead skin is removed from the body. This allows the cells beneath the surface to breathe. Massage all areas of the body with the exception of the breasts and face. Do not use the brush where you have any skin abrasions or irritations. You will feel invigorated after this brush off. Your skin will be tingling and pink with increased blood circulation by the time you are finished.

The dry brush massage is the most effective means of regenerating poorly eliminated skin. Follow this treatment with a bath or shower to further remove the dead skin cells.

*Principles of Bathing:* A bath can be energizing and psychologically nourishing. It also serves to remove the external toxins accumulated on the skin. Urban air is heavily laden with particles of dirt and soot, radioactive fallout and poisonous spray. A bath removes this external collection of debris.

Don't rush your bath. Set aside time for complete peace and relaxation. In fact, rest and bathing can be successfully combined to produce excellent results not possible with rest alone.

Hard water, found in many cities, leaves a dryness on the skin, and only frequent rinsing will remove this irritating film. For this reason, it is recommended that fruits, oils, milk, or bran be used in the bath to counteract the damage that the hard water can do to the body. *Soap* can be very drying especially after the age of 30. It takes the natural oil from your skin put there to keep vitamin C in the system. It is wise to use a liquid cleanser and soap only three times a week.

## RELAXATION BATH

Fill the tub with 100° water, which is just above the body's own temperature. It should be neither too hot or too cold. Once the tub is completely filled, submerge yourself up to your chin.

Next place a rolled-up towel or plastic-covered cushion behind your head. The nape of your neck should be comfortably supported by the padding to promote soothing and relaxation.

Rest for 20–30 minutes in your own spa-bath. Then, take a cold shower for two minutes. The warm water relaxes the adrenal and pituitary glands to help draw tension and congestion away from the inner organs. The spa bath helps the glands send soothing hormones to relax the blood vessels, stabilizing circulation. It also helps send a flush of nourishing red blood to the entire body, forcing it to relax. The cold shower closes the pores and aids the treatment.

Step out of the spa bath and pat yourself gently dry, then ease into bed for deep and tranquil sleep.

## MILK-BATHS FOR DRY SKIN

Milk-baths are particularly good for dry skin. Thirsty pores will be saturated with this calcium covering, resulting in firmer and softer skin. Cleopatra considered milk-baths an integral part of her beauty ritual. Many cosmetic companies have included milk powders in their bath lines. However, the preservatives and other added chemicals make this bath of questionable value.

To prepare your own revitalizing milk-baths, mix one cup of powdered milk and three tablespoons of olive oil in half a tub of warm water. Swish the mixture around, then sit in the water and soak up to your neck. Stretch out while imagining you are bathing in a swan-shaped bath of Pompeii. Conclude with a quick, cool shower to close and invigorate the pores.

At Christmas time, use commercial eggnog. One quart in a bathtub will make your skin utterly silky for days. Think of all the calories you are saving! I have known people whose skin was as parched and dry as the Sahara desert, but after several eggnog treatments, and 1 tablespoon of lecithin daily as a food supplement, their skin became increasingly moist.

## LEMON BATHS FOR OILY SKIN

The lemon is a multi-purpose fruit which acts as an astringent upon the skin. It also helps to restore the skin's acid mantle. Whether your skin is oily, dry or normal, you will find a lemon bath to be refreshing and energizing. Cut up the rinds from five lemons and drop into a lukewarm tub of bathwater. Be sure that the pieces are large enough that they do not clog the bathtub drain. Soak for twenty minutes and imagine that you are the star attraction in your own floating fruit bowl. If your skin is particularly oily, alight from the tub after your beauty bath and pat dry with a Turkish towel. Should your skin be moderately oily, you may choose to conclude your beauty treatment with a brief cold shower.

## LEMON AND VINEGAR BATH

Slice two lemons and add to 1 cup of vinegar. This mixture will help to maintain the pH-acid-alkaline balance of the skin. Combine 1 cup of Epsom Salts and the peels of three lemons. Steep in a covered glass jar for 24 hours, then remove the cover and pour the mixture under warm, running bath water. Fill the tub ¾. Recline and enjoy the sensation of tension dissipating from your body.

## BRAN BATHS FOR ECZEMA

The Swiss treatment for eczema has been bran emollient baths. Bran baths which are very popular in Europe, are used for stimulating the circulation, softening the skin, cleansing face and hands, and enriching the bath. Bran is also used in bags as hot poultices. Reformhaus, a European health food store, sells bran bags. To make your own bran bag, just put one cup of bran in a cheese cloth and securely wrap. Add it to your bathwater and soak. For particularly rough spots on the body, such as knees, elbows, and feet, make a paste of the bran and, before bathing, apply vigorously to the rough areas. Let it harden, then rub it off with a washcloth. Rinse off the bran bath, then pat your body dry with a coarse towel. Many Europeans like to conclude this bath with a dry brush massage for added stimulation.

## BRAN BATH FOR CHRONIC ECZEMA

Chronic eczema responds well to bran emollient baths; however the bath treatment is not enough. The person suffering with eczema is advised by European doctors to stick to a bland diet of cereals, and vegetables, avoiding all meat and soured milk products like yogurt or buttermilk. Liquids in the form of fruit or vegetable juices and ample amounts of water should also be consumed.

## HOW TO MAKE THE BRAN EMOLLIENT BATH

Before bedtime, place two pounds of bran in a porous bag, such as cheese cloth. Soak it in a pan of hot water for twenty minutes, then fill the bathtub and pour the pan of hot water and the bran bag into the tub. Get in and relax. After fifteen minutes, start massaging yourself all over with the bran bag. Keep mashing it against yourself. After twenty minutes, get out and pat yourself dry, do not rub. This will leave a sticky film all over you. Next, place a plastic sheeting in your bed, above and beneath your body, and get in bed and sleep soundly. The next morning, take a warm shower to wash the bran film from your body and note the fine texture of your skin. At the Bads, this treatment is done three times a week for two weeks.

## WHEAT GERM BATH FOR SOFTER SKIN

Like the bran bath, wheat germ is effective in softening rough, red skin. For your own luxury bath, place one cup of liquid wheat germ in warm water. Fill the tub two-thirds full to cover your body. Use another cup of wheat germ in a bag or cheese cloth and rub over the dry-skin areas of the body. Wheat germ is a definite bath-enricher. You will emerge from the tub with glowing skin.

NOTE: Wheat germ can also be used as a facial mask.

Mix wheat germ and water to paste consistency. Pat on your face, avoiding the sensitive areas around the eyes and the hairline. Keep the mask on your face about 15 minutes, or until hardening occurs. Splash off with cold water, followed by liberal dousing with cold water to close the pores.

After your facial-pores have been cleansed via the wheat germ mask, take a freshly peeled cucumber and rub the insides of the skin again your face. This natural astringent is refreshing and soothing to the skin.

## SALTS

Mineral salts are alkalis that soften water, giving it a smoother texture and the ability to suds when soap is added. This softening effect on the skin makes it feel silky after bathing. Salt's antiseptic quality also cleanses the skin surfaces and washes out abrasions.

The most common salts used in bathing are: Sodium chloride, common table or sea salt. Sodium carbonate is washing soda for clothes and skin. Sodium bicarbonate, better known as baking soda, is used to absorb odors, neutralize acids, clean teeth and is used in lotions to relieve itching. Magnesium Sulfate—Epsom Salts, soften skin and can function as a mineral laxative.

## SALT BATH FOR RHEUMATIC RELIEF

Rheumatism responds well to a mixed-salt bath. Add 1 cup of Epsom Salts and 1 cup of table salt to a full tub of water. Soak in the tub for 30 minutes, then take handfuls of table salt and rub all over the body. This is effective when done for several days. Mineral or distilled water should also be consumed during this time.

## BEAUTY BATHS FOR NEW RADIANCE

### Swedish Salt Glow

The Swedish are known for their beauty and their saunas. One of their bath secrets is a salt bath. To prepare your own, use 1 cup of table salt or sea salt (can be purchased in health food stores) and pour into hot tub-water. Sit in your full, hot bathtub until perspiration breaks out on the forehead. While standing, rub the skin briskly with dry table salt until the body is glowing pink. Your blood circulation is energized by this treatment. Follow with a cold shower of about one to two minutes' duration. Rub down with a coarse towel, and get into bed or recline, depending upon your habit. Sleep will be almost immediate. The next morning you will have renewed energy and feel like your old body was repossessed and you have been issued a new model. In short, you will feel rejuvenated.

### Sage Bath for Silky Skin or to Ease Itching

Sage is a plant of the mint family that is used in beauty baths. Most people think of sage solely as an ingredient in soups or dressings. Not so. The French say it is a very effective bath treatment, acting as an astringent with a healing effect upon the skin. Sage can either be used in a bag, as with bran or wheat germ, or it can be used loose in the tub. If used in a bag, place one cup on a cheese cloth and soak it for twenty minutes in warm water. Then pour the mixture and sage bag into an awaiting half-tub of warm water. Should you elect to use sage directly in the water, pour two cups of sage in the warm bath-water. Wait five minutes for it to steep, just as you would with tea. Then, immerse yourself in your French bath and enjoy. After bathing for twenty minutes, you can splash some of the sage water on particularly dry spots to ease itching or for added silkiness of the skin. Rinse in cool water and dry.

### Lagnappe or Lagniappe

Lagnappe is a French word meaning "a little something extra." Along the Cote d'Azur, that little something extra is the usage of oils to lubricate the skin before and after bathing. Such inexpensive beauty treatments as corn, safflower and olive oils, or other unsaturated vegetable oils are used to condition the skin after bathing. These food lubricants are rubbed into the skin, with the effect of increased circulation and a healthy color. Note: as a pre-bath rub for flaky skin, one cup of salad oil is used all over the body.

## SUNBURN-RELIEF BATHS

When most of Europe heads to the south coast of France and Greece for the June and July holidays, many of these baths are taken. Basking in the sun's vibrant rays can leave tender skin painfully red and burning. To relieve this distress, bathe in a tub of tepid water to which two cups of apple cider vinegar have been added. If the sunburn's pain is too intense, sponge a mixture of three tablespoons of vinegar to four cups of water over the affected areas. Also use aloe vera potion. Either cut open the leaves of an aloe vera plant and rub the milky substance on the skin or buy a prepared potion from a health food store. Several applications of aloe vera is very effective to relieve the heat of sunburn.

## WATER THERAPY FOR INSOMNIA

There are many reasons for not being able to sleep at night. Europeans consider that insomnia in itself is not a disease, but rather a symptom of something wrong in the system. It may be due to stress, auto-intoxication, overwork, bedtime eating, poor ventilation in the sleeping room or a host of other problems. To cure insomnia, take a warm bath followed by cold water treading which releases cerebral congestion and make sleep possible.

1. Take a warm bath (90–95°F) for 20 minutes lying in the tub submerged to the chin.
2. Follow this with cold water treading. Fill the tub half-way with cold water, to mid-calf level. Slowly walk back and forth in the water for two minutes.

3. Dry feet and put on wool sweat socks since this will encourage the body to reach its own heat level.
4. Get into your bed in a room well-ventilated with cool air.
5. Program yourself for relaxation. Stretch out and tense every muscle in your body. Hold your arms tightly by your sides with clenched fists. Then, gradually relax your toes, ankles, feet, and progress up the body until you reach the head. Talk to yourself gently saying each part by name. Keep repeating the process until your body responds to the auto suggestions.

## SCHLENZ-BATH

One of the overheating approaches that is used particularly in Austria is the Schlenz-bath, named after Maria Schlenz. Fever-bath is important to strengthen the body's capacity to fight infection and to make the skin a lively organ again. The object of this bath is to totally cover the body with water, starting with a low temperature of about 98°, or approximately the temperature of the skin. Let water run constantly from the faucet, and in 15–20 minutes, bring the temperature in the tub to about 100°. The length of the treatment is about an hour.

The secret to the effectiveness of this treatment is that the body is totally emerged in water. No heat escapes from the body and its temperature will rise to match the temperature of the water.

After alighting from the water treatment, give yourself a dry brush massage, as previously described. The dry brush massage brings the blood to the skin's surface and relieves undue pressure on the heart.

The Bircher-Benner Klinik has an incredible hydrotherapy department. I experienced so many water treatments there I was wondering if I would be all washed up. Some of my favorite footbaths to fight fatigue are the following:

### Footbath #1—Alternating Hot and Cold Water for Instant Energy

This footbath is designed to revive a tired body. Sit on the edge of the bathtub and let hot water run over the feet. The water should be as hot as can be endured. Let the water run for two minutes, then switch to cold water. Alternate hot and cold streams over the feet for about ten minutes . . . and *voila* . . . the feet and body come alive!

### Footbath #2—Mint Footbath to Aid Sleep

To assure a tranquil sleep after a hot day, place a handful of peppermint or spearmint leaves in a container or basin of hot water. Then soak the feet for ten minutes. Pat dry with an absorbent towel and feel the tenseness dissipate from your body via the feet.

### Footbath #3—Epsom Footbath for Headaches

This footbath is helpful in relieving headaches, backaches, cold feet, and congestion in the stomach and pelvic organs. On cold days, soak the feet in a capful of Epsom Salts in a basin of hot water. Feet and legs should be covered to the knees. Follow by patting dry with a towel and relaxation should be yours.

### Footbath #4—Baking Soda for Swollen Feet

After a day of endless shopping or walking a mail route, tired feet can be revived by the following method: pour three tablespoons of baking soda in hot water. Follow this by rubbing with either witch hazel or an alcohol rub. Austrian hikers used to an uphill ascent say this footbath is a good means of relieving body tension.

## FOOTBATHS

### Hayflowers for Foot Gout and Open Wounds

This footbath was frequently mentioned in the writing of Father Kneipps, the renowned herbalist. Take about 3–5 handsful of hay-flowers (stalks, leaves, blossoms, seeds, even the hay itself), pour boiling water over them and cover the pan for 10 minutes. Let the mixture cool to the warmth most comfortable for your feet. You can either skim off the hay and pour the remaining liquid in your footbath or leave them in. Place feet in water for 15 minutes, and if you have a good book to read, bring that along and stay longer.

This footbath is also good for dissolving blisters caused by jogging, marathon-running or just plain walking. Puffiness in the feet, which usually accompanies gout is also relieved, as are sweating feet, open wounds, and contusions.

### Salt Bath for Corns, Calluses and Bunions

Prepare a footbath by adding one tablespoon of salt to three quarts of water. Add one cup of mint leaves, and soak your feet in this mixture for about 15 minutes just before bedtime. After they are thoroughly dried, take a small piece of lemon peel with the pulp intact and place it directly over the corn or callus and bandage. This is left on overnight. You might also want to place a sock over it to hold it in place. Continue this procedure for 4–5 nights. Each night use a fresh piece of lemon.

### Athlete's-Foot Bath and Treatment

Soak feet in mint and saltwater bath as directed above. Dry feet and apply apple cider vinegar to the affected parts of the foot. Frequent application speeds up the remedy.

### Footbath for Sore Feet and to Improve Circulation

Sore feet, calluses, leg cramps and varicose veins (which are a circulation overload) respond well to a footbath of alternating hot and cold water. Take two pans of water and alternately place your feet in first the hot, then the cold water. Do twice, always concluding with the cold. Often when you feel bad, a foot bath can relieve discomfort.

## HIP BATH FOR LOWER BACK PROBLEMS

Lower back problems are helped by sitting in a basin or tub of cold water. Sit for one minute in cold water, get out, and walk around in a warm room. Then, sit again for one minute in cold water. The warmer you are when you get into it, the easier it will be to take it.

## HEADACHE AND EYE STRAIN

Take two wash cloths, one dipped in cold water, the other in hot and wring them out. Place a hot compress on the back of the neck while a cold cloth is placed on the forehead. Leave them on for 5–15 minutes, placing a small towel over the hot wash cloth to retain heat. Increased circulation will result.

## REJUVENATIVE BEAUTY BATH

Young men fell in love with the youthful-looking French beauty, Ninon de Lenclos, even when she was 70. French historians claim that herb baths kept her looking young all her life. To make her formula, take a handful of dried lavender flowers, mint, comfrey roots and thyme. Mix them together loosely in a muslin bag, place in your tub and pour on enough boiling water to cover. Let it soak for 10 minutes, then fill up the tub. Luxuriously recline in your rejuvenative potion for at least 15 minutes.

## SULFUR BATHS

At many European spas, parcticularly St. Mortiz, sulfur baths are a frequent treatment for problems of skin disorders, nervous conditions, neuritis and rheumatic diseases. In small amounts, sulfur can act as a disinfectant for the organs discarding it, such as the lungs, kidneys and skin. As an irritant to the intestinal tract, it increases the peristaltic action of the bowels as they try to rid themselves of it. Although sulfur is very antiseptic for the intestines, digestion may be inhibited by too much mineral bathing.

If you are allergic to sulfur, do not use this treatment. However, if your rheumatic condition is screaming for attention, try the following treatment: to a tub two-thirds full of warm water, add 5 ounces of sulfurated lime, ten teaspoons of zinc-sulfate crystals (make certain all crystals are dissolved by stirring the water), or two ounces of potassium sulfate. Some drug and health food stores carry ready-made preparations for sulfur baths, which you can use according to directions.

As you leisurely recline in your own spa for twenty minutes, think of the money you are saving. In the spa at Tiberias, Israel, you would pay many pounds for this treatment, in Bad Ragez, your Swiss francs would be long gone, and in Bad Nernforf, you would have to shell out many deutsche-marks for a similar remedy.

## ITALIAN OIL BATH—LA DOLCE VITA

Oil baths were the favorite of the Roman aristocrats who reclined in ornate marble bathtubs around 212 A.D. In a later era, they were used by tired, dry-skinned Roman soldiers returning from their daily battles. It was customary to leave three coins in a nearby fountain in gratitude for the healing.

At the present day Trevi Fountain in Rome, legend has it that if you leave three coins in the fountain you will return again to the Eternal City. If the cure doesn't work, you may have to anyway! However, you can make your own Roman bath by using the following:

½ cup sesame oil

½ cup olive oil

1 tablespoon of liquid detergent shampoo

½ teaspoon of your favorite perfume

Pour oil, shampoo and perfume into a bottle. Shake vigorously before you use it. The shampoo breaks the oil into many fine globules that cling to your open pores. Just 2 tablespoons of this mixture in a tub moisturizes dry skin as you bask in your Italian oil bath.

Relax and enjoy your own la "Dolce Vita." If you can't take a "kur" at Baden-Baden, Aix-lex-Chapelle or Marienbad, you can get the same benefits right in your own tub.

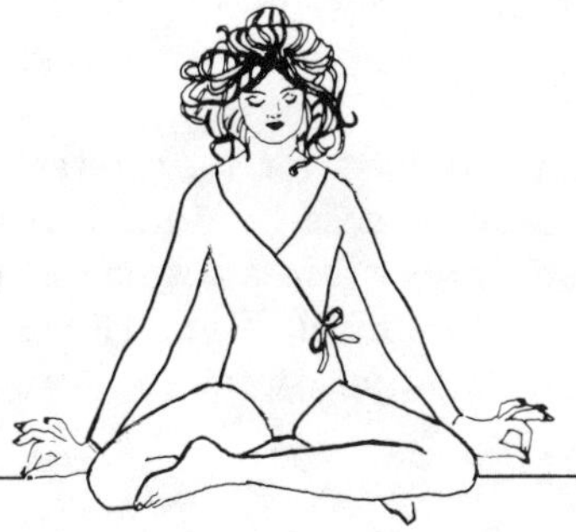

# 5

# Common Ailments and Uncommon Treatments Abroad

*"Human beings possess great powers of spontaneous recovery from illness and other traumatic experiences."*
*Dr. Rene Dubos*

In Europe, food is medicine as are herbs, water therapies and other treatments that might seem absurd to us on the other side of the Atlantic. The use of apples, lemons, potatoes and other foods for healing are standard fare. Who would think that you could eat potatoes all day long and still lose weight? In many spas a "potato day" is commonplace due to the diuretic action of this vegetable which extracts surplus fluids from the body.

Many regions of Europe use plants in minor medical emergencies. I was told that plants are like laboratories in the ground, cranking out healing materials. In fact, many drugs prepared pharmaceutically have their roots in the plant kingdom. Yesterday's folk-remedy is today's cure.

## POTATO AS A DIURETIC

In the seventeenth century, the Irish potato had its beginning as a staple food in Europe. Containing vitamin C, iron, amino acids, protein, thiamine, vitamin G and nicotinic acid which dilates the capillaries, potatoes are an excellent food source. Contrary to popular misconception, they are not high in calories. (Not the potatoes, but the butter and sour cream on them are the fattening villains!) The potato skin has many vitamins and minerals that lie just beneath it, so be sure and eat it.

Many chemical diuretics that are prescribed for fluid-retention have harmful side effects, since they remove excess liquid and badly needed minerals as well. Magnesium and potassium are some of the minerals that are excreted with prescribed chemical drugs. However, potatoes supply minerals while acting as a natural diuretic.

*Menu for a "potato day"*

| | |
|---|---|
| Breakfast: | 2 apricots<br>3 small red potatoes covered with unsalted vegetable broth |
| Lunch: | Sliced cucumbers/tomato<br>3 small red potatoes |
| Dinner: | lettuce—radishes<br>3 small red potatoes<br>(drink Golden Seal tea) |

Want to eat something sweet?

1) Eat sour pickles
2) Eat sauerkraut
3) Eat sweet-sour cabbage
4) Eat stewed tomatoes

## APPLES: ANTIDOTE FOR DIARRHEA OR AS A LAXATIVE

An apple can actually keep the doctor away from diarrhea sufferers. Freshly washed, raw apples, eaten three times a day is Europe's answer to America's Kaopectate. Eat the skin which contains pectin, an important healer which is also being studied for its cholesterol-lowering potential.

If constipation is a problem and you want a natural laxative, grind up fresh apples and eat them in muesli for breakfast and dinner. (See recipe in Chapter 9.)

## CURRANTS FOR SORE THROATS

Currants, which contain vitamin C, calcium, phosphorus, and iron, are an effective means of treating minor sore throats. Simmer, don't boil, two teaspoons of currants in 2 cups of water for 10 minutes. Strain and gargle or add honey and swallow.

## LEMONS FOR STAINED TEETH

In addition to having a high vitamin C content, they are good for dissolving nicotine stains on the teeth. Take a wedge of lemon and abrasively rub against the teeth, then rinse the mouth with clear water.

## GRAPES FOR ARTHRITIS AND OTHER CHRONIC DISEASE

For days or weeks in many spas, people consume only grapes or grape juice to eliminate poisons from the body and to cleanse the system. Drink 1½ quarts of grape juice daily with either mineral or distilled water. Try this for one day a week, then build up to three days.

## GARLIC FOR HIGH BLOOD PRESSURE (AND AS AN ANTISEPTIC OR COLD REMEDY)

Garlic contains an antibiotic called allium that has a reputation for lowering blood pressure. In Russia, where garlic is used extensively for medicinal purposes, people are advised to eat one clove morning and evening.

When crushed and applied to the skin, garlic cures insect bites and stings. When you feel a cold coming on, try chewing a couple of cloves of raw garlic, followed by parsley, which is a natural breath cleanser. Besides its medicinal qualities, garlic has been glorified through the ages. The Romans gave it to laborers to make them strong and to soldiers to give them courage. (Probably in hand-to-hand combat they just breathed on their enemy and the latter succumbed.)

## BANANAS CORRECT EITHER DIARRHEA OR CONSTIPATION

This fruit is a natural regulator of the body, and many European baby specialists make considerable use of thoroughly ripened bananas in the feeding of young children who are constipated or have diarrhea. Bananas are eaten exclusively for three days or until constipation or diarrhea are corrected.

## CARROT JUICE FOR SINUS INFECTION

Fresh carrots possess vitamin A, without a sufficient amount of which often leads to a tendency of the skin and mucuous membrane cells to atrophy. Drink one pint of freshly squeezed carrot juice twice a day to aid in your sinus infection, suggests Dr. Claude De Pris, medical expert. In southern France, carrot juice is consumed to purify the blood.

*Riddle:* *What heals wounds, improves thyroid activity and diminishes body odor?*

*Answer:* *GREEN VEGETABLES.*

Parsley, endive and spinach are only some of the leafy green vegetables that provide a variety of benefits to the body. Chlorophyll, the green color substance in plants, is largely responsible for such curative properties. This little miracle promotes the formation of red blood cells better than iron therapy, stimulates breathing and nitrogen metabolism of the cell tissues, improves protein utilization, normalized blood-pressure and reduces insulin requirements. As if that were not enough, it waves its magic green leaf and body odors disappear. It also heals wounds and improves thyroid activity. These special vegetables deserve a place of honor on any table, so have at least one fresh green salad a day, preferably two.

## OVERWEIGHT SOLUTIONS: NEW WAYS FOR THE MIRROR TO SHOW LESS OF YOU

Attended any free food functions lately? Open houses, wedding receptions or Irish wakes all seem to bring out the vulture in humanity as the food-laden tables are attacked by eager eaters. While one half of the world is starving, the other half is overeating, disturbing their metabolism with excessive food. How often do we really consider that overeating or obesity can lead to an early death?

### *BASIC GUIDE FOR WEIGHT REDUCTION*

1. Europeans generally believe that not only does decreased food consumption aid in weight-loss but also that increased amounts of fresh, uncooked food helps too.
2. Raw foods, such as fresh vegetable salads or fresh fruit should be eaten at the beginning of a meal. Not only is digestion aided, but the appetite is also appeased and your desire to overeat is diminished.
3. Avoid table salt, hot spices and seasonings like chili powder, paprika, mustard, curry and coffee that overly stimulate the salivary glands making you want to eat more. Instead, use vegetable salts (can be purchased at any health food store and some super markets) and fresh or dried herbs like dill, parsley, basil, rosemary, thyme, etc.
4. Limit animal protein to fresh-water fish or low-fat milk products such as cottage cheese, yogurt, buttermilk, Edam, Swiss and other

cheeses. Beware of high protein diets that create an immediate weight-loss that may be a short-lived success, but in the long run, damage your health. Liver damage, inflammation of the large intestine and rheumatic disorders are just some of the after-effects of too much animal protein, says Dr. Liechti von Brasch, renowned European food and health authority.

5. Chew food slowly and thoroughly in a relaxed atmosphere. It's better to sit in a park and leisurely enjoy an apple, than to wolf down a full meal in a restaurant in a few minutes.

6. Have one juice-day a week. This gives your body a needed rest. Ideally, this is best done when you can stay home and rest. If you want to do it at work, then take along either a thermos of juice or buy a quart of apple, cranberry or mixed juice and liberally imbibe them during your coffee breaks.

## HOW HOUSEWIVES CAN AVOID SNACKING AND OVEREATING

When you're at home all day there is a tendency to snack and allow food to become a substitute for emotional satisfaction. It's important to think about the positive changes you can make to overcome your unfortunate love affair with the kitchen. First, you might consider making a room other than the kitchen the center of family activity, so that the temptation to snack is not near at hand. Instead of improving your culinary skills, embark on fun, educational programs with your children, or, try daily running or biking adventures with them. If they are small, put them in the newly designed backpacks and take them along. For years I had one child in a backpack while I biked. Later, I was able to get two bike-seats, one attached in the front and the other in the back, which added balance and safety to an adventurous outing.

Rather than snacking eight times a day, as a recent study indicates the average American housewife does, wait until your small children are napping or playing contentedly before preparing a meal for yourself. Instead of peanut butter and jelly sandwiches eaten amid activity, mix bunches of vegetables in a blender with tomato juice for a quick and tasty gazpacho.

Schedule rest breaks and rewards for the completion of major tasks. Plan to get out of the house on a regular basis so you won't succumb to "cabin fever" and self-pity. When your child is at pre-school or when you can get a baby-sitter or husband to fill in for you, go out and enjoy a sport at a local adult education center or join an exercise class. The more physical activity you experience, the less you will want to eat. Make sure whatever activity you choose is vigorous and lasts an hour at a time if you want to recharge your energy to the maximum degree.

*Want to lose a few pounds painlessly?* Increase your exercise activity by one half-hour to an hour-a-day, says one noted German fitness authority. Go out and jog, run, play racquetball, swim vigorously, bike or play tennis. You will find that the more physical pursuits in your day, the less inclined you will be to overeat. Also remember that skipping meals and eating one big meal late in the day seems to be conducive to putting on weight: morning calories more often go to energy, evening calories go to fat.

## EDEMA-FLUID RETENTION

There are various times when we retain fluids; either premenstrually, through fatigue or during pregnancy. What to do? Initially, try a juice fast for one week.

*Cucumber, pineapple or watermelon* juices all act as diuretics. After a fast is completed, consider a lacto-vegetarian diet of raw and cooked vegetables, particularly green leafy vegetables, seeds, nuts and yogurt. Avoid animal protein and salt. Weekly colonics and daily enemas will help carry away accumulated fluids and toxins, and hot baths, preferably saunas, should be taken twice a week.

Strenuous exercises, jogging, walking, and playing tennis induce perspiration.

Foods to encourage: all silicone rich foods such as young green plants, alfalfa, garlic and onions, parsnips, asparagus, apples, strawberries, grapes, beets, coconuts. Parsley tea also functions as a diuretic.

## HOW TO TRACK YOUR EATING AND EXERCISE PROGRAM

Keep a daily record of your exercise and food intake. You will see that often we do not rationally apply all that we know about good health care.

> *Riddle:* *What can stop momentary depression, low self-esteem and apathy?*
> *Answer:* *Exercise, says Dr. Werner Hess.*

Exercise is effective for fending-off depressed and pessimistic moods that mentally healthy people have occasionally, says Dr. Hess of Baden-Baden. Why? Because exercise produces marked changes in blood-hormone levels. As an example, strenuous exercise causes significant increases in growth hormones, *that bring about salt loss and improved metabolism*. Studies in Europe, as well as those of Dr. Taub at the University of Virginia, indicate that depression seems to be uncommon among athletes, except those who play for high stakes in professional sports.

## HOW TO OVERCOME CRAVING FOR FOOD

Wanting to eat anything and everything in sight is usually an indication of an unbalanced metabolism. To regulate the body's excess cravings can be overcome by a total fast of three to seven days. Thereafter, raw fruits and grated vegetables for two weeks. Such a simple diet provides little in the culinary pleasures, yet natural taste and sensations awaken. Small food intakes will seem satisfactory, and cleansing the system of excess debris is also important. Eliminating excess toxins from the colon via enemas or colonics helps bring about balanced body functioning.

Putrefactive bacteria responsible for many systemic disorders are counteracted by lactic acid. Good sources are yogurt sour milk, buttermilk, cottage cheese, sauerkraut, and sour pickles.

## WHY FATIGUE? AND WHAT TO DO ABOUT IT?

Fatigue, either mental or physical, often comes from a toxic body state. Sluggish circulation and blood loaded with acid debris bring about low-energy days. When muscular activity breaks down fuel to furnish energy, these accumulated wastes cause muscle fatigue and a minimum of oxygen goes to the brain.

To help your body along, you can breathe deeply and get more oxygen flowing to the brain. Take three tablespoons of Brewer's Yeast in juice during the day to provide more B-complex vitamins to your system. Eat plenty of fresh fruits and vegetables, plan periods of rest during the day, or practice autogenic training for six minutes twice-a-day. You will find this exercise listed elsewhere in this book.

## SOME UNCOMMON TREATMENTS

### Fight Urinary Infections with Cranberry Juice

Cranberry juice is used to help fight urinary tract infections like "honeymoon" cystitis and other occurrences of this kind. This plant makes the urine acidic and creates an environment unfavorable to disease-causing bacteria. Two four-ounce glasses of cranberry juice a day for as long as the infection lasts, usually 3–5 days, will help.

## Digestive Problems Answered with PAPAYA

The papaya plant produces a milky juice containing the enzyme called papain, which digests protein much the way the body's own enzyme pepsin does. Papain is very effective for indigestion or overeating. When you have a case of indigestion, take a freshly cut slice of papaya and eat it slowly. Within 15 minutes you should feel relief. Or, as the commercial says . . . Relief is spelled . . . "Papaya!"

Incidently, papain extracted from unripe papaya is the activist in meat tenderizer and is also sold in health food stores as a digestive aid.

## ARTICHOKE, Nature's Own Insulin for Diabetics

Artichokes contain levulose sugars which are helpful for persons with diabetes. Eaten steamed, boiled, stuffed or raw, the heart of the artichoke is the most succulent feature. Cook whole in boiling water for 20 to 30 minutes. Incidentally, in 15th Century Italy, the artichoke was considered an aphrodisiac and for this reason it has been considered as "dear to Venus."

## ASPARAGUS—Potassium Aids the Heart

First used for medicinal purposes, asparagus was not considered a food until the 17th century. Wild asparagus, a much-loved delicacy, is considered to be more tasty than the cultivated varieties. To cook, stand on end and steam until just tender, and serve with lemon butter. Asparagus contains vitamins A, B and C, plus potassium.

## BEETS Help the Liver

Beet greens are a good source of riboflavin, iron and Vitamins A & C. Beet juice is best for cleansing a toxic liver. They can also be boiled, baked, grated and added to salads, and borsch, a soup which is native to Russia and Poland, can be eaten hot or cold with yogurt or sour cream on top.

## Chapped Hands Aid

In Greece, the following solution is used for chapped hands.

1 egg white

1 ounce liquid honey

1 teaspoon glycerine

Knead barley flour to make a paste. Roughened hands will be passé with this inexpensive recipe.

### Burns, Boils & Wounds Treated with Honey

According to Dr. Michael Bulman, a British Medical Doctor, honey is the best surgical dressing for any wounds, particularly burns.

### Halitosis—Bad Breath

The green, chlorophyll-rich juices of parsley, spinach, watercress, comfrey, alfalfa and beet tops combined with carrots and celery are excellent for treating bad breath that is caused by the retention of toxic waste matter in the tissues. Two glasses of vegetable broth a day are also advised.

## HOW TO EXERCISE IF YOU DON'T WANT TO GO OUT AND RUN OR WALK ALONE

If you live outside the city where you work and it's too dark or cold to run when you get home, invest in an exercise bicycle. Try a half-hour every day with stretches before and afterwards. Use it when the weather is bad while you watch the news on TV.

## NUTRITIONAL NEEDS OF BUSINESS WOMEN

Despite the efforts of affirmative action programs, the ride up the career ladder can be bumpy and frought with excess stress. To fight such overt tension, stock up on foods loaded with vitamin C, which helps your system combat stress. Broccoli, tomatoes, oranges, rose hips, strawberries, apples, persimmons, guavas, potatoes, cabbage, black currants, citrus fruits, turnip greens and green bell peppers are some of the natural sources of vitamin C.

If you are like most middle-management women, calories are one thing you have to watch. When you devote a lot of attention to your career, you often tend to overlook your health and your waistline. When ordering business lunches, have a balanced meal of fresh fruit as an appetizer or salad, followed by broiled or baked fish or poultry and a vegetable. Enjoy your food, and eat slowly, as if you are hanging onto your client's every word, which you may be, but you are also aiding your digestion. Concentrate on portion control, and eating smaller amounts. No one expects you to clean your plate. If you've had a heavy business lunch, balance it out with a light evening meal. At cocktail time, consider bottled mineral waters with a twist of lime or a cocktail glass of tomato juice. If you must drink, do so with moderation.

On days when you have to work late and don't have an opportunity to eat till later, take along a thermos of buttermilk, which will provide extra energy as well as a good calcium source to calm your fraying nerves.

## MENSTRUAL DISORDERS AND WHAT TO DO ABOUT THEM

Job and home pressures, coupled with monthly menstrual hassles can leave you feeling irritable, depressed, retaining water, experiencing backaches and fainting spells, cramps, or tension. Many hormonal and metabolic changes occur before and during menstruation, which account for such unpleasant symptoms. Healthy women living close to nature and eating more fresh foods, such as those in Hunza, and parts of Russia and China, do not have the same symptoms of menstrual discomfort as their sisters in western countries. Many of these problems are caused by nutritional deficiencies which lead to improper metabolism of the female sex hormones which abound during menstruation. Vitamins E and $B_6$ are particularly involved, as well as the minerals calcium and iodine.

Sour milk products digest easier than sweet milks. Yogurt, kefir, buttermilk, cottage cheese or sweet milk with a whole lemon squeezed into it and allowed to sour for 20 minutes, will all fill the calcium needs. Brewers Yeast, our old B-complex favorite, plus almonds, millet, oats and other whole grains also supply high-quality proteins and essential minerals and vitamins. Also iron-rich foods like blackstrap molasses, apricots, whole grains and nuts help fight off tiredness resulting from anemic tendencies. It's a good idea to have vitamin C-rich foods, which help absorb iron from food sources. The vitamin C sources listed in the nutritional needs of business women are also good, as are grapes and red beets. Rather than eating 3 squares meals a day, eat frequent smaller ones to prevent low blood sugar which seems to be common during menstruation. In Russia, taking garlic capsules or eating cloves of garlic encourages menstrual flow if sluggish menstruation is your problem. Irregular or profuse menstruation can be aided by one teaspoon of kelp granules added to food every day, claims one French authority.

## HOW TO AVOID MOTION SICKNESS WHEN TRAVELING

Nausea, trembling, dizziness, loss of color, salivation, perspiration are all symptoms that may result from a jolting ride in a plane, train, car or bus. The secret is to prevent these symptoms by resting prior to traveling. If you are overly tired, your chances of developing motion sickness are increased by fatigue. Plan ahead and concentrate on the pleasurable aspects of your trip. Glean adventurous ideas from travel brochures, discuss your exciting plans with your friends rather than anticipating motion sickness. Don't overeat prior to travelling and avoid alcohol, which tends to intensify motion symptoms. Ride up front, if you are in an automobile, bus, train or plane where the motion is less severe. Stay amidship if you are on a boat, says a doctor with the Cunard line. Try to keep your eyes on objects and people inside the vehicle rather than staring at the horizon. The same Cunard physician suggests that you look away from the ocean if you are on board a ship.

Despite all these preventive measures, if you begin to feel discomfort, sit rag doll fashion in your seat and place your head firmly on a pillow or headrest. Close your eyes and keep your movements to a minimum. When in an airplane, turn on the head set to pleasant, soothing music and take your mind off the symptoms, suggests Luftansa airlines.

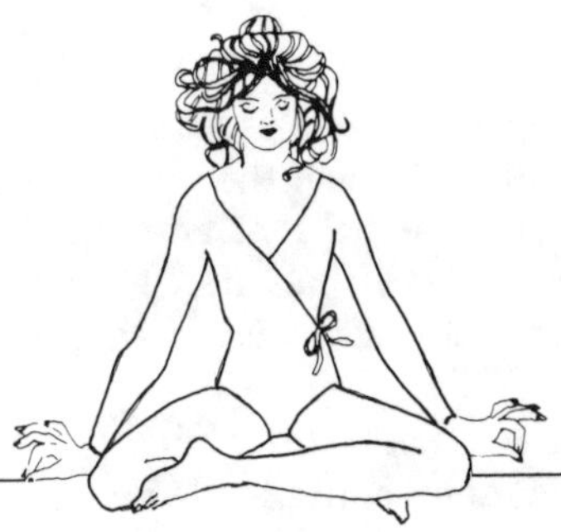

# 6

# Baden-Baden's Answer to an "All-American" Health Problem

*"Health is altogetherness."*
*Dr. Max Bircher-Benner*

In this country, stress is accepted as an inherent part of the American life style, while Europeans try to be more relaxed. Nevertheless, no one, here or abroad, can entirely avoid stress.

From the moment that the alarm clock awakens you, quickly gulped morning coffee and the dash for the bus or subway starts a tension-filled day. Consider the office worker who must submit an important report by five o'clock, or the working mother who is faced with getting children off to music lessons, soccer practice and planning the evening meal before rushing off to an evening meeting. Deadlines must be met . . . a constant race with the clock ensues. Whether you call it tension, anxiety, distress, pressure or stress, the end result is still the same . . . a dragged out body. Such a demanding life style and a diet deficient in nutrients combined with the effect of unrealistic time schedules symbolize contemporary life.

Europeans know, as we do, that tension-induced disorders have become the number-one health problem of the last decade. One standard medical text estimates that 50% to 80% of such diseases as heart attacks, cancer, arthritis and respiratory problems (including bronchitis and emphysema), insomnia and colitis have their origins in stress. Stress is part of the cost of modern living.

Stress, like birth, death and taxes, confronts people on both sides of the Atlantic. No one can avoid the overt tension that is part and parcel of our 20th century life style. People from all regions of the globe experience it in one form or another. Those who are affluent enough to do something about it trek to Baden-Baden to take the Kur. "Entschlackungskur" is the attention grabbing word that is also known in English as the "Anti-Stress" program.

When I first stepped into Dr. Werner Hess's antiseptically white office, his winsome smile and gentle manner convinced me that he undoubtedly was proof of the success of his anti-stress program. Dr. Hess suggests that there are many tensions inherent at work. In order to find the particular stress cause, it's important to know where to look. The first area to investigate is the job itself. Are there frequent deadlines? Is the workload well-defined? Is the personality a type A, or stress-prone individual who will create unreal deadlines, take on extra responsibilities, always impatient and in a hurry? Career conflicts are another source of anxiety. Mismatched ambitions, talents and reality often contribute to stress, as does overpromotion or underpromotion.

New organizational objectives and values resulting from modern technology often find older executives being undercut from their well-defined career expectations. At times, just being a member of a vast organization is a dehumanizing experience. It places restrictions on one's behavior which is often complicated by budgets, filling out forms and compromising one's individuality and identity.

Dr. Edmond Jacobson, initiator of "*Progressive Relaxation*" states: "Business problems can be solved by learning just to be tense enough to solve the problem but no more."

Most life stresses are due to a lack of centering in one's own life. Too often we are like mirrors, reflecting what everyone else wants us to be and not investigating who we really are. Taking time to become acquainted with that inner direction in one's life is vitally important for one's own emotional survival. At many of the European spas there is an effort made to deal with the mind as well as the body. This concept seeks to place a person in harmony with their environment by a combination of the healing efforts of dietetic therapy and changing one's life style.

Presently, the most frequent cause of distress is psychological. Dr. Hans Selye, the international stress authority at the University of Montreal believes that: "stress is induced by not having a code of behavior . . . a lack of adaptability." In an era of rampant change, many people have no roots, and don't seem to get in touch with their own abilities. This problem is expressed by the French author, Montaigne, who said: "No wind blows in favor of the ship that has no direction."

The idea presented at most European spas, primarily at Baden-Baden, Bad Gestein, and Aix la Chapelle, is one that Dr. Selye also advises. That is, make stress work for you. It's important not to exceed one's own critical limit by learning to stop in time before tension sets in. It is possible to get worked-up and simply not be able to slow down and get high, quite literally, on the adrenaline and hormones produced by stress.

An overtense person does not pause to consider whether he is tense. He may be so engrossed in his business that he may fail to realize that success is a variable dependent upon the businessman's maintaining his health thru proper economic and energy expenditures. Suppressing feelings of stress is common. In present society, it is considered normal to tolerate extraordinarily high levels of stress, and there is a martyr-like quality in this attitude which is not healthy.

It's important to become responsible for maintaining good health by learning to identify the major stresses in your life, learning the effects of a situation or person who is affecting you and developing a strategy for dealing with the situation.

After conversing with many stress authorities and tension victims, I was able to compile twelve suggestions on how to make stress work for you.

## POINTS ON HOW TO MAKE STRESS WORK

1. Understand the workings of stress . . . what makes you ill?
2. Whatever situation you come up against, consider first whether it's really worth a fight.
3. Set priorities. Determine what has to be done immediately and what can wait.
4. Space your deadlines.
5. Keep your mind on the pleasant aspects of life and on what you can do to improve it.
6. Stop tension-producing thoughts, e.g., "I'll never get it done."
7. Let go of everything unpleasant and painful that can't be changed, whether these be health, family, personal, or business difficulties. This voluntary mental diversion is perhaps the best way of minimizing stress.
8. Admit that perfection is not possible. Be content to strive for whatever is possible in any given field.

9. Leave buffer times when you're headed for an appointment. If you are going to be late, call ahead to take the pressure off yourself.
10. Nothing helps like success. After a great set-back, take stock of all your undeniable achievements. This will help to restore self-confidence that is needed for future success.
11. Do your own thing. When you do what you *want* to do and what you were *made* to do with your talents, at your own rate, then stress will be reduced.
12. Most important, establish a philosophy or code of life. Know what it is that you value in your life, and, in the word of the stress expert, Dr. Selye, "Know How to Live."

## WHAT TO EAT WHEN SOMETHING IS EATING YOU

The spa approach to relieving tension involves proper nutrition, exercises, rest and water therapy.

Since we do not have the European-quality nutrients in our foods grown in depleted soil, we have to resort to food supplements. During times of stress, it is particularly important to consume foods that will add needed nutrients, vitamins and minerals. Dr. Soliman, a noted nutritionist, says Brewer's Yeast is one of the best all-around nutritional food supplements and stress combatants. "It not only contains all the B vitamins, but is also a cheap source of important trace minerals and an excellent source of protein." Four tablespoons of Brewer's Yeast can be taken daily in either fruit or vegetable juice, buttermilk or water. This provides the much needed B-complex vitamins needed to rebuild health.

Wheat germ, fresh fruits and leafy green vegetables, along with dessicated liver and soy flour, from which the oil has not been removed, add extra nourishment to tired cells.

Vitamins that are particularly needed are vitamins C and E. Adele Davis suggests that 500 milligrams of vitamin C be taken every three hours prior to going to bed. Vitamin E in 100 I.U.'s provides a protection against air pollution, which is one of the major agents of stress in society.

## ON THE MOVE—TO GOOD HEALTH

Learning how to relax the muscles helps to reduce other tensions as well. In many of the European spas, and particularly in the anti-stress program at Baden-Baden, a minimum of two hours' exercise is recommended per day. This can be broken up into several time periods. One hour of hiking in the Black Forest prior to breakfast could be translated into American terms of jogging, swimming or walking to work for the same time period. At midday, walking around the block would offer a reprieve. Daily exercise, whether it be a brisk walk, jogging, swimming, handball or aerobics will do much to dissipate a dragged-out feeling. Yoga is an excellent means of exercising the body with a minimum of effort. The added benefit of it is the extensive oxygen replenishment that occurs throughout the body.

You can get more energy at the end of the day by moderate physical activity. A game of tennis, a swim, dancing or a standard calesthenics program will get rid of tensions better than sitting down to rest.

## EXERCISE FOR STRESS RELIEF

Assuming you have three twenty-minute breaks during the day, you can do any of the following:

At lunchtime, go outside and stretch for about five minutes, then run or jog around the block. At the conclusion of the five minutes, cool down by walking around for an additional five minutes.

If you have to stay inside, consider running in place, climbing stairs, or skipping rope, which can also be done outside. It's reported that ten minutes of skipping rope is equivalent to 30 minutes of jogging.

Other acceptable exercises are cycling, walking and swimming.

Two important considerations about exercising involve the time before and the time after. It's important to warm up the muscles and joints with a preliminary conditioning. Try a slow, three-minute walk, toe touching, stretching with arms extended up to the ceiling, then dropped to the floor. After adequate flexing, begin the actual exercise.

At the conclusion of the exercise the tendency may be to just drop down and relax. Don't! A time to cool down after exercise is as vital as warming up beforehand. Walk around the yard or gym for five minutes. Avoid going from a cool temperature to a warm one right away or vice versa. This could induce fainting or dizziness. (For added physical conditioning refer to Chapter 8 on Yoga.)

Dr. Broino Kieveloff, Director of Physical Medicine, at the New York Infirmary, says "Regular daily exercise may help lower blood pressure and in some cases even replace anti-hypertensive medication." Dr. Kieveloff instructed a group of high blood pressure patients to perform a set of brief isometric exercises, for six seconds each, three times daily. After five to six weeks of this routine, blood pressure was lowered considerably, he reports. Other doctors have had similar success with exercise therapy. Dr. Werner Hess, has his patients hike through the Black Forest for several hours a day. He then checks their blood pressure and correlates it over a period of time. He has discerned a reduction in count as well.

Dr. Hess emphasizes exercise as a tension reduction technique for all his patients at Baden-Baden. When executives come to his clinic, he suggests that they first decide upon the type of sport that they will pursue at home. He particularly recommends an activity that will increase the heart rate, such as aerobics. He says: "The aerobic principles of improving heart and circulation via a good work-out are vital for a meaningful exercise program."

Tennis, swimming, jogging or biking are all recommended by Dr. Hess, but he does not favor golf as an exercise because it requires little overt exertion.

## WATER THERAPY

Dr. Hess feels that it is vital to use the legs and limbs vigorously in exercising. This process is further implemented by the hydrotherapy treatments and gymnastics at Baden-Baden. Such water treatments as the Kneipps are used to improve leg circulation. A slow, exaggerated march through a pool covered with warm water and pebbles, then through cold water three times, followed by rest, is the recommended treatment. (Refer to Chapter 4 for other water therapies.)

## BADEN-BADEN BATH FOR TENSION REDUCTION

Chamomile, a relaxant tea, is also used in a bath to relieve muscular aches and pains. Place ¼ cup of chamomile in a pan of boiling water, cover and allow to simmer for about 10 minutes. Strain the chamomile and place liquid in bathwater. The residual chamomile leaves can be placed, in a cheesecloth, in the water, to be rubbed directly on the skin. Soak in the tub for about 20 minutes, massaging the aching muscles until the body feels a comforting glow of warmth.

To relieve frayed nerves and fatigue after a difficult day at the office, you can try the following treatment:

In the bathtub, place one cup of sea salt (can be purchased at a health food store), then add one cup of Epsom Salts to the tub of warm water. Sit and soak for fifteen or twenty minutes. When you pull the plug, you will feel like your tensions went down the drain along with the water.

## YOU DESERVE A BREAK TODAY . . . REST

During the day give yourself a twenty-minute break twice a day. At this time try any of the following: a nap, meditation, yoga, walking, or creative day dreaming. Try to relax prior to going to bed at night. If this is difficult due to excessive tension, try a Swiss nightcap: chamomile, golden seal or mint tea are used to encourage sleep in Swiss spas since these teas have a natural calming effect upon the nerves.

## RELAXATION—ANTIDOTE TO FATIGUE

While we use programs of progressive relaxation or a relaxation response to learn to relax in North America, our European neighbors experience autogenic training. This approach to relaxation was developed in Germany after World War I by Dr. Schultz, a neurosurgeon who initiated this form of self hypnosis to help a woman who could not respond to anesthesia. He had such success in doing painless surgery on the woman that he began teaching his method. A student of his forty-one years ago, Dr. Joachim Krammerer, currently on staff at the Bircher-Benner klinik, graciously taught me this method.

## AUTOGENIC TRAINING

Lie down on a hard surface, such as a floor or firm bed, making sure that the head, small of the back and heels make contact with the hard surface. Keep the arms bent and put one hand momentarily on the epigastric region, which is one inch below the navel. Then drop your hand in bent fashion to your side. The epigastric region, or solar plexus, is the site of the regulator response of the body.

You are now about to take a mini-vacation. Say to yourself: "When I awaken in 6 minutes, I will feel refreshed." Breathing in and out, feel that the rhythm of your breath is setting the pace for the rhythm of your life. Feel that you are in the arms of Mother Earth and are being supported. This is a time to surrender all problems, cares and anxieties . . . these six minutes devoted to you and your relaxation. You are in control as you breathe in and out. This is the time to gain a rhythm and balance between relaxation and activity. The liver and other organs of the body need this balance.

As you breathe in and out say to yourself: "My feet feel heavy and warm. My legs feel heavy and warm. My torso feels heavy and warm. My hands feel heavy and warm. My arms feel heavy and warm. My shoulders feel heavy and warm. My shoulders are pressed into the floor. My neck feels heavy and warm. My face feels heavy and my forehead feels cool. My eyes are closed. I am relaxed."

Repeat these directions to yourself about three times, saying each word very slowly to mesmerize yourself. The heavier you feel, the deeper will be your state of relaxation. When you do this for six minutes and actually feel the warmth and heaviness, you are on the threshold of sleep. You will awaken and truly feel refreshed. As a practitioner of many different forms of relaxation and meditation I can attest that this is the best that I have experienced.

Six to ten minutes a day, or twice a day, is one of the best gifts of relaxation that you can give yourself. However, it does take some conditioning. You cannot do it for the first time and expect to go into a deep state of relaxation. I have found that it took me about one month before I really experienced deep relaxation emerging as a habit. Now I can lie down at will and be immediately relaxed due to autogenic training.

## Benefits of Relaxation with Autogenic Training

Autogenic training is a cornucopia of benefits. In addition to helping you surrender the excess tensions and anxieties of the day, it helps in building self-confidence. When you realize that this is a segment of time in which you are totally in control and can prevent present and future tensions by using autogenic training, it's bound to elevate your sense of power and self-esteem.

The energy you save is economical from both a health and business point of view. Many people using this method say they have conserved so much energy that they can accomplish twice as much in half the time. At the end of the day, they still have energy reserves for going to the theatre or a concert without feeling excess fatigue. Autogenic training also enables you to detach yourself from your immediate problems; the distance that is gained helps you to understand the essences of the problems more completely so that when you return from your autogenic mini-vacation, you can arrive at more viable solutions to your problems.

## Why Autogenic Training Is Needed

Dr. Joachim Krammerer, the eminent doctor and personification of relaxation, said that depression, anxiety and overwrought people are endemic in our global society. There is a strong need to learn how to relax; we need to discover how to gain balance and control in our lives. Often we feel that we are victims of and at the mercy of society. "Eastern people, including Russians and Indians, tend to be more passive and worry less than western people," says Dr. Krammerer. He went on to illustrate his point with a quote from the late Winston Churchill. When asked what the difference was between socialism and capitalism, he replied: "Capitalism is the unequal distribution of blessings, whereas socialism is the equal distribution of misery."

If you are experiencing unequal distribution of blessings and need to gain a perspective on your life and relax, then autogenic training is the answer. Six minutes a day is a small investment to make in your health.

## How Gerhard Overcame High Blood Pressure

As a manufacturer's representative, Gerhard had constant deadlines to be met and insufficient time in which to meet them. He experienced heartburn and general fatigue after a daily luncheon of beef, alcohol, and hurried business. While at night he was restless and unable to sleep, his day was a mixture of fatigue and tension. Yet, he kept pushing himself to meet deadlines. When he finally checked into the Klinik Stephanie at Baden-Baden, he was beginning to reassess his life. He willingly gave up smoking and drinking. Daily walks in the Black Forest, utilizing the improved breathing techniques he had learned in the anti-stress program, water therapy treatments, a new system of eating smaller meals and avoiding overeating were part of his new life style. Today Gerhard does business during the business day and reserves his lunch time for a jog along the Rhine River, followed by a lunch of fresh fruit, yogurt and herb tea. He concludes with a twenty-minute nap before returning to his work. Gerhard finds that high blood pressure is no longer a problem. He has more energy and is far more productive as a result of his life style.

## FOODS TO EAT TO COMBAT STRESS

A skilled business person may have "know-how," but cannot apply this for results if there is not adequate energy to implement the solutions. On days of anticipated tension, it is wise to start the day with a high-protein drink. Honey and Brewer's Yeast with whey added to juice is a recommended drink at Swedish spas. This provides a combination of minerals and pantothenic acid to help strengthen the ability of the adrenal gland to emit cortisone. Anti-stress foods are easy to digest, and apples, watercress, green beans, bananas, whey, bran, lecithin, apricots, and apple juice are good food supplements. Low fat meats such as chicken, and turkey; fish such as freshwater, sole, cod and trout are beneficial; as are low-fat cheeses, including Edam, cottage, ricotta, and farmer's. Brussel sprouts, cabbage, cauliflower, cherries, cranberries and assorted fresh or frozen berries, without sugar, are all easy on the system.

These drinks are easy to prepare and can be taken to work in a jar or thermos.

### *Hi-Pro Drink*

Add one tablespoon each of the following:

- Brewer's Yeast

- Wheat Germ
- Dessicated Liver Tablets (ground up)
- Raw, unheated honey
- Use either 1 cup of soy milk or 1 cup of buttermilk with fresh fruit such as bananas or strawberries. This drink is an energizer to start the day. It is also beneficial at other times of fatigue or stress.

I know a masseur who drinks about 5 servings of this a day when he anticipates a stressful workday.

A simpler approach to an anti-stress drink is to use:

*Easy Protein*

- 2 tablespoons of Shaklee's Protein Powder with
- 1 tablespoon of Wheat Germ in
- 1 cup of either buttermilk or soy milk.

This is a high protein drink and dynamic source of energy that is easy to digest.

Another stress-tonic that improves gland power is:

*Instant Pep*

- 4 tablespoons of Brewer's Yeast
- 2 tablespoons of raw, unheated honey
- 1 cup of either tomato or pineapple juice
- 3 tablespoons of wheat germ
- ½ teaspoon vanilla or almond extract

Stress is the great destroyer of everything, especially enzymes. Papaya Juice is featured in the enzyme cocktail that Carlson Wade recommends in time of stress.

*Papaya Pep-Up*

- 4 heaping tablespoons of fresh Brewer's Yeast
- 1 - 8 oz. glass of papaya juice
- Fold in 1 teaspoon of tupelo honey.
- Stir vigorously and drink 30 minutes prior to mealtime for better digestion.

Adele Davis suggests a stress-sustainer drink which consists of the following:

- 10 almonds
- ¼ cup sunflower seeds

- 1 cup pineapple juice
- 2 teaspoons Brewer's Yeast
- ⅓ cup alfalfa sprouts
- 2 teaspoons honey
- First grind almonds and sunflower seeds in blender. Add the rest of the ingredients. Blend well and drink. Yield: 1¼ cups.

In several of the European health spas, detoxification drinks are suggested to rid the body of accumulated waste. At Bad Gestein, this cleansing potion is consumed during stressful times:

*Detoxifying Drink*

- 3 lemons
- 3 limes
- 3 oranges
- add the juice of these to ½ gallon of distilled water.

This is to be consumed during the course of one day.

## REDUCE STRESS VIA A HIGH ENERGY DIET

During times of stress, it is important to conserve what energy one does have and replenish the energy that is lost. This can be done with a diet for energy and stress reduction. Dr. Andre Soubirar, a French nutritionist, recommends a protein breakfast, light lunch and moderate dinner. He says that when you have a good breakfast, you are prepared, physically and emotionally, for your day's work. The brain will be clearer, and productivity will be greater. It will be possible to get through the day with a minimum of fatigue because the body is nutritionally sustained.

A further suggestion is that if "hunger pangs" develop, soothe them with a glass of skim milk, an orange, or a wedge of cheese. Drinking two glasses of skim milk daily provides calcium, which fights stress. The drink also helps wash the harmful, metabolic by-products out of the body. Dr. Soubirar suggests the following type of protein breakfast:

- 2–4 oz. cheese
- Fresh fruit, apples, melons, or berries
- Slice of whole wheat toast
- Herb tea
- Parasitic foods as white bread and flour, sugar, jams, breads, cakes, bacon, instant cereal, liquor and coffee should be eliminated to reduce stress.

Dr. Hess suggests a minimum of carbohydrates in the diet and a calorie count of 800–1200. He maintains that a reduction of weight will increase a person's energy level. The eating program he recommends is similar to that of Dr. Neil Solomon, a weight control expert at Johns Hopkins University and author of Dr. Solomon's *Easy No-Risk Diet*.

The rules of the diet are easy to follow:

1. Salt should be avoided since it retains water in the body keeping weight on, and producing stress. This means avoiding salty foods such as ham, bacon, cold-cuts, saltines and pretzels.

2. Animal fats also produce stress because they are hard to digest. This in turn makes one tense and irritable, so avoid high-fat meats such as marbled beef, beef filet, and pot roasts. Instead, eat low-fat protein sources like fish, turkey or chicken.

3. *Eating breakfast* cuts down stress by providing energy throughout the day rather than hunger pangs.

4. *Eliminate junk foods.* They have the same effect as sugar inside the body, triggering insulin and creating stress in the form of lowered blood sugar. Avoid candy, cookies, ice cream and milkshakes. Instead, eat foods rich in potassium such as bananas, oranges, green leafy vegetables and sunflower seeds to help reduce anxiety.

5. Caffeine, found in coffee, black tea and cola drinks, triggers the release of excessive insulin in the body, causing blood sugar to drop. In turn, this creates a craving for more sugar and carbohydrates, and produces more tension.

6. Vitamin C is needed to fight tension. It keeps the walls of the small blood vessels flexible so the blood can flow smoothly. Vitamin C-rich foods are all citrus fruits; oranges, grapefruits, lemons, tangerines, tangelos, and leafy vegetables; spinach, endive, lettuce, cabbage and watercress.

Pharmaceutical tranquilizers and aspirins will drain stores of vitamin C, creating more stress.

7. Constipation causes discomfort and tension. To avoid this problem and the accompanying anxiety, eat plenty of bulk foods such as fresh fruits, fresh vegetables and whole grains; bran, millet, oatmeal, farina or cream of wheat.

8. *Relax* before and after the meal. In Europe it's traditional to rest for at least an hour following a meal. Avoid becoming upset and arguing while eating. If a business luncheon is upsetting, try to conduct the business at another time. When a person is anxious while eating, there is a tendency to eat more, and faster and to improperly digest the food.

9. *Exercise* is essential to this diet. Keeping physically active is a good way to work off bottled-up tensions. An hour a day for jogging, walking, swimming, etc., is ideal. This can be broken up into twenty-

minute segments to accommodate a busy schedule. At Baden-Baden, two hours of exercise a day is normally recommended.

10. Eat the main meal in the middle of the day. Heavy meals in the evening contribute to weight gain.

## FOODS TO EAT TO FIGHT FATIGUE

These foods increase energy but tend to be high in calories. For weight reduction while under stress, consider the high energy diet previously mentioned.

- Start the day with a Brewer's Yeast drink.
- Breakfast should be nutritious as:
  —Homemade granola with bananas
  —Fresh fruit
  —Herb tea, (as chamomile, rose hips, or peppermint)
- Lunch should include fresh fruits and vegetables.
  —Tossed green salad (spinach, alfalfa sprouts, endive, radishes, tomatoes, mushrooms)
  —Yogurt sundae (yogurt with raisins, wheat germ, honey, sesame seeds, lecithin granules and bran)
  —Fresh juice (orange, grapefruit, berry, etc.)
- Dinner can be the main meal or can be interspersed with lunch
  —Fresh vegetable salad
  —Fruit
  —Fish, poultry, veal or liver in 4–6 oz. proportions
  —tea
  —Whole-grain bread
  above all, raw fruits are to be emphasized
- Refreshing herb drink
- Take Golden Seal, bayberry, myrrh. Mix together 1 tablespoon each of these herbs. Take a half-teaspoon in a cup of boiled water one hour before each meal and prior to bedtime. This simple herbal tea stimulates the thyroid and helps create improved digestion.

Health foods and drinks are suggested. However, they provide only a momentary solution. Dr. Hans Selye states: "Although we cannot avoid stress as long as we live, we can learn ways of keeping it at a minimum." A person's ability to take control over his mind and body, essentially holistic medicine, determines his "cope-ability" as well as capability for living. Being aware of times of tension and either coping with or avoiding them will enable one to gain more control over stress.

One last consideration is relaxation; truly an antidote to stress. Transcendental meditation, yoga, biogenics, progressive relaxation and autogenic training all contribute to tension-reduction.

Dr. Krammener suggests autogenic training as "self-concentration for relaxation." He suggests that controlled breathing, being attuned to the rhythm of one's breath and thinking thoughts that build self-confidence, contribute to easing tensions. "Learning to have confidence encourages good mental balance." This balance is what stress-reduction is all about: somehow, amidst the chaos of life, we need to find harmony within our environment.

Dr. Selye's concept of having a stress-reducing code of life is a very real consideration for Dr. Viktor Frankl as well. Dr. Frankl, who spent years in a concentration camp during World War II, has written two books that deal with finding life's meaning. *Man's Search for Meaning* and *The Doctor and the Soul* both provide insights as to how to find a sense of purpose in life. Dr. Frankl, an internationally renowned Viennese psychiatrist, suggested that Socrates' idea to "Know Thyself," was a valid consideration when dealing with stress. He suggests that people write about the things they like about their lives, things they like least, things they want to accomplish in their lives, skills and strengths that they have, who they want to be with, and what they *love* about living.

In my stress-workshops, I too encourage people to write their autobiographies; including where they live, what they have done in life, their major accomplishments, and their character or personality. Try it yourself. Paint a short, detailed picture of what your life has been, and what you *wish* it had been. Often, this written statement is the impetus to change to a more positive way of living.

## FOODS TO HELP YOU DEAL WITH STRESS

Raw fruits and vegetables are good sources of vitamin C which fights infection, repairs tissue and maintains healthy adrenal glands.

- *Vitamin C Sources:* include citrus fruits, tomatoes, strawberries, melons, spinach, endive, watercress, parsley, lettuce, chard, and beet-greens.
- *Vitamin B:* essential because it produces energy, is found in the above mentioned vegetables and high-protein fish, cheese, and almonds.
- *Minerals:* Calcium, nature's own tranquilizer, tends to soothe nerves. It is found in milk and cheese products, broccoli, turnip greens, kale and almonds.
- *Potassium:* sources are bananas, oranges, leafy vegetables and natural cereals such as bulgar, millet and legumes.

- *Iron:* egg yolks, whole grains, vegetables, potatoes and dried fruits.
- *Zinc:* seafood, liver, eggs, milk and pumpkin seeds.

## FOODS TO AVOID WHEN DISTRESSED

Salt—makes you thirsty and can cause fluid retention, bloating and edginess.

Sweets—white sugar, flour, junk foods: boost energy for awhile but within an hour the energy level drops with the blood sugar level. For some, a sugar-overload spurs a hypoglycemic reaction and depression.

Caffeine products—coffee, cola drinks, black tea and chocolate stimulate momentarily but can cause restlessness as the blood sugar level fluctuates.

### Plan for Eating

- Begin each day with a protein breakfast. A good breakfast cuts tension by sustaining your energy level. Have eggs, cheese, cereal, and almonds as protein sources, plus fruit, herb tea, toast, rye or pumpernickel bread, and one teaspoon of raw honey on toast.
- Mid-morning snack—fresh fruit in season or an apple. This cuts hunger pangs and further increases energy.
- Lunch—fresh green salad, yogurt, chicken, fish or cheese; fresh fruit or juice; herb tea; chamomile, mint, or rose hips. (The body digests protein best prior to one p.m. The main meal of the day should be either breakfast or lunch.)
- Mid afternoon snack—orange, banana, peach or any fruit to prevent mid-day fatigue.
- Dinner—turkey, chicken, yogurt, cottage cheese, salad or fruit are all possibilities, but portions should be smaller than lunch.

### Energy Aid

On days of anticipated pressures and tensions, start off with a high-protein drink for more energy and easy digestion. In blender put:

- 1 tablespoon of Brewer's Yeast
- 1 tablespoon of protein powder
- 1 tablespoon of whey

Add either one cup of juice, e.g., orange, pineapple, apple or one cup of buttermilk. Add ½ cup fresh fruit such as strawberries, bananas or peaches.

## COPING WITH CAUSES OF STRESS

There are many ways of coping with life's situations. Sometimes change and the opportunity to cope better than is hampered by old habits that keep us in a rut. Pressures mount when we become inflexible until an insurmountable problem may appear.

You can develop stress-skills that break down rigidity and enable you to stretch your flexibility and diminish pressure.

Basic Approaches for Coping:

1. *Get Organized:*
   By reorganizing yourself, you can use your time and energy more effectively. Decide what is important for you and do it.
   a. List two things that are important to you right now.
   b. Choose two activities to do in the next 24 hours that you have not done before but would like to.
2. *Personal Planning and Goal Setting:*
   Your values are put in action when you plan and act. Setting goals and following through on them is an art that enables progression towards self realization.
   a. Write down one major goal for the next year.
   b. Make a daily plan of short-term tasks.
   c. Divide your large goal into smaller parts to be implemented.
3. *Commit Yourself:*
   After clarifying your values and making plans, you are ready to act. Making a commitment is saying "yes" to yourself and investing your time and energy into making your values and goals a reality. Anything worthwhile in life involves a commitment. Invest in yourself and see what kinds of personal rewards you experience.
   a. Decide on a risk. List all that could go wrong, what you have to lose, and then, if it seems worthwhile, do it.
   b. List time-wasters that annoy you. Commit yourself to changing one each day.
4. *Give In but Not Up:*
   When a situation is not worth the fight, let it go. It is not "giving in" but an acknowledgment that some forces in life are bigger than you are. Surrender can be a strategic retreat in which you may lose a battle but win the war for your own emotional freedom. If a relationship is not working because there are too many obstacles and neither person has sufficient energy to invest, then practice the art of saying "good-bye."
   a. Think about something that you need to let go of.

b. Avoid worrying about problems ahead of time. Plan but don't become anxious.
c. Realize that you and I and life are unfinished and subject to growing pains . . . build tolerance.

5. *Keep a Faith and Belief Going:*
Believe in yourself and that your life will improve. Faith develops as you accept the mysterious and unknown elements of life. Such belief adds depth to life and helps you deal with the larger questions of your existence. Peace of mind can result when you have faith, act upon your beliefs and trust that the future can be yours.
a. Spend some quiet time alone and experience the serenity of silence.
b. Consider that any crisis can be an opportunity.
c. Discuss with your co-workers and friends your belief-system and find out theirs.

6. *Handle Yourself with Care:*
Making unreal demands is often natural in our culture. Instead, be gentle with yourself. Such a healthy attitude will reduce wear and tear on your physical and psychic energy and lower tension.
a. Practice listening to your body . . . do you feel tired or have tension? Take a few minutes to stretch, take deep breaths and relax.
b. Listen to soft music, a symphony, instrumental sounds.
c. Walk in the woods and listen to the silence.
d. Look in the mirror and say "I love you."

7. *Measuring Your Capabilities:*
Often we have more strengths than we know. To find yours, on a piece of paper try listing five strengths that you possess which can get you through a crisis. Below them, list five weaknesses that can prevent you from reaching your goals, and finally, list five attributes that you would like to have and explain why you want them. Finally, record your activities in the previous week, and list things you most enjoy doing. You may be surprised at the results of this self-examination.

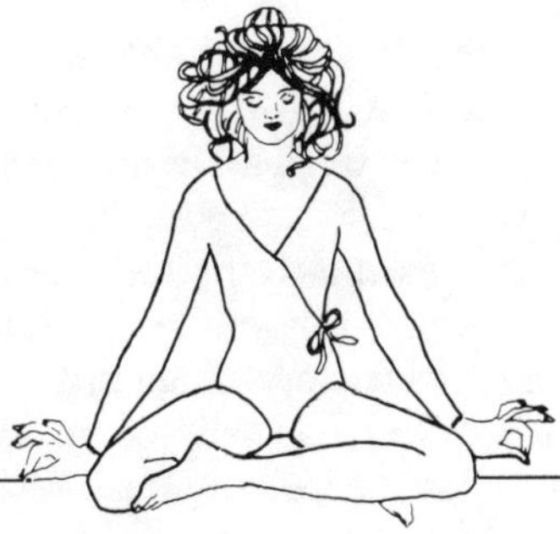

# 7

# An Austrian Version of an Ancient Asian Regimen for Beauty and Health

*"Self conquest is the greatest of victories."*

*Plato*

In America, "bottoms up" usually refers to drinking, but in Europe it is likely to refer to a yoga posture. In yoga, one of the most effective postures is standing on one's head or "upending." Europeans practice various yoga postures and positions for a revitalized way of life.

Yoga probably is India's most valuable export to the western world and has practitioners everywhere. Those followers in the Bads and kliniks of Austria and other European health centers seem to give this ancient regimen a distinct European flavor.

The Indian method of discipline, physical improvement and a controlled aura of well being is often followed by health-conscious Austrians. They like yoga's consideration of the whole person, and its concern with the health and strength of the entire body, and the toning-up of the brain, glands, internal organs, nerves, tissues and cells. Yoga improves respiration, circulation, digestion, and elimination, with its forte being the invigoration of the brain as well as the normalization of the body's metabolism and functions.

The Austrian version of yoga is no longer regarded as something involving Indian fakirs sitting on a bed of spikes. Yoga, the oldest and possibly newest accepted form of healing therapy, teaches that a healthy person is a harmonious integration of body, mind, and spirit. The term is derived from Sanskrit which means "union."

Yoga unites the body and soul with the healing effects of "assanuas" or yoga postures. Accordingly, good health European yoga style requires a simple, natural diet, exercise in the fresh air, a serene and untroubled mind, and a spiritual awareness.

Are you thinking, "Who can do that and earn a living too?" Well, my friend, you can. I say that emphatically. I've tried it and know that it is very effective, especially in our time-conscious society. Yoga provides a mini-cure. Twelve minutes of yoga on a regular basis can accomplish more than comparable time spent on isotonics or aerobics. Despite the fact that these forms of exercise are very good, yoga does more since it provides a complete form of relaxation. So often in our culture we are tempted to use diversionary tactics in order to relax, like lighting a cigarette, changing activities, taking a walk, or talking to a friend.

Yoga relaxes body and mind. When we try to divert ourselves from tension, we get only a momentary reprieve since all we have done is shift our attention to another activity. With yoga, the body as well as the mind sinks into passivity, the antedote of activity.

## YOGA BREATHING FOR IMPROVED RESPIRATION

The basis of all yoga is breathing. In many European spas, this is done outdoors early in the morning or at twilight. Start by breathing deeply. *Abdominal breathing* provides maximum usage of oxygen in the body and helps it perform at optimum levels. In America, we tend to breathe in a shallow, heavy chested fashion. Perhaps it is our innate response to air pollution. Deeper breathing which is not difficult to learn, can become second nature with practice.

- *Inhale, slowly and deeply, expanding your abdomen as you do so.* Be sure to keep the shoulders down. If you raise them—you revert to shallow breath.
- *Then exhale while pulling your stomach in as far as you can.*

This breathing can be practiced in whatever position is convenient; lying flat, standing or sitting erect in a chair. The slower and deeper you breathe, the better it is for control and relaxation.

## BREAK TENSION BEFORE IT HAPPENS/ PREVENTIVE MAINTENANCE

In Bad Gestein, the renowned Austrian spa, I was told the easiest way to relax your body is to acquire the habit of breaking tension *before* it is beyond coping. For example: if you have been sitting too long in one position you should change, stand up, walk around, or go to the water cooler for a drink. Should you be tired from standing on your feet too long, sit down, or better still, stretch out on a rug or couch that is not too soft.

A person confined to a desk and leaning forward while working should remember to do a few backward stretches as often as possible. *Stretching* is always extremely helpful in preventing development of various aches and pains.

## How to Stretch Effectively

Grasp your hands behind your back. Pull up as far as possible. Release. Then grasp hands over your head and move from side to side from the waist. Continue this activity while breathing deeply.

## Stretch Effectively to Relax When Driving

Releasing tension while driving a car:

Are you driving in rush hour traffic with your hands tightly gripping the steering wheel, shoulders hunched, neck tensed, arm muscles taut? Typical tension-building activity! Besides, you are probably staring fixedly at the highway, straining your eyes and inducing fatigue. By the time you arrive at your destination you have built up considerable stress.

*Tension-Breakers*

1. Breathe deeply. Practice deep abdominal breathing. When you stop at red lights, blink your eyes frequently and shut them every now and then.
2. At intervals, preferably at stop lights, do neck exercises as dropping your head forward and backward several times while letting it go completely limp. Rotate your head slowly to the right and then to the left.
3. Shrug your shoulders, loosely moving them up and down. Make rotary movements with your shoulders, clockwise and counter-clockwise.
4. Do the lion posture of extending tongue, and making a noise. This releases tension in the neck, throat, and face. (Once I was doing this while driving down a freeway. Ahead of me was a semi-truck whose driver was looking in his side mirror as I was doing my posture. He did a double-take apparently thinking I was having an epileptic seizure.)
5. Alternately move the fingers of your right and left hands as though you were playing a piano. Also shake your hands loosely as if you were dispelling drops of water from your fingers.

6. After getting out of the car, stretch with your arms extended then drop over in rag doll fashion. Then loosely shake each foot to dispel tension.

When a person is beginning a new habit, and relaxation for most of us is a new habit, it's easy to forget to practice. If you are a note-maker like I am, write yourself a note. "Hang loose," "Relax," "Peace," "Shalom," are all reminders that you can place on your desk, on the dash of your car, the bathroom mirror, or wherever you need tension reduced.

In the Salzburg Therapeutic Center it is said that relaxation is not something you achieve "on cue." When you are truly relaxed, you can accomplish your work with a minimum of energy. Often we develop the attitude that our ordinary work is tedious, tension ridden, and boring at times. When the workday is over, an attempt is made to relax over a drink with friends. However, many people find it more difficult to let go when they are supposed to be relaxing and having a good time because anxiety and irritating experiences tend to stockpile. No wonder it is difficult to let go. So at the end of the day, take a momentary retreat.

## How to Relax at the End of the Day

Go into a quiet, darkened room and lie down on the carpet or a mat. Stretch out. Then, tighten and tense every muscle in your body beginning at your toes and progress to your head. Mentally say each body part to yourself, e.g., "I am tightening my toes, ankles, feet, calves, knees," etc. Tighten and tense each muscle of your body, and hold until you are as tight as a rubber band about to snap. Then gradually relax your toes, feet, ankles, etc. again saying each body part to yourself.

- Feel the tenseness drain from your body.
- Listen to the silence about you.
- Gently say to yourself . . . "I will let all things be healthful, all things be happy, all things be tranquil. I will be sure to count my blessings at least once a day."
- Lie there until you feel ready to get up.

In yoga, this is called a Savasauna and is used at the conclusion of a class. Once while I was teaching yoga, a very tense banker in my class informed me that nothing could possibly make him relax. He did this posture, and before it was even completed he was snoring soundly. When the class was over, everyone had departed and he was still sleeping soundly. Upon being awakened, he commented that was his best rest in twenty years.

## YOGA, HOUSEWORK, AND RELAXATION

Frenzied activity, a small child crying for attention, soup boiling over, the phone ringing, an evangelistic caller knocking on the front door and a salesman at the back . . . I know what you're up against. I've been there, too. Let's face it, despite all the modern conveniences, housework can be drudgery. The end of the day can find you irritated, depressed, frustrated, and just plain tired. How do you handle it?

Have your children take a nap, or give them a creative project like a big roll of paper and crayons for making their own mural. Take the phone off the hook, (forgive me Ma Bell) and retreat to a quiet, darkened room. You owe yourself a few minutes vacation before the evening begins. Lie down and begin taking deep yoga breaths for about five minutes.

- Stretch—do leg over stretches.
- Twist.
- Do a forward bend.
- Do an angled stretch.
- Lie down and do the relaxation Savasauna exercise that was previously suggested.

If more relief is needed, resort to your own Bad. Put Epsom Salts or baking soda in a tub of warm water, and relax. Let tension go down the drain.

### How Laura T. Overcame Her Tension

Laura T. was 45 and experiencing menopause. When I met her at a European Spa, her hot flashes, pounding heart and palpitations kept her in a constant state of tension. She could not focus on any thought. She said she felt as if her mind and body were on a fast-moving train. Mental images were rushing by, faster and faster. Near exhaustion, she enrolled in a yoga session that was being held in the Wienerwald. As she learned to breathe slower, tension and her fast-moving mental images seemed to flee. She began to relax and focus her attention on her breath stream. Whenever she felt hot flashes or could not direct her attention, she would stop and lie down or sit in a chair to practice deep breathing. Laura is still menopausal, but is now in control while breathing and stretching with yoga. Her serene face gives testimony that yoga is working for her.

## HOW TO BEAT INSOMNIA

There is nothing that can deplete your energy as quickly as insufficient sleep. One hour of deep sleep is worth more than many hours of fitful turning and tossing. The key considerations for a decent night's sleep are the following:

- The bed or sleeping surface should be as firm as your body will tolerate.
- The head should be only slightly raised to permit good circulation.
- The stomach should be as empty as possible . . . no eating for approximately two hours prior to retiring.
- Do not read anything stimulating prior to sleeping, instead consider philosophy or spiritual reading.
- Establish a ritual, e.g., bathe, brush teeth, read.
- Do deep breathing and yoga postures such as the back stretch, cobra, headstand (drains blood from the cranial area and induces sleep) or alternate nostril breathing for added relaxation.

When you recline on your pillow, all thoughts should cease. When you close your eyes, if there are no thoughts, there will be no restlessness or anxiety, and deep sleep will result.

### What if Sleep Still Won't Come?

If you have tried all of the above and still can't sleep, here are some added suggestions for surrending into the arms of Morpheus. These "Betsyisms" have been effective in Vienna and elsewhere.

- Listen to quiet music for a half-hour before retiring.
- Write down the day's events. I have found this very helpful when the day has been frought with stress. It's better to have the tension out on paper than in your body.
- Drink herb tea: chamomile, golden seal, peppermint, or sage. These are favorite sleep-inducers in Austrian and Swiss kliniks. Add a teaspoon of raw honey to taste.
- Sit up and read something deadly boring. Reading in bed prevents relaxation so sit in a comfortable chair. My favorite sleeper is a book called, *The Last Days, Death and Funeral of Henry Clay.* Two or three paragraphs of that and I'm ready to hop into bed and sleep serenely.
- Change your attitude.

- Stop worrying about the sleep you are losing. When you remind yourself about how tired you are, you self-hypnotize and reinforce this feeling. Try to be indifferent and sleep may come more easily.
- Try water therapy. (Refer to Chapters 3 and 4 for suggestions.)

### How Evelyn G. Breathed Away Her Asthma

Pills, medical bills, oxygen tanks and wheezing were Evelyn G's constant companions. Her doctor suggested that she spend six weeks at Austria's famous Bad Gestein. It was here that she was introduced to yoga. At first she was a reluctant participant in the yoga sessions, prefacing each breath with the phrase "I can't do it." After encouragement from the instructor, she proceeded to breathe in the deep rhythmic yoga breaths. In time she began to imitate the postures with greater facility, and by the end of the third week, she was no longer taking her medication. Instead she was relying solely upon the yoga breathing. Her doctor approved of this and provided further encouragement. By the time six weeks were up, Evelyn G. was breathing normally, feeling better and returned to Vienna sans oxygen tank. She readily admits that yoga breathing helped her.

## BASIC DAILY PROGRAM

On a daily basis, yoga is a good health investment. Twelve minutes a day will purchase muscle toning, improve the digestive, circulatory, and respiratory systems as well as increase energy-giving oxygen to the nerves and brain. Yoga provides a self-massage, internally and externally. The following exercises will provide a well-balanced program, supplemented, of course, by any other postures particularly good for your needs.

### Posture Instructions

Before eating, in either morning or late afternoon, spread a blanket on the floor in a well-ventilated room or outdoors, as I prefer. Wear loose clothing. Generally, the backward bends should be balanced by forward bends. Never force or strain in yoga: these postures should be performed slowly and meditatively. They are meant to be held in dynamic tension, and should not be confused with vigorous calisthenics which deplete energy, accumulate body toxins, and forcefully constrict blood flow.

### Yoga Postures

Controlling your breathing creates a chemical and emotional balance just as practicing yoga postures strengthens the body. Also, when concentrating on affirmations, you are practicing the power of prayer. The synthesis of all three factors is your entry into the most powerful mystery of healing: the basic harmony of life.

Greater benefit is derived from the postures when you imagine the affected area as receiving fresh blood circulation, oxygen, and massage. For example, if you have diabetes, visualize the healing energies in the pancreas, near the stomach. A person with rheumatism should concentrate on the release of synovial fluid, which dispenses waste matter which can cause joint stiffness.

*Instructions:* Each posture should be preceded by relaxation and deep breathing. Yoga should be done prior to eating, either in the morning or late afternoon.

## Austria's Antidote for Air Pollution Ills

Air pollution, sedentary life styles and lack of movement contribute to increased respiratory ailments. Tight clothing also encourages shallow breathing and cramps the lungs. The purpose of *complete breathing* is to fully expand the air sacs of the lungs, thereby exposing the capillaries to the maximum exchange of carbon dioxide and oxygen.

## How Arthur Controlled His Asthma

Arthur, a 50-year-old Swiss banker, had been troubled with breathing problems for years. Asthma, hayfever and other assorted respiratory ailments kept him in chronic discomfort. While on a ski holiday in Austria, Arthur had an asthma attack, and was sent to nearby Bad Hofgastein, where the doctor suggested he stay for several weeks. He was told yoga and deep breathing would lessen his erratic breathing patterns. By this time, Arthur was ready to try anything, so each day he would faithfully sit in a yogic posture and breathe deeply. He was amazed how well he felt after each yoga class.

When he returned to his home in Basel, he continued doing yoga early in the morning and before bed. Two years have elapsed and he has not experienced another asthma attack and his hayfever has not reappeared.

## Complete Yoga Breathing

(1) Lie down and place hands on the stomach, resting fingertips lightly on the navel. Breathing through the nose, inhale and expand the stomach *only*. (Watch the fingertips part.) Exhale and contract the abdomen. (The fingertips will meet.) Practice this abdominal breathing slowly, without strain, 10 times.

(2) Place the hands on the rib cage and inhale, expanding *only* the

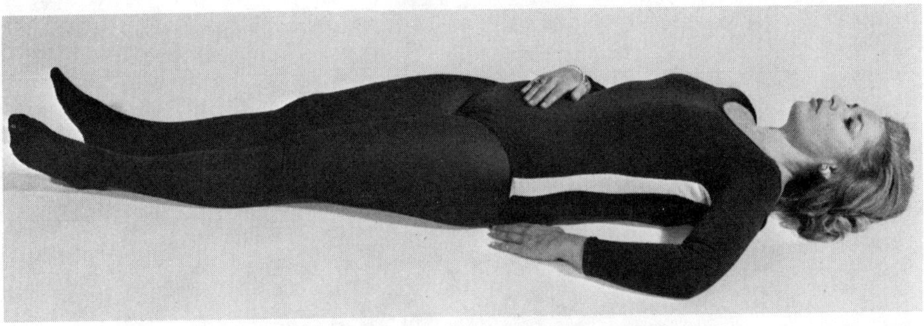

**Photo 7-1.** Breathing yoga breath.

diaphragm and the rib cage. (Watch the fingertips part.) Contract and slowly exhale. Practice this *Diaphragm Breathing* 10 times.

(3) Place the hands palms up beside the body and put these three breaths together. Inhale, expanding the stomach, the diaphragm, and the chest, in a slow, wavelike movement. Hold. Exhale, in the same order.

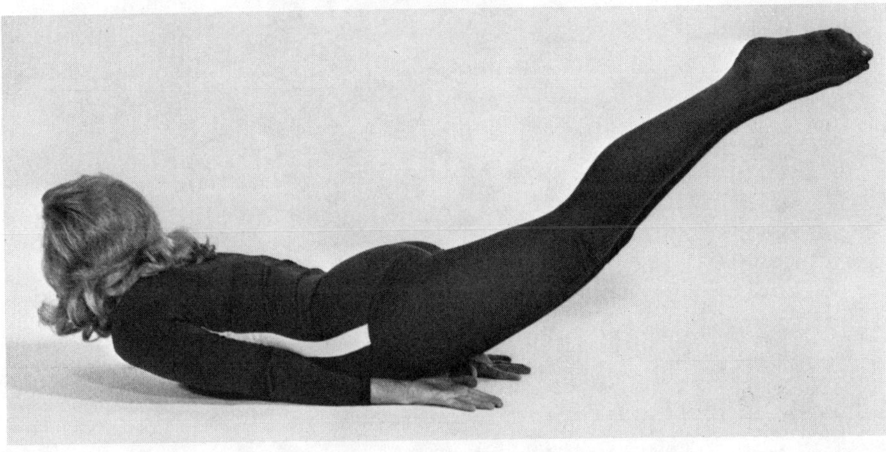

**Photo 7-2.** The bow.

This tones ovaries, uterus, and liver, is beneficial for menstrual irregularities, constipation and limbers the spine.

*Lion.* Sit on heels with palms on knees and stiffly fan out your fingers. Lean slightly forward over hands, and protrude your tongue as far as possible, contracting the throat muscles, and rolling the eyeballs upward. Completely exhale, saying "Ahhhhhh." Repeat 4 to 6 times.

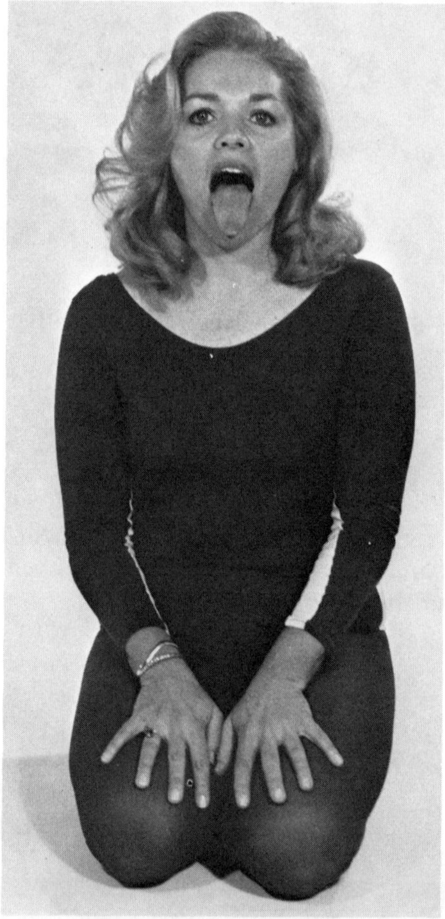

**Photo 7-3.** The lion.

## Neck and Eye Exercises

Sitting upright, slowly nod head forward three times. Nod to the left shoulder three times, to the back three times letting the mouth fall open, and to the right shoulder three times. Slowly roll the head clockwise three times, then reverse. Inhale and shut eyes tightly while holding position. Exhale, open eyes wide and blink rapidly ten times.

### *Eye Exercises*

Opening eyes wide, look in a slow circle. Repeat in opposite direction. Now, look diagonally. Next, look up and down ten times.

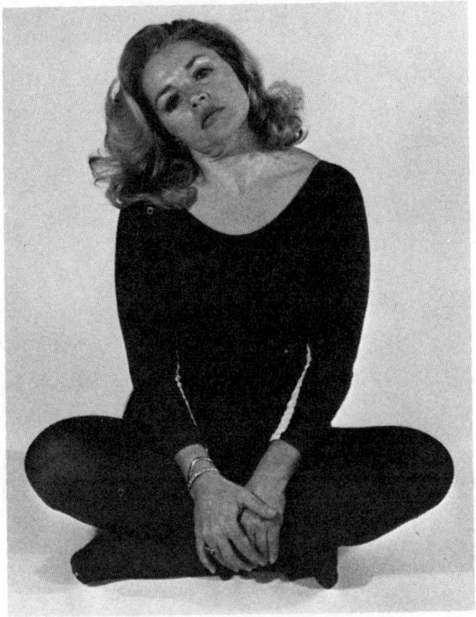

**Photo 7-4.** Neck and head roll.

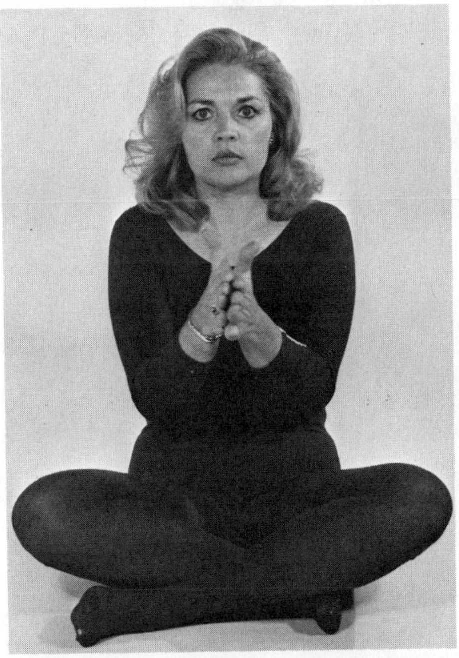

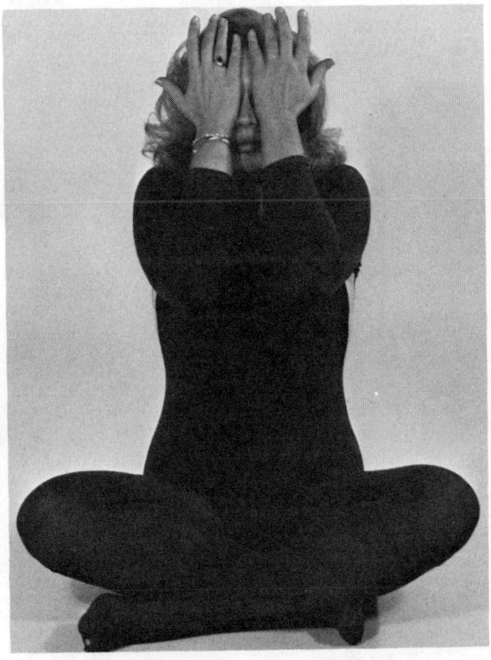

**Photo 7-5a.** Palming-eye relaxation #1. **Photo 7-5b.** Palming-eye relaxation #2.

*Palming for Relief from Eye Tension*

Rub palms together vigorously. Close eyes and cover with your palms, then take five very slow deep breaths, visualizing new energy and brightness into the eyes.

Benefits of Eye and Palming Postures: Relieves headache and eye strain, improves eyesight. Relaxes neck and shoulder tensions.

## Plow

Lie on your back on the floor. Slide arms under buttocks for support and raise the legs. Slowly swing the feet over behind the head until the toes touch the floor. Rest the arms beside the body palms down, then concentrate on relaxing the shoulders, arms, and hands with the legs straight. Slow your breathing. If you can't touch behind the head, let the knees rest on your forehead. Inhale and round the back. Roll out slowly. Exhale and lie prone. Relax.

- Do not force any yoga posture or hold it if it hurts.

Benefits: Relieves headache, hangover, sinus and nasal congestion and has a slimming effect. Rounding the back is very good for tight back muscles. As you relax and practice the abdominal breath, you will be massaging the abdominal organs, and your back muscles will slowly become limber.

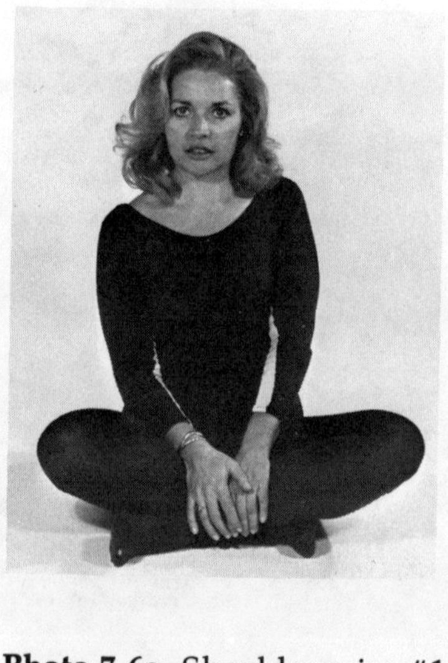

**Photo 7-6a.** Shoulder raise #1.

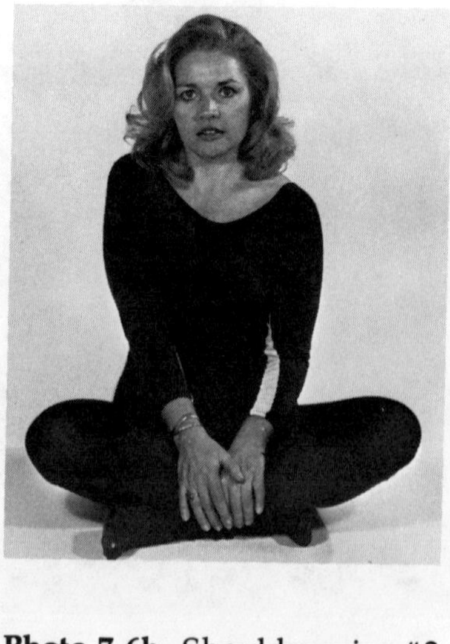

**Photo 7-6b.** Shoulder raise #2.

## Fatigue and Tension Reliever

*Shoulder Roll.* Sitting or standing, roll shoulders loosely forward in a circular movement five times. Reverse. For a great stretch, roll one shoulder at a time.

Benefit: Relieves fatigue and tension in shoulder area.

## Circulation and Digestion Aid

*Shoulder Stand.* Lie on your back on the floor and slide arms under buttocks. Inhale, slowly raise your legs and lift the trunk, hips, and legs to a vertical position. Resting the elbows on the floor, support the back with the hands. The chin is pressing into the chest, the legs are vertical like a candle. Hold this pose for as long as comfortable, but no longer than 15 minutes. Breathing slowly and evenly will help to steady the legs. Concentrate on the thyroid gland which yoga experts claim is stimulated by this exercise.

Benefits: Reduces excess fat; stretches the spine and muscles of the legs, back, abdomen, and neck; tones up the nervous system and improves circulation.

## Twist

Sit on the floor with legs outstretched. Bend the left leg under the right thigh. Bring the right foot across the left leg, placing the foot on the outside of the left knee. The left hand grasps the toes of the right foot from outside the right knee. Inhale and swing the free right arm to bend across the lower back, lower palm turned outward, with the trunk and head twisted right around. Hold the pose for as long as is comfortable, increasing to 2 minutes. Repeat toward other side. Work into the twist easily and gradually.

Benefits: Massages stomach, kidneys, liver, pancreas. (People with back problems should not do this posture.)

Yoga provides the breath of life, it is energizing, and it offers new vitality and self-mastery. Good health is not just a blessing, but an inner virtue derived from self-discipline and courage of the soul. So, go take up your bed of nails and have a deep breath of air. Bottoms up for better thinking and breathing!

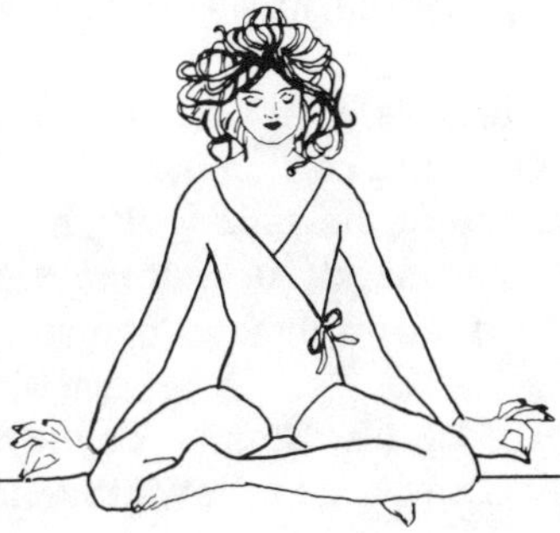

# 8

# Rebuilding Energy as the Scandinavians and Germans Do

*"To be healthy, eat less and exercise more."*

*Dr. David Turner,*
*Canadian Cardiologist*

Exercise is a way of life in Europe, as the parking lots of many industries prove. Bicycles frequently outnumber cars, which is a contrast to the overt number of cars in America's asphalt jungles. In Scandinavian factories, a gymnasium and sauna are part of the work facilities. At midday, workers have the opportunity of working out in the gym or taking a sauna prior to returning to the assembly line. Not only does such a reprive add to their psychic and physical well being but their productivity is increased and employee absenteeism is diminished.

Walking to work, taking leisurely strolls or a lunchtime break for tennis, swimming or running down a nearby street are all part of the day's rigors. Fortunately in America there is a new wave of interest in exercise. In some businesses, swimming pools and handball facilities have been built nearby. However, interest in physical conditioning still does not measure up to Europe's. Dr. Cooper, who brought Aerobics to the American public, freely admits that most Americans trail Europeans when it comes to physical conditioning and fitness.

Dr. Cooper states: "I keep holding up Europe as an example. They are ahead of us in their overall approach to physical fitness." Having personally viewed droves of Europeans exercising in assorted ways, I can appreciate his remark.

Exercise is integral to the European life style. When the sun comes out in the morning so do the walkers, joggers, and early morning swimmers. In France, barefoot runners plow through the sands which were formerly trod by combat boots during the Normandy invasions. Along the Italian Riviera, one can stroll through equally soft sand before sailing, boating, or water skiing.

Exercise is for everybody. In the early 1960's, Denmark's mayors would jog through the early morning streets and urge fellow citizens to run as well.

Dr. Per Olaf Astrand of Stockholm, inventor of the Monarch stationary bicycle, and one of Europe's authorities on exercise, believes that there is a definite correlation between physical fitness and the quality of mental health. He says, "A person whose circulation has improved, giving the brain more oxygen and glucose, is less depressed, less hypochondriac, and will feel more alert and is more ready to handle stresses and challenges."

## WHAT HAPPENS IF YOU DON'T EXERCISE?

"Whenever I feel like exercising, I just lie down until it goes away." In the past, this remark has been a standby for American humorists. It has also given rise to comments by undertakers and admiring relatives: "He never looked better than he does in that coffin."

Heart attacks and other cardiovascular diseases are leading killers in the United States, accounting for 53 to 58 percent of all deaths. Many businessmen, forewarned by doctors about their vulnerability to this disease, head for the nearest handball court or begin some program of physical conditioning. Still others, who consider their financial acumen more important than their physical health ask, "Why exercise?" The reason is that a lifetime of inactivity, on the job and off, takes its toll in several ways.

Muscles shrunken from disuse slow down, and an inadequate supply of blood gets back to the heart. The lungs lose some ability to handle oxygen, so the heart pumps blood less efficiently. Limbs lose their flexibility, girth increases and digestion slackens.

The sluggish heart beats faster than normal even while resting, but almost any activity can cause the rate to accelerate without a corresponding increase in the volume of blood per beat going to the vital organs and tissues.

## PROOF OF THE BENEFITS OF EXERCISE

For over 60 years, doctors have been systemactically trying to answer the question of whether regular exercise can prevent or retard diseases of the heart and arteries.

Twenty-five years ago a study was done in London among bus conductors. It was found that those conductors who walked up and down, and back and forth on double-decker buses in London had fewer heart attacks and less heart disease than drivers who stayed seated all day.

More recently, a California study of 6,351 male dockworkers revealed that those who spent their whole careers doing heavy labor on the San Francisco docks had about one third as many fatal heart attacks as workers who transferred to light work or held sit-down office jobs.

Exercise that increases pulse rate and deep breathing has a number of measurable benefits. After a while, each heart stroke pumps a greater volume of blood, the pounding sensation from exertion diminishes, and the resting pulse rate decreases. By lowering blood pressure and establishing new physiological demands, exercise may improve the circulatory system and even enhance the development of the peripheral or collateral blood supply to the heart.

### How Barbara Found New Energy

Barbara, age 30, was continually nervous and obese. Her teaching position in a middle eastern oil company created many pressures.

Being able to unwind was very important to her. During her stay at a European Klinik, Barbara was encouraged to take daily walks, and participate in gym class. Swimming seemed like an added bonus so she took it up as well. Today, many pounds lighter, and with excess tension gone as well, Barbara resumes her work positively and with more vitality as a result of her daily exercise routine.

### How Andre Stopped Smoking

Andre, age 41, reluctantly participated in the aerobic classes that were held at a North Sea spa. At first he preferred smoking and observing others stretch and sweat rather than actively participating.

Soon, however Andre, a frugal man who spent many guilders coming to the spa, decided to get his money's worth. Each day he would do warm-up stretches—jumping, and kicking in time to the aerobic music, running along the coast line of the North Sea and eventually lying down in the crisp sand and concluding with cool-down exercises.

Soon he was able to break away from cigarettes. After four weeks, Andre concluded his cure. Two things happened during his healthful holiday:

1. He had dropped his reservations about exercising and began to love aerobics.
2. His breathing and energy level increased when he gave up smoking. He decided that his newly toned body was not going to be impaired by nicotine so he forfeited his former habit.

When last contacted in his native city of Amsterdam, Andre reported that he gets up at dawn and runs along the canals for eight kilometers. In the evening, instead of lingering over a glass of wine and smoking, he goes out dancing for more exercise. He reports that his attitude has become more open and accepting after exercise was included in his life style.

## AEROBICS

This brings us to aerobics, a simple conditioning program that causes your body to demand more oxygen over an extended period of time.

Forms of aerobics such as jogging, running, handball and cycling are evidenced all over the continent. The brisk-paced exercises train the cardiovascular system to become more efficient by strengthening the heart, lungs, blood vessels, and figure. The duration for workouts is usually 25 to 30 minutes for three or four times-a-week. Dr. Per Olaf Astrand believes that a person can feel the results of more energy and fitness after eight weeks, while thirty weeks are required for optimal benefit.

Aerobics differ from recreation, isometrics, or isotonics in that you select an activity such as riding a bike, running or rope skipping. Gradually, after several weeks, you build up your body to demand large amounts of oxygen for a sustained length of time.

Should you be more inclined to indoor exercising, stairclimbing, one step up—one step down; stationary running; cycling or using a treadmill are possibilities. Schedule it into your day just as you would a business appointment. Pick three times in the next week on nonconsecutive days to schedule your running time. When running outside, particularly in a heavily polluted area, it is best to run either early in the morning or late in the evening to avoid some of the excessive exhaust fumes. Start out at a slow, steady, long, non-competitive pace. Select a target distance or a target time. You might choose to run a mile or to run thirty minutes a session. If you have a friend who is a runner, go running together. Locale? Try the nearest park, run around the block, or join a local organization that may have a running or exercise program. For those who do not feel comfortable running at first, start out with a brisk walk, gradually increasing your pace until you are running. In any case, the first step is getting out the front door, since making the decision may be the hardest part of a new running program. After pursuing it for several months, you may like to begin reading books on running, buying special shoes and discussing the subject with your friends.

As you build up endurance, you will experience the change of consciousness and euphoria that results as more oxygen enters your system. Dr. Thaddeus Kostrubala, a San Diego psychiatrist and runner, says this about running: "I have talked to many runners—runners who run long, medium, and short distances. I have come to the conclusion that running, done in a long slow pace with a target pulse, is a form of natural psychotherapy. It stimulates the unconsciousness and is a powerful catalyst to the individual psyche." Dr. Kostrubala has reported using running as an effective therapy in his practice of psychiatry.

After months of successful running, you may want to run a marathon. The Boston Marathon is the best known in the United States and is the goal of many runners. That twenty-six miles and some odd yards is a kind of jogger's Holy Grail.

In Europe, running has been a natural part of the life style for years. An early morning run is about the same as brushing teeth or washing faces for many Europeans. My first experience running in Europe was in a German spa that was frequented by important political figures. The first morning out, our instructor explained the course in German, which was of no help to me since I don't speak the language. I decided to follow the leader, who happened to be the Russian ambassador, with his body guards. As he lead the pack through the verdant woods, he was followed by the Minister of Education and his entourage of protection. As we ran down a boulevard of trees, through a meadow and past a stream, I looked around at the group and realized that I was the only one without at least one body guard. I felt naked.

## How to Exercise

*Get a complete physical examination.* Your medical doctor may recommend less vigorous exercise if obesity, high blood pressure, a recent heart attack or other warning signals are present. You may have to walk before you can run.

*Watch what you eat before exercising.* Wait at least two hours after a heavy meal before exercising vigorously. About 90 minutes after a meal, blood is diverted away from the heart and the brain.

*Warming-up or Stretching* is basic to condition the muscles and joints before actual exercise can begin. A person over the age of 40 should do a slow warm-up of toe touching, jumping jacks and bends.

*The actual exercise,* whether it be jogging, swimming, or biking, should last for 25–30 minutes. The exercise should be continued to the point of stressing the heart and lungs moderately. Shortness of breath and an increased heart rate are indicators of moderate stress.

However, *don't overexert.* Some of the signs of overexertion are pain in the chest, severe breathlessness, dizziness and nausea. If you experience any of these symptoms, stop exercising immediately and reduce the intensity or duration of your activity.

The *cooling down* or tapering off period after exercise is still as vital as warming up beforehand. Stroll around the park, gym or yard for about five minutes. Resist the impulse to drop down and rest instantly. Avoid going from a cool temperature to a warm one right away or vice versa. This can induce faintness or dizziness.

Dr. Werner Hess of Baden-Bads goes on to state that noncompetitive exercise is the proper way to build good health. "Endurance is what counts, not speed or strength," says the doctor. Healthy, noncompetitive activities including long walks, swimming, rowing, bicycle riding and skiing are all acceptable, he adds.

## Benefits of Exercise

1. Your circulation will improve, aiding the entire body process.
2. Your body will become more limber and agile.
3. Nervous tension will be released and replaced with new energy and vitality.
4. Flabby tissue will become firm, healthy and youthful.
5. Sleep will be improved.
6. Weight will be normalized if accompanied by a proper eating program.
7. Your complexion will improve.

Since physical and mental health are inseparable, when health is improved, your outlook on life will improve.

The physically fit person is able to withstand fatigue for longer periods of time than the unfit, is better able to tolerate physical and mental stress, has a stronger and more efficient heart, and usually is more alert.

Exercise is said to be everyman's vitamin in Europe.

## Simple Exercise Program

1. Begin by walking one mile a day.
2. Increase the distance to two miles a day.
3. Walk fast so that you can walk two miles in 30 minutes.

Need a choice? Walk the first mile and run the second. If energy sustains, run both miles.

### Rules for Exercise

1. Start slowly with a few exercises, e.g., walking, rope skipping. Don't overdo it. Stiff muscles from overexertion can dampen enthusiasm for exercise.
2. Set a regular time for exercise and make it part of your daily routine.
3. Keep track of your progress. Write down your target or goal for exercising and pulse rate. Note the difference over a period of weeks or months.
4. Remain enthusiastic. Don't get discouraged. You didn't get out of shape overnight, so you can't expect perfection. Take your time.
5. Persevere. Don't quit at the first drop of perspiration. Push yourself to the point of discomfort but not exhaustion.

## STRETCHING

Once, when anyone said the word "stretch," my immediate thought was of a television commercial for a bra or girdle. Repeat the same word to an athlete, and the response is "warm-up" for exercising. Stretching is preparation for exercise which, when done slowly and deliberately, allows the muscles to relax. This can counteract aches and pains in the neck, shoulders, and lower back which result from tension and lack of exercise.

### When and Where to Stretch?

Have you ever watched a cat slowly and deliberately stretch out the kinks when it awakens from a nap? That's a good way to begin the day. When the alarm goes off, stretch leisurely before getting out of bed. Stretching can be done whenever you feel like it. It may be done at the breakfast table, while waiting for a bus or talking on the phone. You can stretch your arms up or grasp in back of you while at work, walking down a path, under a shady tree, or at the beach. Stretching should be done before and after physical activity, when the body and mind are tense. Stretch after sitting or standing for a period of time when poor circulation has set in and before and after sleep. Stretching breaks tension and enables relaxation.

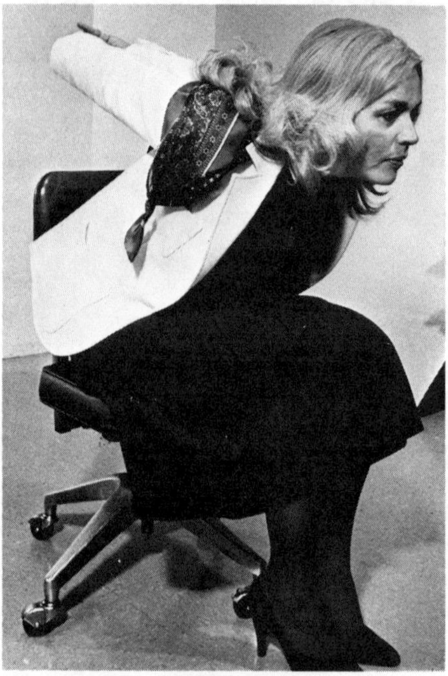

**Photo 8-1.**

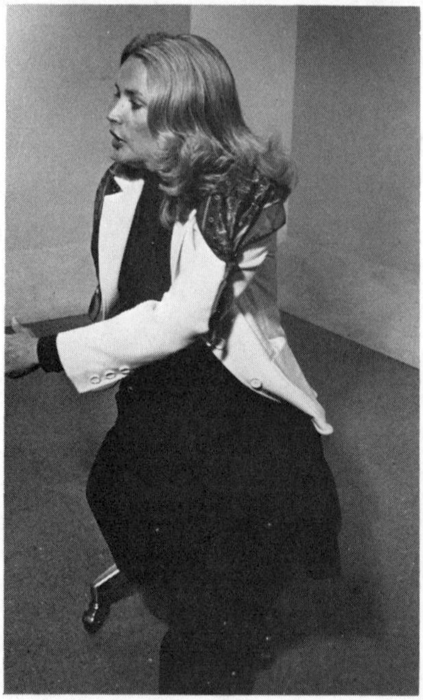

**Photo 8-2.**

**Photo 8-1.** *Stretch back* with hands clasped behind you; then stretch forward. (This relieves tension in the shoulder and neck area—common problemareas for people who work at desks.) Pull back several times until you feel the tension easing. A few minutes a day is a great preventive measure from upper back tensions.

**Photo 8-2.** *Torso twist.* Pull arms across your chest and twist; first to the right, then to the left. This relieves tension in the arms and slims the waist.

---

## ROPE SKIPPING

Skipping rope is an easy, versatile exercise. I carry a jump-rope in my purse and jump for ten minutes or so between business appointments. This form of exercise used to be relegated to boxers in training sessions. Not so anymore. If your muscles feel tight and tense, rope skipping aids in flexibility.

Use a clothesline or buy a professional rope with handles that are weighted with ball bearings. Begin with a long rope and then shorten it to suit your needs by tying knots in it. Be sure to wear good sneakers or track shoes to support and cushion the balls of your feet.

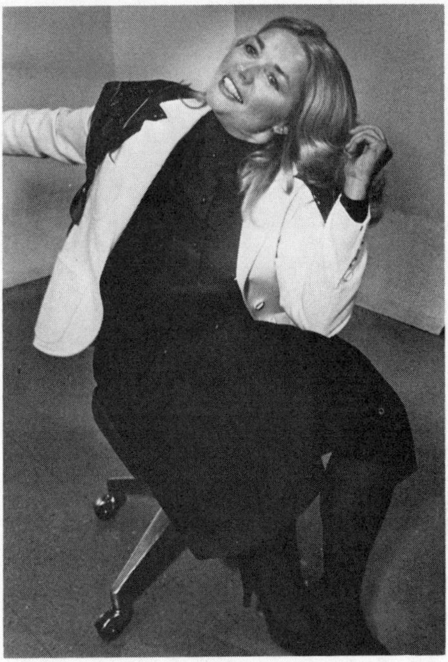

Photo 8-3.

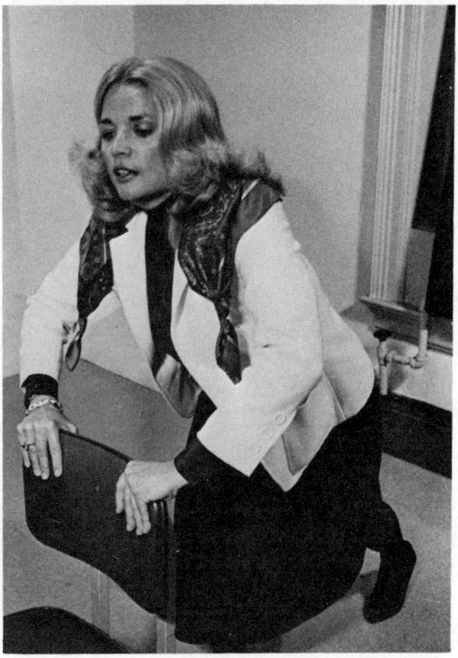

Photo 8-4.

**Photo 8-3.** *Elbow to knee.* Cross left elbow to right elevated knee. Alternate back and forth between left elbow and right knee, and right elbow and left knee. This relieves pressure in the mid-back and is also good for the waistline.

**Photo 8-4.** *Total body pressure release.* Stand with feet spread in a wide gate and hold on to the back of a chair. Push against the back of the chair and then release. After sitting in on a long meeting, this is a great exercise to relieve back pressure.

**NOTE:** All exercises can be more fun if done to music. On your lunch hour turn on the radio and stretch to the music. As you exercise, breathe deeply. Inhale; then on your exhale say "sh-sh-sh." Lift arms on inhaling, lower arms on exhaling.

---

## When to Jump

Plan to skip rope for 10–15 minutes in the morning to boost your energy and circulation for the day ahead. If you are dieting, a five-minute rope-skip before each meal will help control your appetite and burn up calories.

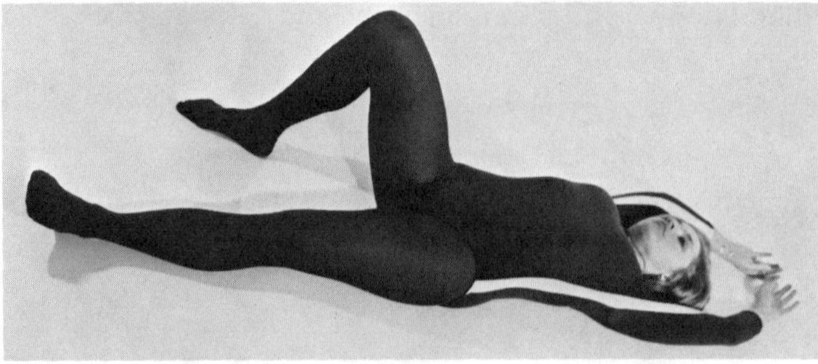

**Photo 8-5a.** Anger release #1.

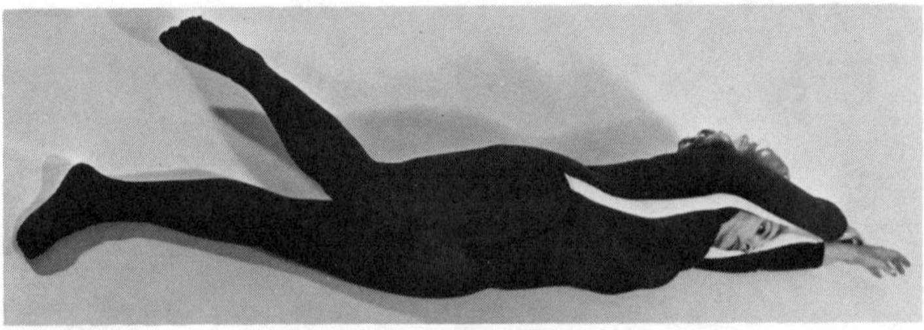

**Photo 8-5b.** Anger release #2.

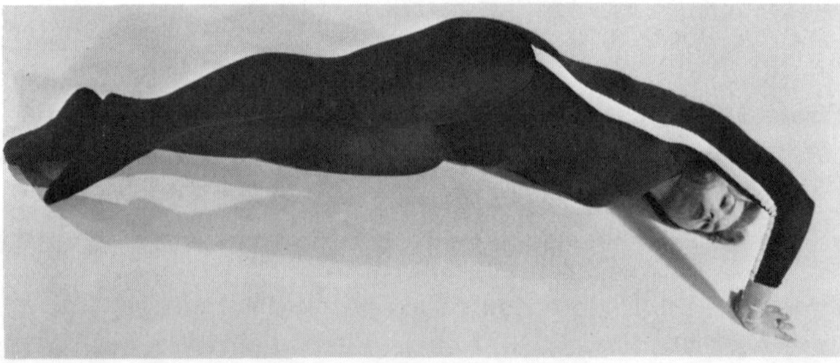

**Photo 8-5c.** Anger release #3.

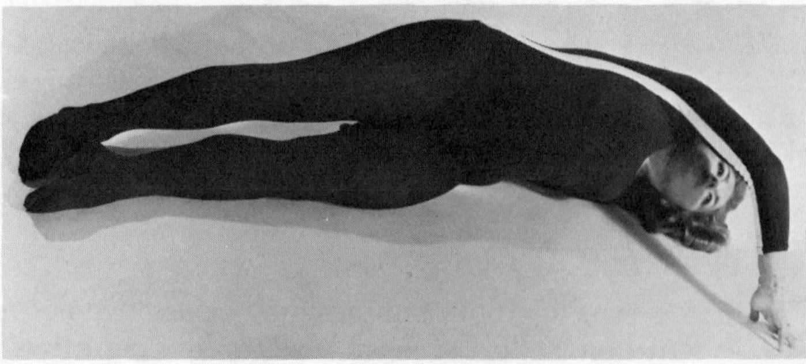

**Photo 8-5d.** Anger release #4.

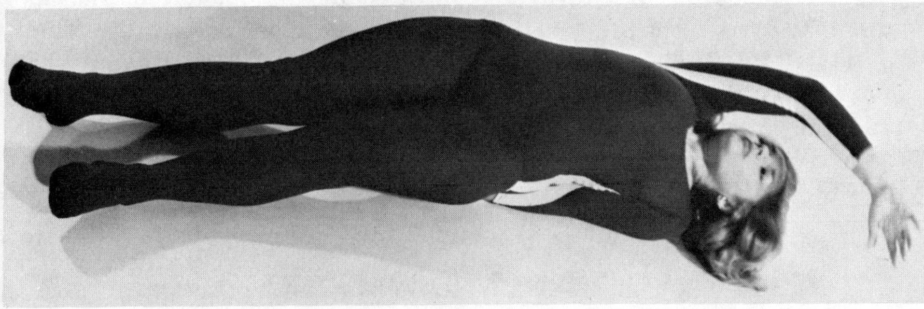

**Photo 8-5e.** Anger release #5.

---

## How to Skip

Hold the ends of the rope and slowly start to skip on alternate feet. Bounce on the balls of your feet and keep your knees slightly bent with arms close to the body. Jump just high enough to clear the rope.

Rope skipping can be invigorating and rejuvenating. It encourages circulation and is healthy for your heart. It also helps to slim thighs, hips, and buttocks.

## TAKING YOUR PULSE

With any aerobic program it is important to establish your pulse rate. The two easiest places to take your pulse are in the wrist, the radial pulse, and in the neck, just under the angle of the jaw, the carotid pulse. You will need to run, then stop for the ten seconds it takes to count your pulse. Practice taking your pulse right now. Use either your wrist or your neck and count the beat for ten seconds. Your pulse while not exercising is called your resting pulse. If you begin a running program today, your resting pulse will be lower six months from now.

Dr. Lawrence Moorehouse, who developed the fitness training program for the Skylab astronauts, suggests the following pulse guidelines;

If you are in *fair* condition, take 170, subtract your age and divide by six.

If you are in *excellent* condition, take 190, subtract your age and divide by six.

For example, if you are in fair condition and age 33, you subtract 33 from 170. Arriving at 137, you divide that by six which equals 22.8. This rounds off to 23. Therefore 23 beats per ten-second intervals would be your target pulse. As your condition improves through an aerobic fitness program, you might aim for a target pulse of 26, which would put you in the excellent category. At any rate, be realistic about estimating your present level of fitness.

## POSTURES AND WALKING

*The secrets of positive walking and posture:* let the arms swing in full sway with your legs. Walk with knees unlocked, smile and breathe deeply. Enjoy the movement of your body and get into your own rhythm. Hum a tune since walking to music, whether your own or the taped variety, helps keep your movements graceful and flowing and makes walking more fun.

### Posture Affects Digestion

If you slump, assimilation of food is affected by the constriction of the body. In a Swiss posture class I was told that the tower of Pisa is beautiful in spite of, and not because of its present position. It was headed for heaven before the weight of the world got it down. Don't let that happen to you. When daily problems upset you, stand up straight and tall and go out and take a long walk. You will find the effect therapeutic.

### Posture

When all the parts of the body are held in their correct position by the muscles, the body is aligned. To check your alignment, stand sideways in front of a mirror, and make sure that the body weight is toward the ball of the foot, rather than the heel.

Edith Risch, a European fitness expert, suggests the following exercises for improved posture and head carriage:

*Exercise 1:* Sit on a stool against a wall with pelvis, upper back, and back of the head in contact with the wall. Place feet a bit forward. Hands rest relaxed on thighs.

*Exercise 2:* Press the entire sole of foot at an angle against floor. This slowly straightens the spine. Neck vertebrae are also stretched. Gently press feet against the floor to aid alignment.

*Exercise 3:* As the foot pressure is released, the small of the back becomes rounded and the neck vertebrae again move slightly away from the wall. The head rolls to the top and the chin rises. The eyes and chin are diagonally aligned. Repeat straightening and releasing feet several times in a slow rhythm and breathe freely.

### Book or Stool on Head for Balance and Posture

The rain was showering its blessings on Zurich when Frau Risch began my posture instruction. Her operatic voice set the beat for me to march with a stool on my head. Feeling like a middle-eastern woman carrying her parcels home from the shuk, I walked to her "tuh run nah nah" beat. Try it. Stand tall, place a book on your head and march around the room. If you need musical accompaniment, turn on the stereo and prance to a John Philip Sousa march. When you master this skill, try perching a small stool on your head, seat side down. And try marching to new rhythms.

## STRETCHING EXERCISES

Flexibility is very important in exercising, and stretching sets the stage for more agile movements. Do some flexibility exercises at the beginning and end of each daily workout. More slowly and deliberately. Do not bounce or pull in an attempt to stretch your muscles. At the first sign of tension, hold the position for several seconds, then release and repeat.

1. *Side to Side Bend.* Start with arms over your head, feet shoulder-width apart and body erect. Bend to the right at the waist. Hold five to ten seconds. Repeat on left side, for a total of five times per side. This is good for trimming the waistline.
2. *Forward Bend—Legs Straight.* Sit erect with arms at side and feet straight in front, toes pointing up. Reach and bend forward as far as you can. Your goal is to eventually bring the chest to thighs with hands grasping toes. Hold five seconds and repeat three times. Repeat another three times with toes pointed forward. This exercise strengthens the back of the legs and the back.
3. *Forward Bend—Legs Apart.* Sit erect with legs apart. Bend at the waist and slide your hands as far forward as possible along your legs. Eventually you will be able to grasp your ankles with your hands. Hold five seconds and repeat three times. This is excellent for legs and back.
4. *Pole-Shoulder Flexibility.* Grasp a pole or broomstick palms down, with your arms spread to about two times shoulder width, and elbows locked. Bring the pole straight back over your head and stretch all the way back. Hold for five seconds. Repeat three to five times. This exercise is good for shoulder agility.

5. *Neck Roll.* Slowly roll your neck clockwise three times, then counter-clockwise three times. This improves your neck-muscle flexibility and removes tension where it accumulates.

6. *Spine Rock.* Sit on the floor and clasp your hands together under your knees, then raise to touch your chin. Rock back and forth five to ten times. This will help to limber the spine. It may be difficult to do at first, but with patience, you can master this exercise which is good for spine and neck conditioning.

7. *Alternate Toe Touch.* Stand erect with feet slightly wider apart than shoulder width. Touch the left foot with the right hand. Stand erect, then touch right foot with left hand. Work up to repeating the sequence ten times. This is good for firming the waistline and stretching the thigh's hamstring muscle.

8. *Waist Twist.* Stand tall with hands on waist. Twist as far to the right as possible and hold for a few seconds. Then twist to the left and hold for a few seconds. Repeat this sequence five to ten times.

## AEROBICS PROGRAM

The object of increasing the activity of your heart and lungs is to keep your heart beating at 65–70 percent of your maximum heart rate for 12–15 minutes. Reaching that goal may take several months. After you maintain 65–70 percent for that period of time, then you will have to exercise harder to stay at 70 percent of your maximum heart rate. Consult the chart below to indicate your age and level. To figure your maximum heart rate level, subtract your age from 220. If you are 35 years old, your maximum heart rate is 185 beats per minute. Your 70 percent rate is 129.5 beats per minute.

| *Age* | *MHR* | *70%* |
|---|---|---|
| 20–29 | 200–191 | 140–134 |
| 30–39 | 190–181 | 133–127 |
| 40–49 | 180–171 | 126–120 |
| 50–59 | 170–161 | 119–113 |
| 60–69 | 160–151 | 112–106 |

## NO TIME FOR EXERCISE? HERE'S AN ANSWER

A fitness program that requires no time? Well, not exactly, but if you can spare *ten minutes a day*, there is an exercise plan for you.

Lufthansa Airlines has devised in-flight exercises for toning the body. They are also adaptable for busy executives whose exercising time is at a premium. "These isometric exercises tense muscles at about 50 percent of their available strength," says Jurgen Palm, the German airline's fitness guru. Despite seatbelts and limited space, overseas passengers practice sitdown rumbas after taking off from Colonge on Flight 408. The exercise program, which aims to relieve the frazzling effect of prolonged jet-travel on the extremities, is the same as that of astronauts. It keeps muscles from going slack, the blood from settling in your legs and feet, and the joints from becoming stiff.

SAS, the Scandinavia airlines, has followed suit with an exercise program with such gyrations as "Jogging on the Spot," "Rowing While Seated," and "Slalom." It is reported that mini-gymnastics aloft may become the biggest benefit of air travel.

*Exercise 1.* Jogging on the spot is a warm-up exercise. It makes sense to warm up properly before strenuous exercise. Use simple, rhythmic movements, engaging as many muscle groups as possible. "Jog on the spot" by raising your heels alternately as high as possible. At the same time raise your arms in a bent position, and rhythmically rock forward and back as when walking. Continue for 1–3 minutes.

*Exercise 2. Raising on the toes* improves blood circulation to the legs. Sit with elbows on knees, bending forward with all your weight pressed down on the knees. Lift up on toes with the heels as high as possible. Drop heels and lift toes. Repeat whole process 30 times.

*Exercise 3. Shoulder rolling* stimulates the joints and relaxes shoulder muscles. Joints thrive on regular motion. Smooth, rhythmic movements "lubricate" the inner joint. Move the shoulders gently and rhythmically, at intervals, making large circles both forward and backward.

*Exercise 4. Head turning and nodding* stimulate joint capsules and cartilage in the upper spinal column. It is important to regularly activate the joints to the full extent of movement. Occasionally do the following: turn the head fully to the right, nod a few times, then do the same toward the left. Repeat the entire exercise six times.

*Exercise 5. Forward bends with stomach in* stimulate digestion, bowels and blood circulation. Draw the stomach fully in. Drop the trunk forward while lifting the front of the feet up high. Place the toes back on the floor, relax the stomach muscles, and raise the body upright again. Repeat approximately thirty times.

*Exercise 6. Hand-turning.* The wrist's cartilage and joint capsules also need stimulation. A good way to achieve this is to turn the hands all the way over and spread the fingers. Return hands to original position and relax them. Repeat 15 times.

*Exercise 7. Foot-rolling* stimulates the ankles. Roll the feet in large circles to the full extent of their movement. This is a valuable joint stimulator. Repeat 15 times in each direction.

*Exercise 8. Knees up against the elbows* done at regular intervals, increases blood circulation by setting to work large groups of muscles.

Drive the left and right knees alternately up toward the opposite elbow—15 times in each direction.

*Exercise 9. Rowing while seated,* a warm-up exercise, uses an imaginary "rowing" action. Stretch the arms forward while bending the upper body forward for a rowing "stroke." Lift the forward part of the feet up, then press the toes down while drawing in the arms. At the same time move the body backwards, completing the "stroke." Repeat the exercise for 1–3 minutes.

*Exercise 10. Alternate knee raising* speeds up blood flow and circulation by lifting the left, right and finally both legs in succession. Grasp the hands together under the legs and "pull." Repeat the exercise 10 times each for left, right, and both legs.

*Exercise 11. "Apple-picking"* stimulates the shoulder muscles and joints by alternately and rhythmically stretching up the arms as if picking fruit from a tree. This exercise is alternated with a rhythmic movement of the shoulders forward and back, holding them in a dropped, relaxed position. Repeat exercise 10 times with each arm and the shoulder.

*Exercise 12. Alternate head turning* stimulates joint capsules and cartilage in the upper spinal column. Bend the head forward keeping the chin against the throat and "bending" the head backwards. Turn the head to the right as far as you can and nod three times. Return the head to the front and repeat toward the left. Repeat the whole exercise 10 times.

*Exercise 13. Rising and sitting* improves circulation and stimulates the passage of blood to the legs. Gently rise upward or attempt to rise, with or without using the hands. Sit down again and lift the toes. Repeat exercise 30 times.

*Exercise 14. Double arm-swings* stimulate the muscles and joints of the shoulders and elbows. Sit with the hands clasped. Swing the arms gently and rhythmically up and back while stretching palms-up. Bring the arms down again and relax. Repeat the exercise 10–20 times.

*Exercise 15. Slalom while seated* improves the passage of blood to the legs and stimulates circulation. Sit with the heels as far out to the right as possible, with both the hands on the same side. Lift the heels right up and swing them all the way over to the left while swinging the arms over in the same direction. Repeat the exercise 30 times.

*Exercise 16. Relaxation. Muscle control.* We often tense various muscles unnecessarily for short or long periods without realizing it. Training muscle control and relaxation techniques help counteract this. Sit fully relaxed and breathe evenly and gently using so-called "diaphragm" breathing. This involves "filling" the stomach when breathing in, which is an active motion. On breathing out, which is a passive motion, the air is slowly released and the body sinks into complete relaxation.

In order to become aware of the difference between tensed and relaxed muscles, which help in avoiding unnecessary tensing, practice alternately tensing and relaxing various muscle groups. Repeat the exercise until you feel heavy and pleasantly relaxed.

## How Camille Found New Enjoyment in Life

When diabetes and being overweight brought her to Bad Pyrmont, my friend Camille had lived a sheltered, sedentary life for 45 years. Her affluence had kept her from any form of exertion and she confided to me that the only thing she did besides read and occasionally travel, was to make yogurt. This, she disclosed, was a divine experience when you place the yogurt maker between mink and ermine coats to get the correct temperature.

Her medical doctor encouraged Camille to walk through the German woods daily with fellow curists. At first she found the experience to be very "pedestrian." However, she became aware that she felt better mentally and physically and also lost weight.

At the conclusion of her stay, her doctor suggested that she select two physical activities to continue at home. Her choice was to walk and bike.

Two years later I learn that she has been cycling through England and Scotland and has a new, joyful approach to life. She says her relationships with family, friends and servants have also improved, and she is looking forward to future bike trips through the plains of Holland.

## Evan's New Sense of Self Respect

Evan was a robust Norseman who took it easy each day at his silversmith job. He liked the leisurely pace, but a sense of restlessness and lack of self-esteem plagued him. At a spa by the Baltic Sea he was introduced to aerobics. His heart and lungs seemed to pound as he daily jogged in place.

He liked the feeling of pushing his body to the limits of endurance. The exhilarating surge of adrenalin felt good. His energy level had never been so high and a by-product of his stay at the Baltic was a new-found sense of self-respect and confidence. His restlessness had also abated. Evan still pedals to work and during his lunch hours you can find him in an aerobics session in the square of Copenhagen.

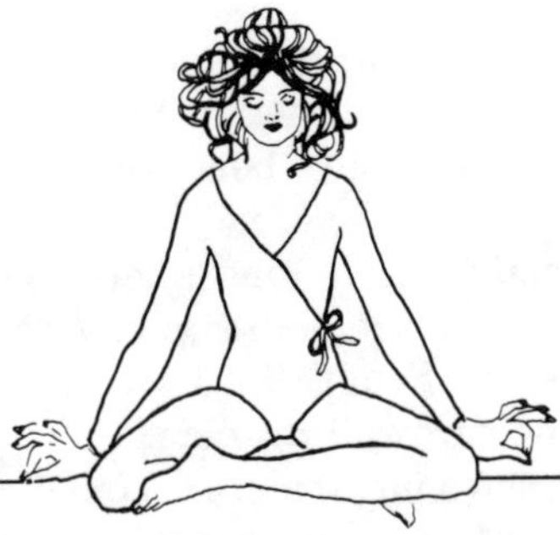

9

# A Wonder Plan for Refreshment

*Chinese medical saying: "All sickness begins in the stomach."*

*Eat your way to good health* is not just an advertising slogan but a truism in many European spas. While investigating numerous dietary regimen on the Continent, I kept hearing people say . . . "Oh, we follow the Bircher-Benner Raw Fruits, Vegetables and Grain Program." After seeing many youthful-looking senior citizens as well as young people with faces that announced good health, I journeyed to the famous Swiss klinic.

Foods that have obtained their energy from the sun, such as fresh fruits and vegetables, proved that life does beget life. The first time I sat down to a breakfast fare of muesli, a fresh fruit porridge, I knew that all those spa enthusiasts were right. Fresh foods not only provide more energy but they taste fantastic. This delicious, fruity breakfast-dish is excellent for metabolic and digestive problems. Lunch began with fresh fruit to aid digestion and prepare the way for further nutrition. Freshly picked green salad, root salad, cooked vegetables and a main dish of rolled spinach leaves cooked in tomato sauce compelled me to keep coming back for more. The marvel of eating fresh food is that your body holds up a stop sign when you have eaten all that is necessary.

This is not true of processed foods of the meat and potato variety that we commonly see in the good old U.S.A. How often have you gone into a fast-foods chain and eaten a sandwich flavored with monosodium glutamate to increase the appetite, and find that no matter what you eat you are never really satisified or full?

Although the processed food looks good, your internal, automatic shut-off valve says no. Natural foods appease the appetite. You get the nutrients that you need and that's it. And you stop because you are pleasantly satisfied.

Food is life surrounded by many social connotations. Major events and milestones in people's lives are customarily remembered by a ritually served meal . . . consider the Passover Seder, the Last Supper, wedding breakfasts, bridge luncheons and farewell dinners.

When people come together to celebrate a meal, more is consumed than food. Symbolically they take each other in by the exchange of words, gestures, smells, sights and sounds . . . a sharing of others. The American theologian, Harvey Cox, speaks of such celebrations in this way: "To remember together who we are."

That "remembering together" expresses an awareness of the relationship between mental and bodily processes. There is a psychological programming that centers around food, which may become an obsessive part of life at times. It is often equated with love, emotional gratification, socialization, repressed sexual needs or relief from boredom. For some people, it is the alpha and omega of life.

Food can be an escape-hatch from anger. What's eating you? And what are you eating in retaliation? Understanding one's eating "modus operandi" is important. It can help you decide which foods are good for you and what is best for your life style.

Have you ever seen a recent convert to gourmet food? Often their faces grimace as they attempt to eat food they don't like but have "learned" is delicious. Why eat something you don't like? If the food is psychologically unappealing, how can it possibly have nutritional value?

In European spas, notably the Bircher-Benner klinik, it's considered that the foods that are best contribute the greatest amount of energy. This nourishing energy source helps you live life more completely and abundantly, and should be able to sustain you when everything around you is draining your energy. The greatest energy-foods are those that are fresh or live close to their original sources: soil, sun, and light. Fresh fruits and vegetables, whole grain cereals and raw nuts provide the stamina needed for daily living.

In America, our foods often are lacking in nutrition or are starkly devoid of nutritive elements. Overt consumption of white flour, white bread, sugar and salt has contributed to poor health and rich doctors and dentists.

Our idolization of convenience foods and quick eateries has deterred us from eating correctly to prevent illness. As a people, we seem to be enamoured of meat and potatoes as well as snack favorites like donuts and coffee.

Fortunately the report by the Senate Select Committee on Nutrition and Human Need (1977) brought the matter of more natural diets to the government's attention. The recommendation was made that Americans should eat more fruits, vegetables, and grains instead of relying on fats and sugars for 60% of their food-energy.

In the report the statement was made that: "Our eating habits may be as profoundly damaging to the nation's health as the widespread contagious disease of the early part of the century." Rapidly increasing fat consumption has "been linked to six of the ten leading causes of death . . . too much fat, sugar and salt are linked directly to heart disease, cancer, obesity, and stroke, among other killer diseases." The report indicates that Americans should eat less meat and more poultry and fish, drink non-fat milk rather than whole milk, and consume fewer high-cholesterol foods. Such a diet would supply vitamins and micro-nutrients inexpensively, and could also reduce the risk of heart disease. It would also normalize the intestinal flora, contain more fiber and lower the incidents of bowel cancer.

This Senate Committee report is very far-sighted, and is the first comprehensive statement by any branch of the federal government on the risks involved in the American diet.

Also quoted in the Senate report is this statement from Dr. Bruno Bettelheim, noted child psychiatrist:

> *Eating and being fed are intimately connected with our deepest feelings. They are basic interactions between human beings on which rest all later evaluations of oneself, of the world, and of our relationship to it. Eating experiences condition our entire attitude to the world, not so much because of how nutritious is the food we are given, but because of the feelings and attitudes with which it is given.*

High protein diets are considered the ultimate in American eating. The popularity of various weight-reduction diets emphasizes how consumption of meat and accompanying weight-loss have contributed to the pro-beef mentality. However, the fact remains that the body does not store protein as it stores fat and sugar. Excessive proteins create uric acid, which overloads the liver and contributes to an accumulation of toxic material in the body.[1]

Dr. D. Mark Hegsted of the Harvard School of Public Health has underscored the problem: "There is a great deal of evidence which strongly implicates, and in some instances proves, that the major cause

---

[1]*U.S. Senate Select Committee on Nutrition and Human Need, March 1977.*

of death and disability in the United States is related to diet and the foods we eat. This includes coronary artery disease, which accounts for nearly half of the deaths in the United States, several of the most important forms of cancer, hypertension, diabetes and obesity."

The Senate Committee has suggested several important goals:

1. Eat more fruits, vegetables and whole grains.
2. Consume less meat and more poultry and fish.
3. Decrease foods high in fat and partially substitute polyunsaturated fat for saturated fat. (i.e., fresh, cold-pressed oils, margarines, etc.)
4. Substitute nonfat milk (also acidified milk and buttermilk) for whole milk.
5. Don't consume so much butterfat, eggs, and other high cholesterol sources.
6. Eat less sugar and high-sugar foods, and less salt and high-salt foods.

Fruits, vegetables and whole grains are good for you and combat heart disease.

The diet recommended in the Senate report is akin to that of the Bircher-Benner Klinik, with the exception of eating poultry and fish. The eating regimen at the Swiss center is widely accepted throughout Europe. As I trekked from spa to spa, I was continually amazed at the number that featured a traditional Bircher-Benner fare. The most exquisite hotels of Europe, such as Brenner's Park in Baden-Baden, included the well-known Bircher-Benner muesli on their menu.

The lactovegetarian diet, which consists of fresh fruits and vegetables, grains, nuts and dairy products, is the pièce de résistance at the Bircher-Benner Klinik. All the negative aspects of dieting, counting calories, martyrdom and guilt, need not be part of this regimen. As one noted doctor said: "It's time to get off a diet and on to a healthy way of living."

When you eat a balanced food program consisting of raw fruits and vegetables, the body regulates itself, and hunger pangs disappear. While eating natural foods, you seem to have an internal control that says, "enough is enough." Besides sound nutrition and weight reduction, this program has been very effective as a means of stabilizing weight. Dr. Ralph Bircher said: "We know of no panacea contributing more to the restoration and conservation of fresh and youthful vigor than a correctly planned uncooked diet with whole grain and green-leafed food. We also know of no diet that conquers obesity better—not even the high protein diets."

The Bircher-Benner plan is not as rigid as you might think. It has various types of programs: the normal diet, the raw food diet, fasting on juices and fruits, and the reducing diet. The *normal diet* offers the cooked vegetable and raw foods counter-balancing each other. It is composed of two small meals, one in the morning and one at night, both with muesli. The large meal is served at midday and always begins with fruit.

The *raw food diet* is recommended one or two days weekly. At the klinik it is usually advised to have one week of raw food in the spring and the fall. This is a preventive measure for people predisposed to high blood pressure, cardiac and kidney conditions, disturbances of the liver, migraines, and chronic constipation. It is also valuable as a general preventive measure, for increased resistance to infection and, for chronic rheumatic conditions. The raw food diet is composed of all sorts of uncooked fruit berries, nuts, hazelnuts, or almonds, raw vegetables such as tomatoes and cucumbers and the leaves and roots of finely-grated, raw vegetables in season. While eating on this plan, the metabolism and entire digestive system are freed to begin the internal cleansing and healing of the body.

*Fruit and juice fasting days* are used in place of complete fasting. They are seemingly as effective as complete fasting, but the side-effects of total fasting are not as evident (Refer to section on fasting in Chapter 5). Chronic cardiac and circulatory disorders, rheumatism and particularly obesity respond well to a juice diet taken as needed for one day at a time or as long as 10 to 15 days. A juice or fruit day is best followed by a raw food day.

*Diet for reducing* involves essentially the same foods in restriced quantities and consists mainly of raw ingredients.[2]

## THE BIRCHER-BENNER FOOD PLAN

When the established way of eating is overindulgence, the Bircher-Benner food plan of systematic undereating may just seem to be Spartan. Although this Swiss food plan seems bland by American stands, you will discover that after two weeks, your body will adapt to the aromatic, natural tastes and smaller quantity, higher-quality portions. You will not be inclined toward richly seasoned foods. Patients at the klinik said that when they have attempted to eat regular food again after this fare, it tasted overly seasoned and unpalatable. They stated that they are completely satisfied with less food of simpler nature.

---

[2]*See* Keep-Slim Nutrition Plan, *a Bircher-Benner manual available at: Harcourt Brace Jovanovich Bookstore, 757 Third Ave., New York, New York 10017. (Staff of Bircher-Benner Klinik, 1973)*

The body has a marvelous way of adjusting to its own needs so that it can self heal. This is evident in so many ways, but particularly in the instance of foods.

You might presume that this diet is designed for sedentary occupations only. However, exhaustive scientific research carried out at the klinik indicates that athletes, manual workers, and those involved in physical labor also do well. In fact, their energy levels and endurance are increased on this program.

The Swiss feel that there is more to life than sitting at a dinner table. The Bircher-Benner plan is nourishing, delicious, economical and simple to prepare. Chef Steiner of the klinik says that it is important to go out and enjoy life rather than spend hours cooking in the kitchen. He suggests leaving the cooking area on days of fatigue or stress. Take a picnic of fresh fruits, wedges of cheese, rye bread, and juice and go off to a park or mountain. He has encapsulated some hints for cooking the Swiss way.

## Six Food Secrets from Chef Steiner's Bircher-Benner Kitchen:

1. Begin each meal with fresh fruit. This lessens the appetite and prepares the body for digestion by stimulating enzymes within the system.
2. Follow the fruit with two salads: one of greens which get energy directly from the sun, such as spinach, endive and lettuce, and one of vegetables grown below ground, such as carrots, radishes and turnips.
3. Vegetables can be grated or cut in bite size pieces. They have to be carefully chewed to be readily digested.
4. Avoid salt. Instead season with herbs, such as thyme, marjoram, basil, dill and caraway.
5. Any seasoning or herb should be used sparingly. If a vegetable is organically grown, it will have its own rich flavor and will not need much seasoning.
6. Prepare as much of the food as is possible immediately before serving it since it begins to lose its nutritional value within 10 minutes.

*The Bircher-Benner Plan*, in particular, is one that normalizes the body. You eat and are satisfied. Period! Whether you want to eat for weight loss, nourishment, vitality, economics, or all of the above, the food program touches upon your needs. Breakfast and dinner are light meals, with the main meal at midday, allowing time for digestion. In a normal diet, the raw food is served with a cooked vegetable. The two counter-balance each other.

Here is a summary of a day's menu:

- *Breakfast*

  Bircher muesli

  Whole wheat or rye bread and butter

Nuts, such as hazelnuts or almonds, ground or whole

Weak herb tea (rose hip, mint, peppermint or blackberry) served at the conclusion of the meal.

- *Midday Meal*

  Fresh fruit, such as apples, grapes, strawberries, grapefruit, oranges or bananas

  Raw salad; celery, spinach, lettuce, tomato, cucumber, carrot or cabbage, etc.

  Vegetable soup or cereal soup

  Cooked dish; mixed vegetables—carrots, tomatoes or any other in season.

  Brussel sprouts, whole rice, baked potatoes, buckwheat, etc.

  Light dessert; (only brown sugar or honey used)

- *Evening Meal*

  (This should be early in the evening, between six and six thirty so that digestive processes do not disturb the first important hours of sleep. This simple menu is very good after a difficult day.)

  Bircher muesli or fruit with yogurt, brown bread, butter or cottage cheese

  Salad Nicoise or other raw vegetables

  Beverage of vegetable broth or herb tea (chamomile, linseed or golden-rod)

This approach to eating encourages you to drink your beverage at the conclusion of the meal. Drinking while eating interferes with digestion. One cup of tea, sipped slowly after a meal is ample. Besides, you will feel hardly any thirst when the meal begins with fruit.

The Bircher-Benner food plan is economical. Muesli is a complete meal, which is satisfying, nutritious, quick to prepare and costs less than a TV dinner. The added attraction is that in an era of instantism you get all the nutrients in one economical bowl.

This miracle food generates much energy, and if you try this regimen you will find out for yourself. You will have surplus energy because the food you are eating is directly from a sun source. The main part of the muesli, the apple, is raw; its purest energy state. That same energy is transmitted to you when you eat it, unlike a quarter-pounder and french fries which lack this sun source.

Beginning to heal yourself can be a creative adventure. Years of improper eating can leave the body devoid of vitamins and consequently exhaust the tissues and organs. A surplus of acidity with accumulated metabolic wastes further impair the system. The prerequisite for healing is detoxification and a crisis to bring about self healing.

Two days of raw foods will begin the process of purging wastes from your system. You can eat all kinds of fresh fruits, and vegetables, green herbs and some nuts including walnuts, hazelnuts and almonds. After two days, if you wish you may remain on raw foods; however, you can add cooked vegetables to supplement your meals.

All foods must be chewed thoroughly. They can be chopped, grated, or finely cut for easy absorption into the system. The French speak of "matiere vivante," or living matter, as the foods that provide nourishment. Sungrown foods, uncooked and undenatured by meat, provide the initial energy needed to sustain health.

So you're convinced you want to try this approach to eating. Question: *What foods do you eat?*

Nature has provided a rich choice of delectable foodstuffs. Here is a list of your energy sources:

1. Fruits: apples, pears, oranges, grapes, cherries, plums, apricots, peaches, bananas, pomegranates, lemons, grapefruit, pineapples, figs, dates, etc.
2. Berries: strawberries, raspberries, blackberries, red and black currants, cranberries, gooseberries, etc.
3. Vegetables:
   a) fruit of the plant—cucumbers, pumpkins, melons, tomatoes, artichokes.
   b) leaf of the plant—lettuce, endive, spinach, watercress, dandelion leaves, white and red cabbage, savoy, chicory, celery, fennel.
   c) root of the plant—carrots, beetroot, radishes, black and red, celeriac, onions, garlic, kohlrabi, horseradishes.
   d) flower of the plant—asparagus, brussel sprouts.
   e) leguminous plants: peas, green beans, soya, green grains, buckwheat.
4. Cereals: bran, millet, oats, bulgar, wheat, rice. (eaten soaked, raw, grated, cooked, or sprouted)
5. Nuts and olives: almonds, walnuts, hazelnuts, pine kernels, Brazil nuts, coconuts, sweet almonds. Commercially pickled olives are good. The oil is the most valuable part of the olive. Peanuts are not recommended. According to research conducted by Bircher-Benner, the peanut produces too much uric acid. Sorry, Jimmy Carter!
6. Vegetable spices: caraway seeds, fennel seeds, capers, chervil, tarragon, chives, parsley, garlic, etc.
7. Milk, milk products and eggs: sour milk forms offer the best digestive aids including yogurt, kefir, buttermilk, ricotta, cottage cheese, sour cream.

8. Raw honey: recommended to aid taste of food. Also fruit concentrates, such as "Birnel", fructose, lactose.

## What Cooking Utensils Are Needed?

Good intentions about eating right can be dissipated by using the wrong utensils in food preparation. Stainless steel saucepans are best, and foods containing acids should not be used in aluminum. Enamel saucepans are good except for roasting and baking. Iron and glazed, steel pans are good for cooking fruits and vegetables, but they may crack. Pyrex cookware is also very good since it is porous and preserves the food aroma and does not retain flavors. Be especially careful with fruits and vegetables containing acids. Don't leave them in containers made of copper, zinc, tin or silver plating since the acid may dissolve the metals.

Next you would want to consider:

## How to Prepare Foods for Greater Nutritional Content

There are three important questions to ask yourself in food preparation:

1. *What is the nutritional content?* Are the fruits and vegetables fresh, or wilted from storage in the refrigerator for several days?

2. *Is the food clean?* Fruits and vegetables need proper cleansing in warm water.

3. *Is your food fresh and wholesome?* No food will ever be perfect. So cut off the parts that are not absolutely fresh. Lettuce leaves, endive, spinach and other leafy vegetables should be soaked in salt water, then carefully washed under running tap water. Apples can be washed and dried with a clean cloth and then cut in half to be sure there are no worms inside. Pits and core should be eaten with the apple. Roots, like carrots, radishes, kohlrabi, etc., should be carefully washed in running water, then scraped. Cut off any hard, woody parts.

# THE AESTHETICS OF EATING

It is just as important to make mealtime an enjoyable experience as it is to make sure foods are nutritional. Realize that this is truly a sensuous time. Does the food look good? Is the color of the food balanced? For example, slivered red beets look more appetizing next to a pale green cabbage salad. Next time you sit down to eat, ask yourself: "How is the food served?"

In Europe, much attention is given to the appearance not only of the food but of the surroundings for food as well. I still remember the lovely, ornate, brown tea cup served on a silver tray in a Northern German fasting-klinik. The service was so attractive that I momentarily forgot that this was not a complete meal. I also recall a hand-painted blue china service with a bud vase of flowers in another spa. Just the appearance of your table heightens the appeal of the mealtime adventure.

Another important aspect of aesthetics is your attitude toward mealtimes. Come to the table with the idea that you will enjoy sharing this time with your family or friends, and make mealtimes pleasant occasions. Bringing up grievances is enough to create ulcers, so don't eat with people you do not like. Business lunches during tense negotiations will most likely encourage indigestion.

Set the scene for eating: arrange the table colorfully, use flowers or a centerpiece for interest. Play background music and, try candlelight!

We all dine alone at one time or another, and it is easy to forget that principles of the aesthetics of eating apply here, too. Take your food out of the kitchen and into more appealing surroundings.

In Bad Hofgastein, individual food trays are taken outside to dine amid foliage and flowers. You can sit on the floor in front of a roaring fire and listen to classical music in the background. Make your dining time special: you deserve it!

No matter what, anything you do three times a day is bound to get dull once in a while, so add life to the day-to-day routine of eating.

## HAVE A VITALITY DAY

Spend an occasional day eating only fresh fruits and vegetables. Eliminating starches from the diet will produce a laxative effect, and raw fruits and green, leafy vegetables are ideal for cleansing the colon. Also, the high chlorophyll in the green leaves acts as an antidote to all the lead in the air. In the body, lead affects oxygen transport and creates fatigue—urban dwellers take note!

Baked and stewed fruits are good too, but are less effective. Try a new herb tea at the end of a meal. Is golden rod or rosehip appealing? Parsely tea is good for the liver, and sage, chamomile, yarrow or ferungreek are all healthful drinks.

During your vitality day, schedule time for a half-hour walk and rest after the midday meal. You will find this day is a time to replenish your strength. On the following day be attuned to your feelings and observe how your body responds after a vitality day.

There are food situations that require special consideration: Social occasions and business lunches, pressured times and lonely times. The following are just a few situations that add to food-frustration and consequently to overindulgence.

## WHAT TO EAT WHEN

*You are snowbound with pre-schoolers and the TV goes out.* Anxiety, confusion, fatigue and frustrations are probably with you. The temptation is to eat or drink something terribly fattening to placate the ego, but have faith; it can be overcome. If you feel that a food reward is necessary, take fresh fruit and place on your best china. Tell your little ones that for twenty minutes you need to be alone. Go into your dining room and turn on relaxing music, and imagine that you are at Maxim's in Paris, Brennan's in New Orleans, or whatever place appeals to you. If fruit is not your idea of a treat, try mineral water in a goblet with a twist of lime or orange. Consider any of the pudding or dessert dishes found at the end of this book, or make muesli as a dessert—use two fruits and add yogurt and honey. This is a delicious treat.

*You are a speaker on the Chicken a la King circuit.* To all those who have been confronted by this standard casserole with frozen peas and candied apples, our condolences. This fare is unappetizing, fattening, and not as nutritious as other possibilities. I have handled this situation by calling the restaurant or hotel in advance and requesting that a cottage cheese and fruit plate or chef salad be substituted. Most restaurants are accommodating and will comply since this food substitution usually is less expensive than the original menu, so their profit is increased and your waistline is not.

*You attend a banquet.* Again, call ahead and get a food substitution. Or, eat at home, save the cost of the dinner, and come to socialize or hear the after-dinner speaker.

*You are at a cocktail party.* Here's a challenge. Before you is a sea of unknown faces. Nearby is a plate of typical hors d'oeuvres. There is security in the familiar and you feel inclined to take some. Take a few, if you must, but consider the natural types, such as stuffed celery instead of pastry wrapped around a fattening filling. Would you like a drink? Order a glass of tomato juice which is usually available as a base for a mixed drink. Club soda with a twist of lime looks authentic yet has no calories. Or, bring your own mineral water, a practice quite in vogue in Europe. When dining in Europe's finest as well as moderate restaurants, you can have a choice of Perrier, Vichy, or some of the local waters. These waters can be purchased at health food stores.

*You want a complete meal and have no time.* Hypocrates, ancient physician of 500 B.C., dined on this fruit mixture. He treated patients for digestive problems with a mixture of raw fruits, natural honey and goat milk. Dr. Bircher-Benner rediscovered this nutritious, economical and quick food which is eaten either at the beginning of a meal or as a meal in itself. You can use it as a featured meal by adding several fruits instead of just the apple.

Bircher-Benner Muesli

- Ingredients for 1 serving:

  1 tbsp rolled oats (or 1 tbsp medium oatmeal) soaked 12 hours in 3 tbsp of water

  1 tbsp lemon juice

  2 tbsp yogurt

  1 tbsp honey or "Birnel"

  1 large apple (or 2–3 small ones)

  1 tbsp of grated filberts or almonds

- *Directions:*

  Mix lemon juice, yogurt and honey into a smooth cream. Add to oats, stirring thoroughly. Grate a washed, organic apple into the bowl, with pits and core, stirring frequently to prevent discoloration. Sprinkle grated nuts over the top for added protein and serve immediately.

- Other fruits can be added to this mixture—bananas, blueberries, apricots, cherries, currants, or strawberries, as well as dried fruits.

The big health advantage of this food is that it is easily digestible, provides nourishing enzymes, vitamins and minerals to feed the cells. It is an excellent energy source.

Muesli, fresh fruits and vegetables offer new vitality. When you eat these natural foods, you can forget about dieting. Your body will take care of its own nutritional requirements. Throw away your calorie charts. You are in a new era. Live!

Go out and appreciate the day. You have more time because food preparation is minimized. Consider a new sport . . . tennis, anyone? Take up yoga, dancing, pottery, or get involved in an organization. New vistas are open to you. When you eat right, you have the energy and zest to do more and think positively. Enjoy yourself. . . for life is a banquet.

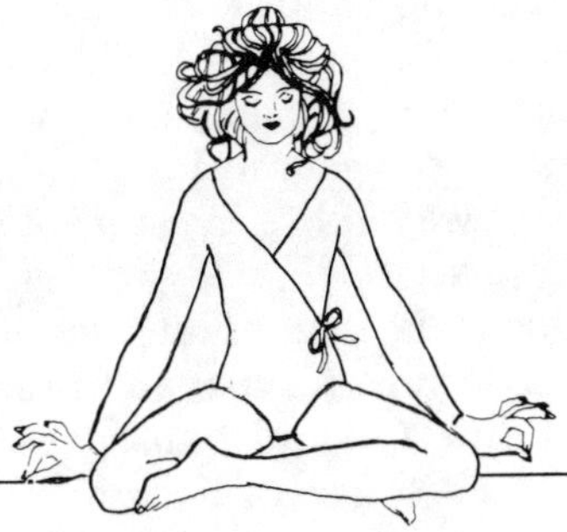

# 10

# The Swiss Way to Treat Arthritis

*"With Health Everything is a Source of Pleasure."*

*Schopenhauer*

Poets and humorists on both sides of the Atlantic have joked about how we all want to go back to the womb, where it's warm, nurturing, and caring. Returning to the Bircher-Benner Klinik, as many do year after year, is the closest thing to returning to the womb. Here, you step into a loving, caring environment in which unconditional support assists in your business of healing.

As a private klinik, somewhat between a hospital and a diagnostic center accommodating 70 people, it is small enough to know everyone intimately. Here a person is seen as a complete human being. Many people report that after many travels from doctor to doctor, this personalism is a first.

The klinik staff, whether it be the doctor you see every day, the nurse who invests time to discover your uniqueness, the cleaning woman who bursts into your room twice a day with a cheerful "Gooten Tag," or the gardner who picks fresh flowers for your room and selects the perfect fruits and vegetables for your repast, all express interest and concern for you in varying degrees.

Where else could you receive a bouquet of flowers and a personal note from both your physician and nurse on your birthday than at

Bircher-Benner? In the United States you would probably get a bill for medical services rather than such a thoughtful gesture.

Bircher-Benner Klinik is nestled in a comfortable neighborhood of villas and gardens above shimmering Lake Zurich. The healing ambiance is accentuated by individual diet programs, physiotherapy, water treatments, healthful life style considerations, and gaining insight about viable changes conducive to a more vibrant way of life are some of the residual benefits of being in this healing mecca.

For some people, part of the attraction is the long list of celebrities who have taken the "kur" there. Princes, royalty, performers and swamis have all graced the klinik. Yehudi Menuhin, Gaylord Hauser, Golda Meir, Eugene Ionesco and Emilio Pucci are some of the prominent personages who come to mind. One wag stated: "Bricher-Benner Klinik has attracted the rich, the famous and the desperate."

People come from all corners of the world and spend either five days for a medical check-up or three weeks detoxifying the body and learning more healthful ways of living.

The healing stage that is set at Bircher-Benner becomes contagious among the patients as well. A spirit of community and comeraderie prevails among the patients as well. Like children away at camp for the first time, friendships of deep intensity are formed. Age, culture, and life experiences are no barriers to intimate relationships that facilitate healing. Sitting down to a meal together, comparing treatments and courses of illness while strolling through the woods for a morning walk, or basking in the sun. The sharing of personal aspects of one's life occurs, the likes of which one would never experience with most friends at home.

Was it because we had disrobed our psyches as well as our bodies while sunbathing that freed us from entanglements? The last time I was there I discovered a best friend 26 years my senior and even more light years apart in economic and social life experiences, yet, like school girls comparing first dates, we developed a bond of friendship that has transcended time and klinik.

The present ambiance is exactly what its founder, Dr. Max Bircher-Benner envisioned when he established his klinik in the late 19th century. His concept of a klinik taking into account the whole person, body and soul, not just the patient's disease, and using an intelligent patient as a co-worker in a total, therapeutic effort, was radical at the time. He wanted people to get in contact with their own "internal physician," thc healing force and system of the body, to self heal. He created a therapeutic climate of dietetic therapy and encouraged a balanced life style as the basis of a total health plan. His niece, Dr. Liechti von Baasch, a most competent physician and compassionate human being, adroitly functions as present-day medical director.

## EAT FOR HEALTH

The secret weapon in Bircher-Benner's disease arsenal is a fruit porridge called muesli.

Muesli is made fresh just before serving and is often combined with other fresh fruits of the season, such as pears, bananas, berries or even dried fruit. A complete meal in itself, this fruit dish has received global rave reviews. Henry Ford was said to have been a devotee of Muesli; a Milanese professor offers it to his guests as Dolce Sorpresa or "Sweet Surprise", and in England it is called "Swiss Breakfast" and can be found on many restaurant menus.

There are many variations of this famous dish. You can find preparation suggestions for it at the end of this book.

Will you have the self-discipline to be different from other people by eating naturally, taking rests and actively pursuing good health? That is the question!

Dr. Max Bircher-Benner once said: "Live from within rather than from without." This dedication to self healing is evident at the Bircher-Benner Klinik in many ways. The medical professionals cooperate with the self-healing faculties of the patient.

When a person is ill, not only one area of the body is affected; sickness is systemic, involving the whole body but manifesting itself in the weakest area.

According to statistics at the University of Zurich, rheumatism and arthritis are 35 times more prevalent and cause an annual loss of work corresponding to $1300 million in purchasing power of the United States.

Sickness is a luxury few of us can afford, so eating right with fresh fruits, vegetables, grains, seeds and herb teas, while having an ordered life, is vital for health.

Dr. Bircher-Benner has stated that a main objective at his klinik is to regenerate the body (via a re-ordering to gain new vitality or growing energy.)

Water therapies and a dietetic program beginning with raw fruits and vegetables are integral parts of the therapy. Here, patients are encouraged to forfeit their old eating habits which originally produced their illnesses. They substitute a healthful plan of fresh foods, raw nuts, and herbs, gradually enlarged with cooked food of harmonious composition, organic quality and highly palatable preparation. This enables the body to begin its remedial work.

While many people are killing themselves slowly by eating too much, consuming the wrong foods and ignoring the natural rhythms of their bodies, Bircher-Benner offers a healthful alternative.

The concept that health is harmony between the body, mind, and soul is nurtured via the various therapies. When people do not live in harmony with nature's rules and with their destiny, then the body becomes distressed and illness invades the system. The basis of the treatment at the Bircher-Benner Klinik is regulation therapy; putting order and a routine into a person's life is the beginning of recovery.

Dr. Bircher-Benner has stated: "The only way in which a real recovery can be effected is via regulation therapy. This involves a new way of life which follows life's own rules of order and advances the vital regulative power of body, mind and soul."

1. *A Regular daily schedule*
   a) Rising at a specified time each day—exercise, either walking or running, offers a time to commune with nature or build strong friendships with your walking partners and begins the conditioning before breakfast.
   b) Have a frugal and light but delicious breakfast with fruit muesli or with main dish, eaten on time, and consequent meals eaten at the same intervals each day with lunch as the main meal, and a frugal and light dinner like breakfast.

It is important to note that activity is balanced between mental, physical, active and passive pursuits.

2. *Rest*
   a) Midday rest after lunch. At the klinik, the scheduled time is from 1:30 p.m. to 3 p.m. Heavy emphasis is given to relaxation and rest—it's a welcome reprieve.
   b) Nightly rest; 8:30 p.m. is the prescribed bedding-down time at the klinik. It is emphasized that the sleep before midnight is the most beneficial. The rationale is that without regular sleep and rest, all metabolic processes and healing are impaired. This is often difficult to accomplish since there are many cultural pursuits every evening.
3. *Exercise:* Two walks a day are advocated, with the early morning walk an exercise must. According to the klinik handbook, "The morning walk establishes a relationship with nature, assisting the recovery of your body by stimulating blood circulation, digestive processes, breathing, and the supply of air. You will feel not only more lively and active afterwards, but physically fitter than after sleeping on into the morning." An afternoon or evening walk should also become a habit. Weekend hikes with gradual, increased activity, but without strenuous performances are also recommended. Morning gymnastic classes offer stretching and isotonic movements to classical music. The class

is taught in 4 languages, so after a month, whenever I heard someone count in German, I automatically would stretch both arms to the ceiling and reach down and touch my toes from such conditioning.

4. *Deep breathing techniques:* Respiration helps to consciously affect body regulation. Steady, deep breathing can achieve a considerable lowering of blood pressure when weakened pressure regulation is involved. Several times a day, a person is encouraged to deeply breathe in and out to promote adequate ingestion of air and exhalation of carbon dioxide. Intense deep breathing, like in yoga, originates from the abdomen and should be done while maintaining a natural posture.
5. *Relaxation:* Autogenic training is taught by Dr. Joachim Krammer, who studied with Dr. Schultz in Germany 41 years ago. Autogenic training is done twice a day for 6 minutes (for specific instructions refer to Chapter 6).
6. *Meals should be eaten on time* to regulate and enhance the total conditioning of the body. Foods need to be chewed slowly, and discussion of unpleasantness is forbidden.
7. *Skin care* regulates waste removal through the pores. A morning dry-brush massage and wash with cool water helps rid the body of dead skin and enable it to function better. This circulation boost is an energizer as well.
8. *Hydrotherapy:* Assorted water treatments are part of the regimen. Usually a patient receives one in the morning and one in the afternoon, which are always followed by a period of rest. After the cold water treatments, the body relaxes and rest or sleep seems to come quickly.
9. *Mental orientation:* Patients are encouraged to avoid discussions and situations that lead to irritation and tension. The avoidance of late night activities aid in coping with the stresses and unresolved problems that a patient may bring with them. Taking one hour a day to be alone and organize thoughts and consider feelings is important. Conscious attention to constructive and happy thoughts helps to regulate the mind and enhance healing.
10. *Sun:* This energy source for healing is also part of the therapy. Sunbaths, starting from a five minute minimum and progressing to fifteen are valuable for restoring verve.

Regulation therapy puts the body on a timetable to allow the principles of natural order to become effective in the preservation of health as well as in the prevention of illness. These principles apply not only to food: breathing, exercise, rest, air, water and sunshine have effects on the system and the entire rhythm of the day. This ordering reestablishes and maintains health.

The basis of food regulation at the klinik is the life enhancing/promoting quality of food energy as found undiminished in fresh, raw vegetables.

Dr. Bircher-Benner has stated that the deeper you sense life, the more it approaches wisdom and health. He goes on to say: "If I could grasp life in its deepest sense, life in itself, I would know that it is the same as wisdom and the same as health. I need not become sick nor remain sick. I can recover as soon as I understand life." . . . "I then gradually would understand that there are crooked ways and straight ways." Recognizing the crooked ones by which I went becoming sick, and going the right way I can recover; working with my life for the evolution of the spirit and giving Him back with my life and what He gave me."

In our rush toward the 21st century, we have forgotten how to live. Professor H. Schipperges of Heidelberg who has done extensive investigation on international health services, predicted at the 1968 German Medical Association, that "as things were going, before long one third of the population will have to sustain the other two thirds, half of the invalids." In 1975, Professor Kirk Enrich at the Davos Medical Symposium in Munich predicted the moment when health costs will absorb the national income. Health insurance costs have risen dramatically in the industrialized countries with the introduction of more intensive and costly treatments.

Preventive medicine presents a plight and a challenge since it calls for a turnabout in viewing and treating health problems. A new kind of medical profession is needed to engage in teaching a new way of life and a change in the industrial structure and values. Irresponsible consumerism, demanding everything from the medical services and nothing from themselves, must have an end. We need to work towards an "all-togetherness."

"We need to become hale and hearty enough to be able to confront the oncoming flood of new problems, dangers and hardships. We will need a much higher life potential in order . . . to right ourselves up again and again . . . to bounce back after unusual stress."

We also need to recognize the full extent of prevalent "inbuilt" diseases which are well documented but far from being generally acknowledged. It means that the great majority of those commonly thought to be healthy are harbouring hidden disease and that these masked pathological disorders can be manifested in years or decades, despite apparent good health.

The claim "there is no cure for arthritis," and its subsequent treatments merely mask symptoms. In the United States, the familiar treatment is aspirin, cortisone, and gold injections, which mask the symptoms and do not treat the cause, prolonging the illness and adding to it. Consider the residual problems that occur from cortisone and gold injections, both of which can cause kidney damage and create an illness worse than the original arthritis.

## Fashion Designer Overcomes Arthritis with Raw Food

When Agnes, a 27-year-old fashion designer from New York City first entered the klinic, she was crippled and defeated as a result of a severe injury to her right leg from a car accident a few years earlier. Thereafter, arthritis set in as did monumental medical bills. Madison Avenue doctors gave her the maximum dose of cortisone, but her condition continued to worsen until the pain became unbearable. The doctors then prescribed morphine which created a momentary "edge" on the pain but soon wore off. Whatever the dosage, Agnes's pain seemed to grow to such an unbearable degree that she considered suicide. Just as she was about to take her own life, a friend came to visit. Agnes broke down and admitted that she could no longer live with unremitting suffering. Her friend wisely took her to a drug-rehabilitation program, since by this time Agnes was addicted to morphine. It was during her rehabilitation that she heard about the Bircher-Benner Klinik and decided to visit it.

When I first met Agnes at the klinik, she looked pale and old. Immediately, however, she began the raw foods regimen eating no animal foods, such as eggs, milk, butter or cheese. (No meats or fish are served at the klinik). This natural regimen helped the body cleanse itself of retained wastes and sluggishness in the digestive organs.

Agnes also ate *muesli* regularly—a food that is as Swiss as cuckoo clocks, watches and Heidi. Centuries ago it was eaten by peasants. It is a hearty mash consisting of fresh fruit; cereal: whole grain oats, wheat or barley; milk: fresh from the cow, and a sprinkle of nuts on top.

When Bircher-Benner revived this food at the turn of the century by which time people had forgotten its merits, he modified the original recipe to make the dish more palatable. His modern version of muesli is refreshing and complete in itself, containing all the nutrients in correct proportions for a balanced meal. The crucial ingredient is fresh fruit, prepared immediately before serving to guarantee freshness.

*Food as Medicine* the most important rule of the klinik, is starting each meal with raw food. Begin with fresh fruit, such as pears, apples, grapes, or any regional fruit in season. Then comes uncooked vegetables like chard, lettuce, carrots and cucumbers, all cut up in fine pieces. Next comes any cooked food. Agnes followed this rule closely.

The virtue of raw food, the klinik believes, is that it's the easiest food to digest because it contains its own digestive enzymes.

Dr. D. Liechti-Von Brasch, the Klinik's Medical Director, acknowledges that cooking can often destroy important vitamins and minerals. The great blessing of raw food is that it prevents "digestive leucocytosis," a molutization of white corpuscles in the intestinal walls that always occurs when cooked food is eaten, but not when it's served after raw food. Raw food also includes the micro-electric tension in the cell-tissue that results in better cell metabolism, respiration and regeneration. The best food combination, Dr. Liechti-Von Brasch insists, is a raw piece of fruit and a whole wheat dish as muesli. The vitamins of one supplement the other, and together, they produce a high-energy food that satisfies the appetite.

Agnes discovered that the uncooked foods supplied all her necessary vitamins and minerals as well as the natural enzymes that are easily digestible for healthy bodily functioning. She began to discover that the condition of her health was related to the naturalness of her food. Her treatment also consisted of rest and water treatments. Agnes was also given homeopathic compounds of herbs to remove the cortisone that had lodged in her tissues and had impeded her metabolism as well as other bodily functions.

After about six weeks, I saw her in New York. She was jubilant and told me she could walk with only slight assistance from a cane, and she was able to resume her work. She had even taken on some fashion assignments on the side. Most importantly, she knew that she did not have to be ill, and that arthritis would not overcome her. She had altered her life style, just as the klinik suggested.

Agnes now sleeps regular hours at night, and despite an erratic schedule, exercises daily. After lunch she lies down for ten minutes before resuming work, and while others are drinking alcoholic beverages at cocktail parties, she sips Perrier with a twist of lime. She has said farewell to devitalizing foods such as coffee, sugar, salt, chocolate, soft drinks, sweets, pastries and pies. She used to smoke two packs of cigarettes a day, but has completely given up smoking and breathes deeply.

Most of all, Agnes is happy and has been able to exercise some control over her life. She has developed the healing attitude that is paramount to health, and also confided that as a result of taking control of her health, she had developed a degree of assertiveness that has fared her well professionally and socially. She now has more fashion designing jobs than ever before, socially, she thinks about whether or not she really *wants* to be in a particular situation and whether she has the necessary energy instead of going just for the sake of getting out of the apartment.

Arthritis is a systemic constitutional disease which always affects the whole body. It is not an unrelated localized disease of certain joints.

*Cause:* Metabolic disorders and systemic disturbances which effect the pathological biochemical changes in all body tissues, specifically in collagen.

The biochemical changes cause inflammatory and degenerative changes in the functions of joints and their surrounding connective tissue.

Underlying causes for these systemic disturbances and pathological changes are found in prolonged abuse the body has been subjected to, such as faulty nutritional patterns, overeating, nutritional deficiencies, lack of sufficient exercise, severe emotional and physical stress. These health destroying factors eventually result in diminished vitality and lowered resistence to disease, intestinal sluggishness, *autointoxication* and impaired elimination.

The current observation of many European doctors is that the patient usually suffers from general health deterioration in the form of sluggish organ functioning incomplete digestion and foods assimilation, impaired elimination of metabolic waste and a weakened nervous system and circulation.

Sedentary life with its resultant impaired circulation and anoxia; constipation; smoking and drinking; contaminated air and water; emotional and physical stress; lack of adequate rest all contribute to bodily deterioration.

The biological treatments are directed at normalizing and strengthening the functions and the vital organs, reestablishing capillary integrity, revitalizing glandular activity and generally rebuilding and strengthening the general health of the patient. Fasting water treatments, exercise, such as walking and resting will all assist the process; then the body's own curative powers are given a chance to take over and bring about an actual cure.

Dr. Bircher-Benner has often stated that . . . "A state of disorder is a state of disease." Maintaining a state of inner-balance that promotes health in a person is the primary concern, rather than only removing disease. Through the curative diet (as mentioned in Chapter 9) and life style changes, not only arthritis but other degenerative diseases as well, can be healed.

## CURATIVE EATING THE BIRCHER-BENNER WAY

When Eve gave Adam an apple, she may have had no idea of the power that was in her hand. This same fruit is used today as medicine. Muesli is standard fare at the klinik. You will find details on how to prepare this mixture in Chapter 9, the Wonder Plan. Basically apple muesli is a food that is easily digestible and provides instant enzymes that aid the sluggish digestion that often accompanies arthritis. This hardy dish is easy to prepare and is a meal complete in itself, providing all the needed nutrients. At the klinik, it is eaten for breakfast and dinner, with fruits and nuts and a hard cracker and butter. The true nutrients are the ingredients in the muesli which is prepared differently for breakfast than for dinner, when currants, blueberries or raspberries, are added, whereas in the morning it can include apples and bananas. Don't underestimate this food. It's a powerful source of energy.

## BATH TREATMENT FOR ARTHRITIS

Bathing in common table- or sea-salt is an effective means of relieving joint pain. First, rub the body with wet salt, then bathe in a tub of lukewarm water. Sit for 10–20 minutes then take a brief cold shower and lie down to rest.

## HOW TO EAT AWAY ARTHRITIS

To correct or eliminate the factors that caused the disease, have periodic days of fasting. To help the body's own healing process in normalizing all the metabolic processes; cleansing the body of the accumulated toxins and wastes, strengthening the function of all vital organs, revitalizing glandular activity, establishing a chemical balance in the tissues, and rebuilding and strengthening the general health of the patient.

*Eat raw, uncooked fruits and vegetables* for the first 2 weeks. (Bircher-Benner excludes all cooked foods during the first phase of the treatment as well as all foods of animal origin, meat, fish, eggs, milk, butter and cheese.)

*Therapeutic Fasting*—Biology-oriented doctors in Europe consider fasting to be the single most important curative measure in treating arthritis. Some of the doctors disagree as to the length of fasting, but all use fasting in their programs.

Rheumatoid arthritis and osteoarthritis are responsible for over 90% of all arthritis in the United States.

- *Symptoms:*
  painful joints
  pain that disappears for months then reappears again
  swollen, inflamed or creaking and cracking joints
  digestive problems and constipation for many years prior to the actual arthritic symptoms.

Arthritis is not just a local disease that affects one specific area of the body but instead reflects an overall disorder. Years of abusive treatment to the body via improper health habits may have occurred prior to the illness being manifested.

- *Prior Symptoms Before the Onset of Arthritis:*
  general fatigue
  physical and emotional stresses
  lack of sufficient rest
  poor diet and nutritional deficiencies
  glandular disorders of the endocrine system
  unchecked infectious diseases.

All these symptoms often occur long before the final joint pains show up.

## UNDERSTANDING THE TREATMENT OF ARTHRITIS

It's important to realize that if arthritis is to be successfully treated, the systemic nature of the disease must be recognized and the abnormal body conditions and disorders corrected. Unless the close relationship between the individual's general health and his/her arthritic symptoms is fully recognized, all attempts to cure arthritis will be futile. Because the Bircher-Benner plan takes into account the whole person in its healing approach, it is the best place to consider such treatment.

## BAD RAGEZ AND ARTHRITIC TREATMENT

The ever-efficient Swiss trains chugged into the Bad Ragez station right on schedule. I alighted from the train and saw before me the most beautiful backdrop of mountains in the Engeden range midway between St. Moritz and Zurich. Bad Ragez offers not only arthritis cures, but a magnificent scene of natural aesthetics too. The corridored street that leads from the train station to the Kur-house is bordered by stone flower pots that seem to emerge through the cement.

As you walk into the immaculately clean Kur-house and swimming pool, the sun accommodates spa visitors with its healing rays. Water is a definite treatment here, with two swimming pools. One is therapeutic with strong jets of water cascading out of the side wall. While emersed in the water, you gingerly wade to the jets and let their powerful stream cascade against your afflicted extremities. Circulation and skin tone are supposedly improved by this method.

In a nearby glassed-in pool, arthritics are encouraged to float around with flugels, the German word for fly, which are inflated plastic arm bands which you can place on either your arms or legs to enable you to float, kick and fling your arms for improved mobility.

Flugels are now available in the United States and can be purchased in swim wear shops and sporting goods stores.

Several people told me that daily workouts in the pool greatly relieved the swelling in their aching joints and improved their mental attitude. On the hour, artificial waves are pumped into the pool. This added pressure is good for the legs; I noticed people twisting about as the waves would break against their body. One of the clinicians said that this kind of movement is very difficult for most cases of severe arthritis. Often the only time that the arthritics can approximate this twisted movement is in the waves.

## SIDE EFFECTS OF CORTISONE OUTLINED

Later, while conferring with the Kur Director, I was told that the treatment here is more natural than the American counterpart. Cortisone, which is widely used in the United States, has so many side effects that it is considered dangerous.

Peptic ulcers; osteoporosis, a softening of the bones with spontaneous fractures; mental disturbances; psychosis; neuropathy or the degeneration of nerves; hypertension; and retention of salt and water in the tissues, with resultant strain on the heart and kidneys, are just some of the side effects that can be experienced with this miracle drug.

## HEALTHFUL ALTERNATIVE TO CORTISONE: CURATIVE DIET AND LIFE STYLE CHANGES

Like the Bircher-Benner Klinik, Bad Ragez too advocates an eating program based on raw fruits and vegetables and life style changes. Rest and exercise, in a healing atmosphere and an ordering one's life are also essential to bring about a cure. Exercise in the form of walking; terrain cures, which consist of walking up different elevations; gymnastics, done outdoors in the invigorating fresh air, water exercises and taking up a new sport are some of the life style adjustments they recommend. I was told that exercise and improvement of circulation are very important as antidotes to constipation, which usually plays a significant role in arthritis.

### How Franz Regained His Health

Franz, age 45, had operated his own delicatessen in Munich for years. For an equal amount of time, he had eaten many of his famous sausages, strudel and dumplings. He paid a high price for his eating: chronic constipation, gas and intestinal cramps plagued him, along with periods of depression, fatigue, and arthritis. In time Franz became so disagreeable that his customers joked about his open-door employment policy. A waitress or waiter could usually take only a week of his volatility before quitting.

At Bad Ragez Franz was advised to begin eating raw fruits, vegetables, grains and to rest. He was told he could prevent future flair-ups by staying on a raw-food regimen, taking hot and cold showers and hot compresses on the nape of the neck and cold ones on the body. He also should then use a one-quart chamomile enema to remove excess body-wastes, and take epsom salts (1 ounce) in the morning on an empty stomach.

After 21 days, Franz experienced relief and has continued his natural diet.

## CONSTIPATION, ARTHRITIS AND THEIR TREATMENT

Many arthritics have a long record of chronic constipation preceding the first signs of arthritis. Constipation can impair the function of the gall bladder, liver, kidneys and other vital organs. Moving the bowels only once in three days constitutes severe constipation. The solution to this problem is to eat finely cut fruits and vegetables that are minced into such small pieces that they are almost predigested. Chew the food thoroughly, taking small, meditative bites, and do not drink with the meal. However, at the conclusion, you can have herb tea or a salt-free vegetable broth which prevents fluid retention. During the day, consume 6–8 glasses of liquids: water, either mineral or distilled; fresh fruit and vegetable juices; herb teas or vegetable broths.

Avoid constipating foods like meat, white bread, processed cereals and refined carbohydrates such as cake, cookies and ice cream. You can supplement your diet with one to three tablespoons of any of the following which are all natural laxatives: Brewer's Yeast, whey powder, raw honey or plain yogurt.

Above all, be sure to begin and end the day with an hour-long walk. This not only improves circulation and eases the pain in the joints, but it prepares the body for digestion as well. Lack of sufficient exercise is one of the main causes of constipation.

### Helmut Walks Again

One illustrious 62-year-old German businessman, Helmut (a fictitious name) had suffered severe stress and brutality while held captive by terrorists for many months. He had been confined to a small room and when he was transported from hiding place to hiding place he was locked in the trunk of a car. The anguish, tension, poor nutrition and immobility took its toll on Helmut's health. When he was finally abandoned on a Dutch village street in the wee hours of the morning, he could not walk. Helmut attempted to stagger to his feet several times, but collapsed to the pavement.

An early-rising cyclist saw him and helped him to the nearest farmhouse for assistance. Interpol, the international police force, notified his family and they had a joyful reunion. Thereafter, they took him to Bad Ragez to begin treatment. In addition to the daily Kneipps therapy of marching over stones in alternating hot and cold water for improved circulation, Helmut was given actual physical therapy in which his legs were manually manipulated. He spent many days taking air-baths and breathing in the fresh Swiss air which seems curative in itself.

A fruit and vegetable juice fast was followed by a daily fare of fresh fruits, vegetables, grains and nuts. When I first saw Helmut, he was a handsome man standing erect in the therapeutic pool where cascading jets of water were pulsating against his legs. He looked tanned and healthy, but there was a tinge of sadness in his eyes. As he alighted from the pool, I noticed he walked with a limp, dragging his left leg. He confided that he felt like he had more energy than in previous years and was grateful for the rest and revitalizing regimen that he had encountered at Bad Ragez.

His physiotherapist projected that within a few months even the limp would be gone. Helmut said that he had always had such a busy life that he had never gone to a *Bad* before. He would always send his family but he didn't have the time to go himself. Now he would take time. He said that when he returned home, he would continue to eat naturally and put more order into his life. As he said "It's good business to schedule health into your daily plan. In the long run, it's a good time management investment." So says a German industrialist who has learned that good health is efficiency as well as good business.

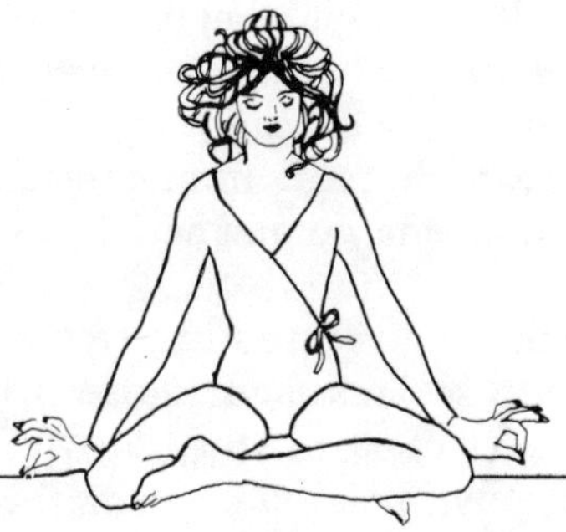

# 11

# The Bulgarian Formula and Other Secrets for Rejuvenation

> *"You ought not to attempt to cure the eyes without the head or the head without the body . . . the body without the soul . . . For the part can never be well unless the whole is well."*
>
> *Plato, 339 B.C.*

The mid-20th century marks the time when we changed idols. In Biblical times, golden calves were idolized. Today they are the bronzed bodies of youth. Modern men and women are searching relentlessly for the way to prolong youth and prevent the aging process: we dye our hair and wear stylish clothing in our efforts to appear more youthful. Medical science pursues gerontology to discover the secret of prolonging life.

Romania's Dr. Ana Aslan offers Gerovital Therapy to stop the signs of aging, while throughout Europe, various countries offer potential methods to arrest age.

## ROMANIAN REJUVENATION

Bucharest has become a mecca for those pursuing youth. Ana Aslan, an octogenarian herself, is responsible for the rejuvenation therapy of Gerovital, on KH3 therapy. This treatment is one of the most popular in Europe.

Dr. Aslan discovered quite accidentally, in 1956, that procaine, an anesthetic agent, has age-retarding properties. She injected specially designed dosages of procaine into patients showing signs of physical degeneration and mature aging, and observed that stiff, immobile joints became flexible, pain disappeared and new energy and vitality were evident.

Dr. Aslan has treated arthritic, high blood pressure and psychiatric patients with equal success. Perennial youth-seekers begin the Gerovital treatments at the age of 40. Between the ages of 40 and 60, Gerovital is taken in tablet forms and after 60 is taken by injection.

According to Dr. Aslan, aging processes start when the body's ability to produce new cells and replenish the old ones is diminished. Gerovital helps the body to regenerate new cell production, which is why it has a rejuvenating effect.

At 83, Dr. Aslan is proof of her own regimen. She looks considerably younger than she is. Her face is free of wrinkles and she has the enthusiasm of a considerably younger person. Celebrities come from all over the world to her institute and her office contains memorabilia of former patients—Khrushchev, John F. Kennedy and Mao Tse-tung, to mention a few.

The treatment costs are fairly nominal, due to socialized medical subsidies from the government. In American money, the cost for such treatment, plus a six-month supply of tablets, is only about three hundred dollars. It is possible to arrange a tour from New York for a 15-day, all-inclusive trip for $1,400.

## REJUVENATION A LA ROMANIA

Selma and Gordon, Frances and Franz, four people from Detroit, have experienced rejuvenation "a la Romania." It seemed like a long flight from Detroit to Bucharest. Selma and Gordon were celebrating their 35th wedding anniversary with rejuvenation treatments in Romania. Frances and Franz, their best friends, accompanied them to see if the Gerovital treatments would help Franz's bursitis and Frances' arthritis.

They all checked into a hotel rather than the sparsely furnished klinic rooms and promptly began the treatment. Their hometown medical doctors had given them complete physicals prior to their departure which they presented to the clinic and experienced more testing before they were prepared for their daily dosage of the "youth serum."

They were instructed to eat and exercise moderately and rest before fatigue became cumulative. When not receiving treatments, they toured the verdant Romanian countryside and frequented the beaches.

Three weeks later they returned home with a six-month supply of Gerovital which they take on a daily basis. Both couples report new energy and the reduction of aging symptoms: their faces look younger and their eyes are brighter.

Frances' arthritis has been arrested as has Franz's bursitis. They report that the experience was helpful and they would go again should there be a need.

## SWISS REJUVENATION

While many youth-pursuers are travelling to Romania, others are headed for Dr. Niehans in La Prairie, Switzerland. This klinik is especially known for its treatment of impotence as well as for rejuvenation. Marlene Dietrich, Greta Garbo and King Ibn Saud are some of the many celebrities who have tried the sheep-embryo-cell (Cell Therapy) injections. One Cell-Therapy treatment is enough for a lifetime if the accompanying diet is strictly observed. The recommended diet consists of raw or boiled vegetables, fruits, rice, barley, enriched farina cooked with water, and weak herb tea. Colonics are recommended for regular intestinal evacuation. Forbidden foods are: alcohol, salt, cooked milk, fruits with pits, spinach, breads, tomatoes, pastry, sugar, coffee and all fatty foods such as butter, oil, eggs and cheese.

## IS CELL THERAPY SAFE?

Infection at the site of the injection is of primary concern. Absolutely sterile conditions must be maintained to guard against absesses.

People who have just received serums or have been vaccinated up to 6–8 weeks before should not receive Cell Therapy. There is danger of transmitting infectious disease from animals to man. Dr. Niehans has pointed out that this is reduced to a negligible quantity when the animals are grown under carefully controlled conditions.

In summary, the patients' health and well-being when undergoing Cell Therapy appear to depend on 4 factors: (1) aseptic preparation of the cells from healthy animals and, in the case of live cells, speedy transmission of them to the patient; (2) aseptic conditions surrounding the injection of the cells; (3) the absence of recent vaccinations in patients and, (4) the diagnostic tools and skills of the physician in rendering the appropriate types of cells for individual needs of the patients.

If you put yourself in the hands of a superbly equipped medical facility, the expert and highly skilled staff can deal with any eventualities in the administering of Cell Therapy.

However, after the avalanche of publicity following Dr. Niehan's success in treating patients, in 1954 some unknown physician in Germany attempted the cure, causing many casualties.

Cellular Therapy insists on the giving up of all other remedies—no hormones, no toxins (e.g., concentrated alcohol, medicine or vaccine). Avoid X-rays, radioactive waters, and healing treatments by saunas, Turkish baths or sunbaths.

I have interviewed many people who have experienced this treatment, most of whom were in their seventies and appeared at least twenty years younger. A woman by the name of Hannah who was particularly impressive took the treatment in 1958 with her husband. She said that since then, their energy levels have increased considerably and they have not experienced arthritis, rheumatism or the usual problems of aging. Hannah has few wrinkles on her face, her eyes are clear. She talks and walks at a clip. While other septuagenarians are playing card games on the Italian Riviera, she is actively travelling around the world for her import business.

Cellular Therapy is definitely for the affluent!

## RUSSIAN REJUVENATION IDEAS

Dr. Nodar Kipshidze, a Russian cardiologist has said that there are four basic principles for health and longevity. They are practiced in Soviet Georgia, where the people live long. The Russian Rejuvenation suggestions are:

1. Plenty of physical activity every day.
2. Never overeat.
3. Get enough sleep. Go to bed when it is dark and awaken at dawn.
4. Do something that has meaning for you. Find purpose in your life and enjoyment will follow.

## THE DOUBLE THERAPY SURPRISE

At age 66, Hannilore began to feel and show signs of aging. Arthritis seemed to flair up at unexpected times and her sex life with her husband Friedric, had waned.

She checked into the La Prairie klinik for Cellular Therapy while giving strict instructions not to let her husband know.

Ironically, Friedric M. had the same plan in mind and also checked in, but was placed in a room on the opposite wing of the building. For weeks their respective secrets were guarded. However, at departure time, they were surprised to encounter each other in the klinik's vestibule.

Hannilore later said that they decided to take a second honeymoon on the Cote d'Azur, which was a great success. Their marriage has been enhanced by Cellular Therapy and her arthritis is a thing of the past. Today, she has more energy to put into her Munich tapestry business.

## GERMAN REJUVENATIVE AIDS

Europe's interest in staying young longer is evident in every country. Germany's newest interest in this regard is *Ginseng*. This strange herb, a most potent rejuvenating plant, has been used for over 5000 years by Orientals as an effective aphrodisiac, rejuvenator and general panacea. Now almost every pharmacy and Reformhaus (health food store) in Germany has a display of it in their window.

Ginseng grows in radioactive soil. Its roots contain radioactive properties that strengthen the heart, revitalize the nervous system and stimulate cell growth and activity. The latter information has been substantiated by medical and scientific research.

This remarkable herb is sold in health food stores in powdered, tablet or capsule form. Ginseng can also be purchased as a tea, with a pungent flavor, which takes time to cultivate a taste for.

Germany is advanced in the medical science of the future—biological medicine. Over three thousand German medical doctors are biologically oriented. They do not use drugs but adhere to the naturopathic methods of natural healing.

The German people also consider their numerous Bad hydrotherapy treatments as means of preventing aging. The varied mineral baths, hot springs, and wet wraps improve their health, prevent aging and illness, and provide treatment for three million people annually. (For more information about the *Bad* program, refer to Chapter 4.)

Consumption of fermented foods is also considered a means of living longer. Sauerkraut, sour-milk products, schwartzbrot (black rye bread), sour pickles and pickled vegetables are medicinal as well as nourishing. They have been reported as cures for arthritis, ulcers, colds, digestive disorders, and cancer. Johannes Kuhl, M.D., a cancer researcher, explains why fermented foods are so effective in preventing and curing disease: "Natural lactic acid and fermentive enzymes which are produced during the fermentation process have a beneficial effect on metabolism and a curative effect on disease." Fermented foods are pre-digested and easy to assimilate even by persons with weak digestive organs.

The most significant German contribution toward maintaining good health and longer life is juice fasting. Fasting has been practiced throughout history, but Germany has accepted fasting as a spring and fall ritual.

Why is fasting regenerative? Since the main cause of disease and aging is the accumulation of toxins and metabolic waste in the body, fasting, turns the body inward and begins to eliminate the dead and dying cells and builds up new tissues. Juice fasting stablizes and rejuvenates the entire system.

### What the Strange Herb Did for Erma

Erma despite her 22 years, looked 20 years older. She had worked hard since 16, struggling to help support her 3 younger brothers who had been orphaned by the death of her parents in an automobile accident.

Fatigue and tension were her vigilant companions along with her attitude of hopelessness for the future. The foreman in the factory where she worked suggested she talk to the company doctor about her chronic fatigue. She did so and he suggested that she go to Badenweder for the cure, which would be paid for by the company.

A regimen of natural food, exercise and daily cups of ginsing tea revitalized her. She no longer looks older than her age and her perspective for the future has become more positive. She has learned how to conserve her energy and live with a more natural approach to eating, exercise and thinking.

## SWEDEN'S APPROACH TO YOUTHFULNESS

Like Germany, Sweden considers fasting a youth-giving treatment. In fact, fasting is considered the national past time. Health enthusiasts around the country as well as medical practitioners in hospitals and clinics abstain from food during the spring and summer months for three days to approximately three weeks usually. However, there are reported instances about abstentions of up to 140 days. During fasting times, people continue to lead active lives, and in fact, they often pursue great physical feats.

Fasting marches, Swedish style, are comparable to our Boston marathon in distance. These people walk with gusto rather than eat, as they prove their strength and endurance.

Sweden's other life-giving secrets . . . whey and sex, also contribute to a long and healthy life.

Whey (of little Miss Muffet fame) is the liquid left over when cheese is made from milk. Curd, the solid part, is removed and the remaining liquid, whey, is used as a popular food. Its claim as a rejuvenative aid comes from its action as an intestinal cleanser and antidote to constipation, which is an ager. A person with such an elimination problem can be spotted as having poor skin tone, blemishes and eczema. The breath is foul because the overworked body is trying to purify its blood via the lungs. Swedish women are renowned for their flawless complexions, and the daily consumption of whey is responsible for their beauty. Whey is standard fare on every table. It is dehydrated and made into whey cheese, (mesost) and whey butter (messmor).

Whey can also be obtained in tablet or powder form. I prefer using 1 to 2 tablespoons of it in juice or milk, or poured over cereals.

Mention rejuvenation to someone in Stockholm, and they will respond with the word "sex". An active sex-life contributes to healthy glands, a glowing complexion and acts as a deterrent to aging. The Swedish people are quite frank in their discussion of this topic. They view it as an integral part of health as much as a nutritional meal.

## BE YOUNGER—FINNISH STYLE

Sweden's northern neighbor, Finland, uses heat for rejuvenation. Overheating therapies have the greatest potential for curing any disease, according to Finnish medical authorities. Two thousand years ago, the ancient physician, Parmenides said: "Give me a chance to create fever, and I will cure any disease." The people of Finland took that philosophy to heart and created their own overheating therapy—Finnish saunas.

The Finns are a rugged people, known for their vitality and endurance. They also have a low incidence of such degenerative diseases as cancer and arthritis. Their exceptional health is credited to their usage of overt heat.

The Finnish sauna, unlike the dry variety that we see in the United States, has a moist steam heat which is created by throwing water over hot rocks. The traditional Finnish sauna is a small structure of about 12 x 18 feet. It is divided into two parts . . . a dressing room and a steam room. The dressing room has several benches where a person can recline during cooling-off periods. The steam room has a large oven built from stones, which are heated by a wood fire. A bather sits on a bench in this room while the temperature progresses to about 212 degrees Fahrenheit.

As sweating occurs, the Finns take fresh birch branches, *Vihta,* to hit themselves with and further increase the effect of the heat and induce more sweating. They overheat their bodies, then immediately roll in the soft snow in winter, or briefly swim in a lake or river in summer, before returning to the hot steam. Finns cool themselves gradually by taking a long rest on the dressing room bench and allowing their bodies to gradually return to normal temperature. This is significant since the healing and rejuvenating effects of the sauna are largely due to the raised body temperature.

The youth-giving benefit of the sauna is that it stimulates the metabolic processes, removes toxins from the body via perspiration and enhances the body's own curative processes to prevent illness.

## LONGEVITY IN BULGARIA

Centenarians abound in this eastern European country. In fact, there are Bulgarians who live to be over 100 years old; 15–20 years longer than in any other civilized nation. These people are known to appear young, despite advanced age and the virility of Bulgarian men is legendary.

A natural diet of fermented foods including kefir, yogurt, sour milk, sour black rye bread, plus honey and sunflower seeds sustains these people for many years. A Russian scientist, Ilja Metchnikoff, studied the Bulgarians' eating habits. He discerned that the abundance of sour-milk products, notably kefir, yogurt, and acidophilus milk help to prevent putrefaction in the colon. Constipation and self-poisoning are thus halted. Dr. Metchnikoff's theory that life can be prolonged by preventing autotoxemia and the growth of poisons in the colon was exemplied by the Bulgarians.

Bulgarian yogurt is made from sheep or goat's milk. The protein and mineral composition of this milk is closer to that of human milk than is cow's milk. Reportedly, goat's milk contains anti-cancer and anti-arthritis factors.

Bulgarian people adhere to a simple, healthful way of living—following a rhythm of working, eating and sleeping. They are involved in heavy physical work and because of economics, they do not have the luxury of overeating. Undereating is integral in their daily lives and contributes to their longevity.

## NUTRITION, APHRODISIACS AND AGING

Our ancestors throughout history sought various aphrodisiacs to prolong their amatory abilities. The local application of herbs and potions or the consuming of various natural foods were attempts to enhance sexual prowess. There was an awareness of the linkage between a person's nutrition and his or her physical ability to love. Scriptures, folklore, and tradtion recommend certain foods for making one immortal for the moment. Honey, milk, sesame seeds, fish liver oil, kelp, raw nuts and seeds are some of the foods that have been used for thousands of years as natural aphrodisiacs to help the glands reach the peak of healthy activity.

In the wake of the sexual revolution of the past decade, European as well as American doctors have begun to consider sex as a legitimate scientific inquiry. Results of studies validate the fact that many sexual inadequacies such as impotence, frigidity and sterility originate in nutritional deficiencies.

According to Dr. Paavo Aerola, international nutritionist, vitamins A, C, E and $B_1$ and lecithin are involved in stimulating the sex glands and increasing sex hormone production. The mineral zinc is essential for the health of the prostate gland. These food substances coupled with adequate nutrition are the basis for sexual vigor.

Eating natural fruits, vegetables and a low animal protein diet add to health and increased longevity. Bulgarians, the healthiest people in the world, attribute their good health and longevity to a meatless diet. An active life of exercise balanced with rest and relaxation is also essential to the quality of life.

Coping with elimination problems via the consumption of sour-milk foods such as yogurt, buttermilk, or kefir, are important for the functioning of the intestinal tract. Fermented lactic acid foods such as sauerkraut, sour pickles, dark sour dough bread or whey also contribute to a free-flowing system. Periodic cleansing of the colon with fasts or taking colonics or enemas is also important. Living longer requires a continuous reduction of autointoxification by removal of waste products from the intestine.

A fulfilling love life is related to overall good health and longevity. The hormone production of the endocrine and sex glands has a powerful influence on the total well-being of a person. Premature aging and senility occur as a result of diminished hormone production and an inadequate diet.

## HOMESTYLE REJUVENATION

Don't think that you have to spend a bundle to have cellular therapy in Switzerland or journey to Romania for Dr. Ana Aslan's gerovital treatment. You can do the same for yourself at home.

Once a week go on a fruit juice fast. (Select any fruits listed in Chapter 9.) For one period during the month, fast for three days. This might be accomplished better during a weekend and one other day, eg., Friday, Saturday and Sunday, or Saturday, Sunday and Monday. The other days of the month, include as many raw fruits and vegetables in your diet as possible.

What happens in your body during a homestyle rejuvenation? A natural juice such as apple, apricot, peach, carrot, spinach, or parsley accentuates the deterioration of over-aged cells and brings about the growth of new young cells in the subsequent dietetic rebuilding and intensive raw diet effect. Result? These young cells become as "alive" as possible from the beginning. Fasting requires the body to live off itself, so that a large number of overaged tissue cells are reduced. As a result, an intensive stimulation for new growth is produced.

The process begins first with detoxification, then with the rejuvenation stimulus and finally, with nourishment that is gradually increased when you change from juice fasting to a regimen of fresh fruits and vegetables.

What happens in the intestine? Another kind of rejuvenation results from the affect of raw food in the intestine. The abundant bacterial flora normally colonizing the intestine, if it is healthy, fulfill the task of aiding digestion and making certain that vitamins are available. Completely healthy intestinal flora are relatively rare due to the general use of popular foods. Unhealthy intestinal bacteria live parasitically on the food in the human body and harm it by depriving it of vitamins.

Fresh food has proved to be the simplest and surest means of salvaging unhealthy intestinal bacterial flora.

It is our responsibility to heal ourselves. We often choose our sickness when, through neglect or illness, we allow it to spread within ourselves.

The body wants to renew itself, but in eating poor quality food we interfere with the revitalizing of life, thereby encouraging illness and premature death. Nature always gives the best treatment. OUR JOB IS TO UNDERSTAND ITS WAYS AND CONDUCT OUR LIVES ACCORDINGLY.

Just as wrong food is the cause of disease, so good food is the best medicine.

## DETOXIFYING YOURSELF

During a curative process, you actually feel worse. This condition of headaches and dizziness is a sign that health is being restored. At this time you may feel disoriented, worried, and have difficulty making decisions. Often, first-time fasters, not realizing that health is close at hand, resort to eating or pain killers to suppress the pain and unknowingly retard the cure.

When you change from a diet of eating meat, dairy and processed foods, the body experiences a discharge that often begins with pain.

During the elimination of toxins, pain progresses through the body in ordered stages.

When pain occurs, allow it to run its course rather than alleviating this discomfort with drugs or aspirin. Be sure and resist any cravings for bad foods. Whatever food you crave is normally that which you are eliminating, e.g., chocolate or ice cream.

## HOW SEPTUAGENARIANS LIVE LONGER

While travelling throughout Europe, I had numerous occasions to interview people at the many spas. It was delightful to learn of the zest and gusto that many of these older people shared. So many of them appeared to be twenty years younger than they actually were. Frequenters of the Bads usually live very productive lives despite the advance of years.

When talking to the spa regulars, I was reminded of a phrase that is attributed to George Bernard Shaw, the English playwright. "People talk about age when they have nothing else to talk about."

Working full-time, despite being in the mid-seventies and upward seemed to be ordinary rather than unusual. To the question, "How to live a healthier life," I received the following replies:

—"Enjoy your work . . . avoid stressful situations and quarrels," says a youthful 78-year-old woman who works a sixty-hour week and commutes between New York and Paris.

—"A natural diet of raw fruits and vegetables—the elimination of salt and sugar," was also a frequent response.

—"Daily exercise is a must," says a virile man of seventy who appears to be twenty years younger. He jogs through the woods twice a day, and swims and works out in the gymnasium of a health spa.

—"Keep an active sex-life," replied an 86-year-old.

—"Participate in activities that interest you . . . sporting events, theater, ballet, opera, outings to the mountains or the sea and art shows."

—"Develop a large circle of friends," was important to many people. Those who were younger also added "family ties must be strong."

—"Take frequent rest breaks to ward off tension," says a successful 80-year-old African diamond broker. He takes twenty-minute naps between negotiating international business deals.

—"Activity, interest, moderation," were all words that were used by many people when speaking of continued good health.

—"Regularity via bran and fruits, mon cherie," was the response from a 78-year-old French importer who works a full week. She added

". . . joy and happiness must be your attitude toward life, and health will flow from that."

—A Homberg lawyer says, "Balance between work and recreation, happiness and sorrow . . . get a good night's sleep, start the day with a wink and a smile, and be grateful you are alive!"

## SUMMARY OF HOW TO LIVE . . . HEALTHY

Enjoying good health is important at any age. Your chance to increase your prospects of living a long and active life may be increased by considering the following suggestions:

1. Attitude: be positive and grateful for the gift of life.
2. Develop a sense of humor. Keep smiling and laughing to reduce tension and prevent premature aging.
3. When feeling tense, tell your body and mind to relax. Take regular relaxation-breaks. A twenty-minute nap or a five-minute shower can help you enjoy better health.
4. Develop a circle of friends and family associations.
5. Be interested in what you are doing. Get involved with work and activities that fill you with satisfaction.
6. Cultivate new interests; in sports, community affairs, cultural activities, arts and craft groups.
7. Your daily diet should be well-fortified with fresh fruits, vegetables, protein sources and herb teas. Restrict your intake of hard fats and high-calorie foods. Eliminate salt and sugar.
8. Regularity is important to good health. Constipated? Boost your intake of fibrous foods, including bran, whole grains, chewy vegetables and fresh fruits.
9. Avoid stressful situations when possible and develop coping skills for dealing with difficult times.
10. Be aware of the beauty around you . . . be sure to count your blessings at least once every day.

*To become younger means to be healthy.* By building health-promoting eating habits, you can add life to your years. Here is how the Bulgarians do it . . .

1. Eat only when you are really hungry.
2. Eat slowly and in a relaxed atmosphere.
3. Eat several small meals instead of a few large repasts.
4. Systematically undereat. This is a prime longevity secret. Amazing as it seems, the less you eat, the less hungry you feel. Reason?

The food is more efficiently digested and better utilized than it is when you overeat.

Studies of centenarians show that they have been moderate eaters all of their lives. So, eat less and live longer!

Another dimension to staying young is the state of mind. It is expressed by a 93-year-old woman I met in Munich. To my question "What is your secret of living?" she smiled wryly and replied: "I stay young by knowing these words from the Bible, 'They who wait upon the Lord shall renew their strength; they shall mount up with wings as eagles; they shall run and not be weary, and they shall walk and not faint.'"

Recapturing youth is a quality of the imagination; a vigor of the emotions and spirit; and a courage to live life fully with all the inherent risks. It is hanging onto your dreams and implementing them. It is viewing each day as spring: a time for new beginnings. Staying young is a realization that the Fountain of Youth is within you!

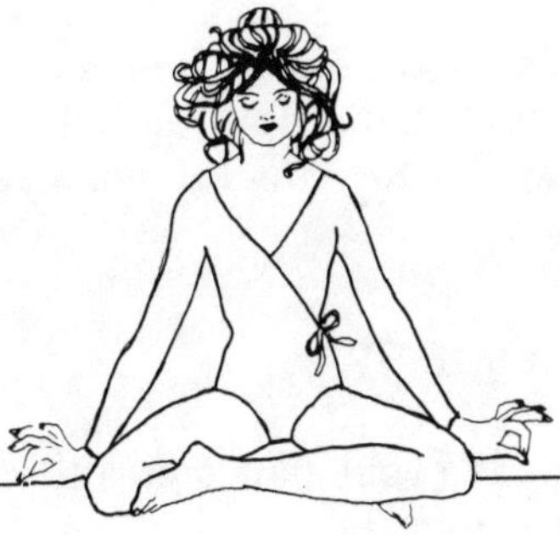

# 12

# Home Spa

*"The end is only the prelude to the beginning."*
*Dr. Max Bircher-Benner*

It's not difficult to set up your own European "spa" at home: create your own unique Bad Bad Gastein, St. Moritz, or Vichey. The first thing to consider is the atmosphere of your present surroundings: what do you see? smell? observe? This sets the stage.

In European Spas, a healing attitude prevails. You can create this attitude in your home as well. Consider the idea that illness is a disharmony, either physical, mental or spiritual, caused by a lack of rhythm. Thoughts of anger, dissention and frustration can make surroundings unhealthy, as can overexertion, the food one eats, the way one lives, the people with whom one associates. There is no doubt that, under the same conditions, one person may be ill and another well. Generally, however, quietness, order, beauty and space to do your living in are all necessary.

The real secret is that there is no better remedy for ill health and exhaustion than nature, rest, repose, exercise, quiet, proper breathing, balanced foods and someone to treat the ill person with love and understanding. Thought power . . . it is your attitude of mind, your willingness to be cured, your desire to get above your illness, and your inclination to fight against disorder which will help you to health.

## HOME LIFE AND HEALTH

Health also depends upon the quality of the family life, and how people relate to others around them. In simple terms, it is difficult to be healthy in an unhealthy home. People who live together influence each other's health.

## AMBIANCE OF A HOME SPA

The quality of your daily life is related to your state of health. Spa physicians ask their patients the following questions:

1. Are you interested in what you do, in your relationships, in the world out there and your interior life? Your health is dependent upon your quality of aliveness. The wellness scale could also be called the aliveness scale. Interest, aliveness, motivation and enthusiasm are all contributory factors to your state of health. When you are interested in your life, you are less likely to overeat, overdrink or overtax your energy level or continue with living habits that destroy health. Resistance to disease is high when you are positive and enthusiastic about life.
2. How do you spend your time, where do you spend your time? Do you waste time or do you invest it in worthwhile hobbies or pursuits?
   Where you spend your time also contributes to the quality of your health. Smog, noise, pollution, lack of space, chaos and disorder all create a disharmonious atmosphere that has a negative effect on your health.
   The space you set aside for living should be quiet, relaxing, comfortable and a place where you can get away at times without being interrupted. This helps balance out the more stressful aspects of your life.
3. What is the quality of your relationship with friends, family and co-workers?
   A bad relationship is as destructive to good health as the lack of an essential nutrient. Whether you are living with someone or attemping to establish a meaningful relationship with friends, it takes work, dedication and open communication for the relationship to be healthy. Without communication there can be no real relationship.
   Do you spend an equal amount of time being nurtured as well as nurturing?

4. Do you have a focus or center in your life? In our frenetic American life style, it is often difficult to make a commitment to someone, something or ourselves. A constant seeking of novelty, adventure and variety needs to be balanced with security and freedom from hassle; otherwise we can find ourselves caught up in utter chaos without focusing enough to reach the heart of anything, whether it be a relationship or a pursuit.
A healthy life seems to be a delicate balance between newness and tradition.

## HOME LIFE AND HEALTH

Mental health as precursor of physical health depends strongly on good interaction within the family. Health does not seem to be strictly a matter of internal health for the individual, but also depends on how the individual relates to his environment and the people in it.

Social sciences have talked for years about the effects of home— its roles and relations with the individual and upon the integral unit. In Europe one sees far more togetherness and solidarity than we have in America. We disperse the various age groups either to nursing homes (if advanced in age), nursery schools, teen centers, and homogenious groupings in the suburbs while our European neighbors, for the most part, are gathering in rather than dispersing to the winds. Some basic ideas are:

1. People who live together influence each other's health.
   A. Do you actively listen and communicate with those around you? Is there a sense of love and caring that enables all family members to grow and be unique? Are household tasks clearly understood and completed by a certain time? Are times of joy and sorrow spent together? Do you have family rituals? How do you celebrate together?
   B. When a family member is ill, how do you relate to him? Is he relegated to a distant room to care for himself or do other family members assist? To recover health, a person needs the cooperation and support of the family. What is done in your home? Do you offer loving assistance or tolerate the illness?
   C. Keep a family log and write down the significant changes you make individually and as a family. Did someone get married, go off to summer camp or did you move away? Write it down, along with your reactions to the move. Enclose a picture as an illustration. Many years hence you can enjoy your own family history that you personally wrote.

2. A member who is in poor health depresses the quality of health for the family as a whole. To recover health, a person needs the cooperation and support of the family.
3. Family health is an on-going process that changes as the members change and fluctuates with environmental pressures.
4. Move from a position of strength in dealing with problems. For instance, a family that has good communication skills can discuss and reach decisions about reducing stress if they have been under much tension during the past year. Other solutions are to change the diet to more natural eating, do relaxation training for a reprieve from tension, and involve more people for emotional support.
5. There is no better remedy for tension and ''nerves'' than nature, rest, repose, quiet, proper breathing, proper nourishment, and someone to treat the patient with love and understanding.
6. How to be cured . . . it's the attitude of the mind, the willingness to be cured, the desire to get above one's illness and the inclination to fight against disorder which help one to health.
7. The best remedy is belief or faith coupled with love.
8. Health and vitality can be limited only by our ability to love. We can create barriers against receiving love because we believe we are not worthy of it.

## RELAXATION IS VITAL FOR HEALTH

Balancing the flow of energy in the body to counter the body's reaction to stress is the role of relaxation.

The body's reaction to stress is contingent upon the mind's response. The mind reacts to stress based upon how it has learned to relax. The relaxed mind is the key to fighting stress.

The mind and body indicate stress and reactions by means of dream images, overt verbal expression (You're a pain in the neck; Don't get up-tight) and pain. A chin thrust forward may mean future or goal orientation, causing chronic neck tension. Rounded shoulders "protect" the heart from the impact of a hostile environment. If you "don't get it off your chest" your breathing becomes shallow.

Look carefully at your goals, attitudes, behavior patterns, physical condition, environment, and relationships. Do you sit down to eat a leisurely meal? Do you read while eating?

A balanced life includes proper breathing and awareness.

Get in touch with your body, mind and emotions. Discover your hidden tensions and their manifestions. Set aside time alone for meditation or just being quiet. Establish priorities. Balance work and play.

*Affirmations:* Positive statements about oneself or one's situation are used in creative visualization to focus the attention and the will on a desired end. They may be precise and specific or quite general. (e.g.: Write a positive statement for yourself, such as: I ________ deserve success in ________.)

*Passive Concentration in AT (Autogenic Training):* An AT technique in which one focuses awareness on a particular part of the body, repeats the appropriate phrase (such as my legs are heavy) to oneself, then simply observes what sensations or emotions are brought to awareness.

*Visualizations:* Creative means for *developing imagination to positively transform any life-situation.* This is the process of forming images and thoughts in the mind, consciously or unconsciously, and then transmitting them to the body as signals or commands.Visualization is the process of forming images and thoughts in our mind, consciously or unconsciously, then transmitting them to the body as signals or commands.

1. It's important to learn to use it *consciously*.
2. Use imagination to create a mental picture of what you want in your mind. Focus regularly on the idea, giving it positive energy, until you achieve the desired effect.
3. Imagine yourself calm and relaxed, and visualize yourself in a successful situation.
4. Use visualizations for: physical health, self image, relationships, forgiveness and release and goals.
5. In this process you may see how you are holding back, blocking yourself from achieving satisfaction and fulfillment because of fears and limited concepts.

## LIFE STYLE

Most current health problems are related to the way we live. Nutrition, fitness, stress control, and self-responsibility for health are important dimensions of personal health care that relate to life style.

## EVALUATION OF YOUR STATE OF HEALTH

Which of these statements matches your own feelings?

- I feel relaxed
- I feel inner tension
- I breathe shallowly
- I feel tired

- I balance work and play
- I enjoy unstructured time
- Overeating and drinking interfere with my health
- I relax during the day

## ENVOURAGING A FAMILY TO PARTICIPATE IN A HOME HEALTH PROGRAM

1. Establish an attitude that we each can take responsibility for our own health by the following means:
   a. positive mind set
   b. daily exercise
   c. nutritious foods of 70% raw fruits, vegetables, nuts and grains.
   d. Adequate rest
2. Include all of the family in food preparation
   a. Put all the ingredients out for a specific dish, such as *Muesli*. Let each person try making it.
   b. Set aside 1 day for cooking experimentally—e.g., Sunday. Plan the menu and purchase the necessary ingredients. Make it fun—not boring routine.
   c. Prepare the table in a festive way, with a good tablecloth, and cut flowers.
   d. Sit down and enjoy the meal together. Don't allow phone calls or other interruptions to disturb your tranquility.

## ENCOURAGING CHILDREN TO ENJOY FRESH FRUITS AND VEGETABLES

In Europe, gardens abound everywhere. For people dwelling in a high-rise apartment house, they have the option of renting a plot of ground for raising their own garden produce. In the Netherlands, for example, the government provides unused land along the railroad tracks for garden cultivation. A little hut adjoins the plot so people can stay overnight to tend it. There is a sense of community that develops from such effort.

In some areas in the States, community gardens are developed on vacant lots. In the area of Denver where I live, Botanical Gardens provides plots for community usage. A sense of comradery develops from such an effort.

Create an attitude that this is a special adventure; that in growing a garden, you will be sharing together. When my children were young, I took them to the store and let them select the packets of vegetables that they wished to grow. I told them that whatever they chose they could prepare and eat in all sorts of wonderful ways. The garden was their special project to love, care for, weed and water.

The sense of responsibility that a child learns through tending a garden and seeing something grow from the fruits of their labor is a feeling of achievement that eventually builds self confidence.

My children began to love such exotic varieties of vegetables as kohlrobi, chinese lettuce and swiss chard. Your children can too. Provide cookbooks that show simple sauces they can make as dips for their fresh vegetables.

Plain yogurt with fresh dill, parsley and grated onions provides a favorable dip for fresh broccoli, cauliflower, turnips, beets, cucumber or any number of fresh vegetables.

## INVOLVE THE NEIGHBORS

Encourage your neighbors to also have gardens for their children. Once a month the neighborhood could get together for a "dip party". Each person can bring fresh vegetables from their garden along with a dip. The host family could provide juice or herb tea to drink. A complete meal could be had from one's own efforts in the garden.

The sense of achievement that comes from a child growing their own food is better than any class in self-esteem and building confidence. The added bonus is that the children learn to appreciate good fresh vegetables on their own, without a mother or father nagging them at the table to "Eat, Boobie, it's good for you." The children will have experienced goodness on their own and will not need anyone to tell them about it.

## BLOOMING ENVIRONMENT

History and legend indicate that woman and mankind have always derived great pleasure from the delicately scented perfumes of flowers and herbs. In 570 B.C., Nebuchadnezzar insisted that flower beds of fragrant herbs be placed in the famous Hanging Gardens "so that the breezes may spread perfume far and wide." When the tomb of King Tut was opened, an albaster jar of perfumed oil was found with 100% potency after the passage of 3000 years.

You can give yourself a psychological boost and enhance your own environmental aesthetics with hanging plants, containers of herbs such as roses, lavender, sandalwood, or various combinations of your own choosing.

## OVERVIEW OF A HOME SPA

One of the key ingredients in the health spa concept is centering, or finding a place of peace within one's mind and body via relaxation, breathing and bioenergetics and within the home via serene surroundings.

No matter what your income, it is possible to establish an oasis for yourself. I have seen the poorest European homes that still had a sense of tranquility. For them it was often a window box of geranimums and old, but clean, lace curtains at the window.

Decide on colors that add to your calmness. Earthtones, of camel, brown and tan are appealing for some. Greens, like spring green with shades of yellow, or forest green reminiscent of nature, are more appealing for others. Blue provides an appeal for cerebral pursuits, says Faber Baren, color psychologist, while offering a good backdrop for paintings and plants. If you have enormous space to camouflage, black or shades of gray may be a viable option.

Plants like ferns, Boston and otherwise, ivys such as Baltic, Swedish, and English all are hardy and offer a minimum of maintenance problems. Small fruit trees such as lemon and orange also add atmosphere.

A sense of freedom is experienced by space. Remove as much unnecessary clutter from the rooms. If it means something to you and contributes to the atmosphere, then by all means keep it, but there is much psychological gain to be had from a sense of openness.

Art work—although we all can't collect works of the masters, a few well chosen water colors, prints or works by unknown artists whom you appreciate further add to the aesthetics.

Create a mood with music . . . if it's harpiscord, jazz or pure instrumental, you can enhance the tempo and feeling of your home via music.

Fresh cut flowers and fresh fruit and nuts are inviting as a table centerpiece. Such additions enhance the health-giving qualities that you may want in your nourishing atmosphere.

Two key rooms in the home are the kitchen and bath, although the bedrooms and living areas are equally important. If you want to stimulate appetites, consider furnishing the kitchen in shades of red or orange. Restaurants have discovered that these colors add to their cash receipts. However, if you want to subdue the appetitie, consider greens and blues, although I don't think that blue delftware has done much for depressing the Dutch appetite. Time-saving measures offer more opportunities to enjoy life instead of being burdened with endless household tasks. The following suggestions are time savers to put order in your home as well as your body.

### *Management*

- Have a home "business center" which will invite you to plan.
- Have a convenient file for sales slips, bills, cleaning hints, garden records, cleaning labels and care instructions.
- Keep a pad and pencil handy at the phone, in the kitchen and living room.
- In a handy spot, keep a box of supplies such as gummed labels, string, gummed paper tape, tags.
- Use a bulletin board for notes to yourself and others.
- Have jobs planned and posted for children or others to see when they come in.
- Post lists of "must" and "may" jobs on the bulletin board.
- Establish "business hours" for telephone calls. Notify friends and organization officers of them.
- Do not putter.

### *Shopping and Marketing*

- Make as few trips to the market as possible.
- Shop when markets are least crowded. (Those who can, should shop when employed women are at work and should leave the markets free to serve those whose time for shopping is limited to peak hours.)
- Serve yourself as much as possible at the market.
- Make out shopping lists and menus before going to the market.
- Keep memos on the bulletin board to add items onto as they come to mind or as stocks are running low.
- Keep in your purse a list of clothing sizes for different members of the family.

### *Meals*

#### *Planning*

- Keep file of quickly prepared menus and tested recipes.
- Check supplies in the refrigerator before planning menus and market orders.
- Check the items on your list for prices before going to the supermarket.
- Plan meals over a period of a week.

*Preparation*

- Study and improve the placing of small equipment in your kitchen to save steps and movement.
- Keep knives sharpened.
- Assemble in one place the equipment and supplies for lunch boxes.
- Select the best utensils for each purpose.

*Serving*

- For busy days, serve meals buffet style and on trays.
- When family has early after-dinner appointments, serve dinner picnic-style, using paper plates and cups.
- Eat meals in the kitchen.
- Use paper, plastic or other place mats which do not require laundering.
- Use paper napkins.
- Cook and serve in the same containers.
- Serve directly from the stove to the plates.
- Use a tray for setting and cleaning the dining table.

*Cleaning Away*

- Ask each person to carry his own dishes to the kitchen and scrape, rinse, and stack them.
- Rinse all cooking utensils after use and soak if necessary.
- Arrange the most convenient plan for doing dishes in your kitchen.
- Do dishes only once a day whenever possible.
- Scald dishes and leave to dry without wiping. When possible, leave dishes in drainer until next meal. Caution: Boiling hot water should not be used on fine china and glass.
- Have paper towel holder at sink.

## *Cleaning*

*General*

- See that all equipment is kept in good operating order for immediate use.
- See that handles of equipment are the right length for good posture while using them.

- Use oil cloth on unpainted or unfinished shelves.
- Wax wood surfaces such as window sills and around door handles making them easier to care for.
- Schedule window washing to be done a few at a time.
- Keep windows dusted to reduce the need for washing.
- Use a basket or paper shopping bag for cleaning supplies, brushes, and cloths, which you can take from room to room. Store in the basket until next use.
- Proceed with one operation until finished.
- Pack away silver which requires extra time for polishing.
- Put silver away in chemically treated cloths or boxes to reduce the amount of polishing necessary.

*Storage*

- Avoid stacking utensils except those of like sizes.
- Arrange shelves of graduated widths to simplify cleaning, to utilize all the space between deep shelves, and to avoid breakage.
- Store those utensils used less frequently in the places which are harder to reach.
- Have a safe stepladder convenient for reaching high shelves.
- Have no unlabeled containers in use.

*Vacuum Cleaning*

- Do all the vacuum cleaning at once.
- Spread furniture out to make the rug easier to clean.
- Use a vacuum cleaner to remove dust from a dry mop.

*Ordering*

- Put away extra knick-knacks which require too much care.
- Gain cooperation of family members in putting things where they belong immediately after use.
- Put living room in order at night before retiring, all hands helping.
- Keep a "tote basket" for things to be taken down from upstairs or to the basement.
- Keep a wastebasket in as many rooms as possible.
- Have materials convenient for children to use when learning to do things for themselves such as towels, washcloths, and combs.

- Provide low hooks for small children and make it easier for them to keep their things in order.

*Laundry*

*Washing*

- Use textiles which are easy to launder but do not require frequent laundering.
- Place a laundry bag or hamper in every bedroom, the bathroom and the kitchen.
- Sort laundry on a table to avoid bending.
- Use a cotton sheet over a blanket to protect it against dust.
- Avoid letting articles get heavily soiled.
- Take clothes immediately out of the dryer and hang on hangers to avoid ironing.

Consider convenience in the kitchen. Hang frequently used utensils in the kitchen. Use clear glass canisters which are inexpensive but very attractive to display grains like oats, soya, noodles, herbs and nuts.

Lighting is very important. Needless energy can be drained by straining to read a cookbook while preparing a meal. Use lighting above all food-preparation areas and the dining table. Use dishes that are complementary colors to your surroundings. At times, give yourself a reprive from washing dishes and invest in paper products. Cups, plates and bowls are found in attractive colors and are not too expensive when you consider the money saved on detergent and water.

Plan as many raw food dishes as possible. It will be more nutritious and you will have more time to enjoy life rather than "slaving over a hot stove."

The bathroom offers the "pièce de résistance." Here you can plan your own private Bad. You can go wild with colors, or be sedate. Splash surrelistic wallpaper or recreate Roman baths and ruins. All are possibilities. Be sure and have a good supply of herbs for the bath. (See accompanying list of herb combinations.)

A loofah sponge and coarse towels are a must for your home spa along with a vegetable brush for a daily dry-brush massage. A pumice stone is good for removing dry skin on the feet. If you can afford a shower spray attachment with extra strength, then by all means, get one. It's great for trying a Facher Douche for improved circulation and new energy on dog days.

Now comes the bedroom. A firm mattress is a prerequisite for a good night's sleep. I prefer the heavy foam variety that is so popular in the Scandanavian countries, but a good inner-spring or waterbed could serve your needs as well. A firm pillow is also important. Goose down is good as are several dacron pillows stuffed into one pillowcase for thickness. I prefer this variety since it's the closest approximation to the horsehair pillows that provide such comfort in Europe.

Good ventilation is important so open a window to give you a good night's fresh, well relatively fresh, air. A night stand that will accommodate books and a good light is also a needed accroutrement, as is a chair with a nearby lamp that can be used for reading, should you have difficulty reading in bed.

## HOME SPA EQUIPMENT

Slant board, jump rope and bicycles are all standard fare. Luxury items could be a redwood hot tub, jacuzzi or whirlpool. These are non-essential but very nice additions.

## HOW TO CHANGE OVER TO A HEALTHIER LIFE STYLE

The attitude of all the family is very important. Often when Americans return from making a "Kur" in Europe they have a missionary zeal to convert not only family but friends as well. This is usually met with great resistance by everyone. From my experience and that of others who have made the transition, it's better to do it gradually. Drastic overnight changes often don't last. When a change is made over a period of time, the results can be more lasting.

1. Sit down and talk with your family. Mutually discuss the importance of this program to each of you. What I found to be effective was telling my family that I discovered a more natural way of eating that enables me to have sustained energy and feel healthy and that I would like to continue to feel at an optimum level and therefore I am going to eat mostly fresh fruits, vegetables, grains, nuts, seeds and herb teas. Grains are a good supply of B-complex vitamins.
2. Enlist your family as part of your support system. Explain that food can be a good medicine. Eating fresh fruits and vegetables offers a live, life-promoting nourishment that cannot be obtained from cooked foods. In addition, fresh air, exercise, clear water, relaxation and a positive approach to life are all essentials of good nutrition. Just eating the right foods alone won't assure you of solid nourishment.
3. Rather than creating voids in your life by removing food that your family has been accustomed to, merely substitute a more nourishing alternative:

| | |
|---|---|
| instead of white flour | rye, pumpernickel, barley, whole wheat, or soya flour |
| " " white sugar | use raw honey, molasses, fructose |
| " " coca | carob powder |
| " " iodized table salt | sea salt or vegetable salts |
| in place of salt, pepper, chili powder, curry and other tart seasonings | try herbs & spices such as dill, sweet basil, thyme, marjoram, parsley, cloves, rosemary |

*More Transition Eating.* If you're overweight or concerned about your cholesterol level, and you are looking for ways to lower your intake of saturated fats and still keep the satisfying taste of fat in your diet, you can replace the saturated or "hard" fats with unsaturated or "soft" fats.

1. To "butter" a baked potato or slice of toast, dip a clean pastry brush in vegetable oil and apply liberally. The taste of fat is there but most of it's unsaturated.
2. A recipe calling for sour cream can be replaced with plain yogurt. Yogurt liquefies easily so add it carefully. Do not beat or stir it too much and do not overheat.
3. If a baking recipe calls for whole milk, substitute low fat or skim milk, or fruit juice.
4. Brown onions, mushrooms and other foods in soy sauce instead of butter or oil. This fat-free food is delicious yet has no fat and less calories.
5. Remove skins from turkey and chicken to eliminate half the fat and calories.
6. When a baking recipe calls for 1 cup of butter or solid shortening, substitute ⅔ of a cup of any vegetable oil.
7. Preserve vitamin E and essential fatty acids by refrigerating oils after opening them. This will also preserve proper taste and smell. By following these hints you'll feel healthier and look thinner.

## WHAT TO DO ABOUT DINING OUT

Restaurants usually offer salad plates, vegetable combinations, or a fresh fruit plate with cottage cheese or yogurt. These are all very nourishing. A baked potato and a green salad is ample for nutrition when the meal is preceded by fresh fruit as an appetizer. Should you desire fish, select trout, cod, halibut, or pike, to mention a few. You could also consider an omelet.

The main thing is to avoid beef, highly seasoned foods, rich sauces, and foods containing excess additives and preservatives, e.g., smoked cheese, pickled foods, preserved, processed or chemically fed meat, fish or fowl.

In 1977, the Senate Select Committee on Nutrition and Human Needs has urged a change in American diets based on studies done by leading cancer specialists. They are now finding out what Europeans have known for years. That is:

1. There is a relationship between colon and rectal cancer and a diet high in red meat. Mormons, Seventh-day Adventists, and vegetarians who eat little or no meat have much lower rates of cancer. Their diet, which consists primarily of vegetable proteins high in dietary fiber (roughage), protects them from such forms of cancer common in America as breast, rectal, colon and uterine.
2. In Japan, prior to World War II, the population's diet contained little meat and almost no dairy products. Cancer, of the colon and breast were uncommon, while the reverse is true in the United States. However, now that the Japanese have adopted a western diet, cancer has dramatically increased and equals that of Americans.

What do you say when someone says "You can eat this ham, just once." Ask them what they mean by "just once?" Is it once in a lifetime, if so, say you've already done it. Make no concessions if you have made up your mind to change. However, if you are not quite sure you want to make such a full committment, then stop. Rethink your priorities before you come up with a spontaneous answer.

At work when someone says, "You're not one of us since you don't have donuts and coffee in the morning or stop for a beer after work," point out that you enjoy conversing with them, if indeed you do. Suggest that you get together to do something that is not food-related, e.g., racquet ball, tennis, movies, or some other outside interest.

Eliminate all foods that contain additives or preservatives. Become a label reader. When you do, you will be amazed at the number of chemicals that are in the foods you eat. Gradually decrease buying canned goods and frozen foods. Fresh fruits and vegetables offer twice as much nourishment for the money.

Start a root cellar. Set aside some part of your basement where you can store root vegetables like carrots, potatoes, onions, turnips, parsnips and squash that will keep for a long time.

Instead of packaged convenience cereals, mix your own. More nutrition and less money will be your pay-off. Make delicious hot cereals with oats, buckwheat, cornmeal millet, barley, bulgur wheat. Either use one alone or mix several.

Gradually break away from meat. Replace it with poultry or fish.

Buy organically grown fruits and vegetables in season. You can be assured of full vitamin and mineral content when the foods are fresh and in season and the price should be better. If you cannot purchase organically grown foods, then be very selective about the fresh fruits and vegetables that you do buy. Avoid overripe or unripe fruits particularly. You can do just as much harm to your body with unripe foods, like eating green bananas. They are usually sprayed with a considerable amount of sulfer to retain their shelf-life and consequently can create stomach pain.

Juices should be consumed slowly for digestive purposes. Gulping merely creates unneeded gas. When possible, make your own fresh, but if that is not possible, buy unfiltered juice in glass containers. Often tin cans react with the acids in the juice and taint the flavor.

Fresh juices can be enhanced with various combinations. Carrot and spinach with 1 tablespoon of cream aids digestion. Carrot, celery, and apple tastes like a meal in itself. Cucumber, which acts as a diurectic combines well with pineapple. Beets, fennel and 1 tablespoon of yogurt is also good.

In place of packaged salad dressings that often contain harmful preservatives and additives, make your own with a few drops of sunflower or safflower oil with lemon juice and grated onion or garlic. Substitute skim milk for whole milk.

## HEAL YOURSELF WITH THE HELP OF FRIENDS

When you want to change your life style or eating habits, call for help. Mutual support systems and self-help groups, from Alcoholics Anonymous to organizations for the handicapped, retired, divorced or overweight, to persons suffering from an endless variety of physical, mental and emotional distresses, encourage you to reach your goals. Zooming memberships in these groups total about 15 million Americans. Interestingly, this emerges at a historic time of isolation, detachment and alienation. Many Americans are turning their backs on customary forms of support; namely the family, community, neighborhood and church. Dr. Alan Gartner and Dr. Frank Riessman, co-directors of the Manhattan-based, National Self-Help Clearinghouse, say that "self-help group proliferation reflects the inadequacy of the formal care-giving institutions in meeting the needs that arise in the absence of these bonding institutions."

If you want to change your life style and would like to live either collectively or communally, consider placing an ad in the paper or making inquiries at Holistic Centers in your region.

With the energy crisis there are more people moving to rural areas or small towns. Emotional support as well as economics are influencial factors for banding together.

*Sample Menu for a Day*

| | |
|---|---|
| Breakfast: | Apple or pear<br>Tahini and honey (sesame seed puree—often called Halvah, a good protein source) or millet, wheat germ and brown rice cereal cooked together. Serve with milk. Or rice, cinnamon, honey and milk<br>Midmorning: fruit of season—e.g., oranges, bananas or peaches |
| Lunch: | Fresh fruit; grapes, plums or apricots<br>Mixed green salad with tomatoes, carrots, fennel and cucumber with dressing made of olive oil, lemon, parsley, chives and dill<br>Brown rice and fresh mushrooms with mineral salt, basil and thyme for seasoning |
| Dinner: | Strawberries<br>Stuffed tomato with avocado, grated carrot and millet flakes, with a filling of grated beets, lemon and mineral salt |
| Breakfast: | Sliced pears and millet cereal cooked in milk<br>Chamomile tea |
| Lunch: | Diced fresh peaches, carrot-spinach salad, polenta (corn meal), luccini, spearmint tea |
| Dinner: | Plums or apricots<br>Vegetable soup<br>Schwartzbrat bread<br>Linden tea |
| Breakfast: | Applesauce and pancakes<br>Yogurt<br>Peppermint tea |
| Lunch: | Apricots or almonds<br>Cauliflower salad<br>Spinach souffle<br>Ginseng tea |
| Dinner: | A banana<br>Slivered beets<br>Assorted green salad<br>Sesame potatoes<br>Alfalfa mint tea |

| | | |
|---|---|---|
| Breakfast: | Grated apple, yogurt and cinnamon, chamomile tea | Kefir, Cottage cheese pineapple, golden seal tea |
| Lunch: | Grapes, swiss chard sliced potatoes, peach coupé | Nectarines, radish and chickory salad, corn pizza |
| Dinner: | Apricots, kohlrabi and carrots, tomato soup | Peaches, millet and tomatoes, potato soup |
| Breakfast: | Muesli | 7-grain cereal, soaked in apple juice with almonds |
| Lunch: | Carrots or cucumbers cheese souffle, tomato soup | Spinach salad, broccoli garnish |
| Dinner: | Vegetable platter, assorted cheeses, apricot souffle | Carrot soup, peach cream, goldenrod tea |

Breakfast: Fresh papaya or juice, oatmeal, rose hip tea

Lunch: Assorted green salad, fresh sauteed mushrooms (1 lb. mushrooms, 3 tbs. butter, wash mushrooms, trim off stems and saute)

Prune whip: 1 cup dried prunes, 1 cup dried apricots, honey to taste, 1 tsp. almond milk, 1 tsp. sunflower seed meal. Soak fruit overnight using enough water to cover fruit. Blend in blender until smooth, adding water if necessary to keep mixture moving. Add honey and top with almond milk and sunflower seed meal. Serves 3.

## BREAKFAST MENU IS LIMITLESS

- Yogurt, fruit
- Muesli
- Poached eggs on bran muffins with hollandaise sauce made of yogurt, buttermilk, cornmeal, dill, parsley and mineral salts. Good for Sunday brunch.
- Swiss breakfast rolls: ricotta cheese, honey, slivered almonds, cinnamon, mixed up with plain yogurt or buttermilk to thin. Place on raisin bread with thin slice of pineapple or banana for added flavor. Put in broiler for 10 minutes and voilà, you have a pièce de résistance.
- Millet, a good breakfast energizer, with honey and cut fruit
- Bulgur wheat
- Cheese grilled on pumpernickel or rye with fresh tomato and dill sprinkled on top

- On the run: to one 8 oz. glass of fresh juice, add 1 tbs. of protein powder, 1 tsp. Brewer's yeast, 1 tsp. vanilla extract to cut taste of Brewer's yeast, and honey. This will provide all the energy you need and send you out the door with a positive attitude.
- Fried tofu is a good substitute for scrambled eggs and has less cholesterol.

Be sure to begin each meal with a fresh fruit or vegetable. Slices of apples and wedges of cheese are good energizers. Yogurt with banana slices, slivered almonds and currants. Cottage cheese with chives and pineapples or guava. Grapes with any cheese, as Camembert, Edam, Swiss or Gruyère. Bowl of fresh fruit with oranges, bananas, grapefruit and kumquats with wheat germ on top and wedge of cheese on the side.

## BROWN-BAGGING IT CAN BE FUN

Carrying your lunch to school or work can be a challenge to your creativity. There are many combinations that you can make to add more zest and variety to your eating. Some of our favorites are the following:

- Grated Swiss cheese on pumpernickel or rye with alfalfa sprouts, and mayonnaise mixed with dill and grated onion.
- Thermos of homemade soup such as tomato, bouillon, onion, vegetable or lentil
- Egg salad with lettuce on bran bread.
- Ricotta cheese with honey, nutmeg or raisin bread with slices of bananas.
- Avocado with lemon, ground almonds or cashews with alfalfa sprouts on seven-grains bread.

---

- Drink: apple, pineapple, orange, or grapefruit juice or herb teas as chamomile, linden, rose hips, either cold or hot. Also a favorite summer drink is peppermint tea mixed with lemonade and strawberries.

---

- In a thermos, take some yogurt dips with fresh broccoli, carrot, celery bets, cauliflower, or cucumber wedges.

---

- Tofu, which is ground soybeans, can be used in many ways. Use it as egg salad. Grind up and add diced celergy, fresh dill, pickles, mayonnaise, parsley, mineral salts, dried onions and garlic.

- Bake it like a patty adding kelp (pepper substitute and good source of iodine), mineral salts, fresh dill and parsley.
  Pudding: put it in a blender and add honey, cinnamon, allspice, nutmeg, almond extract, and either plain or flavored yogurt. It adds a zesty conclusion to the meal.

Create an unhurried life style with room for humanism.

## LOW ENERGY DAY

Begin by stretching before getting out of bed. Slowly get up and make your way to the bathroom. For your water recharge of the day—a Faucher douche. This is a very good water treatment for improving circulation and renewing energy. (See Chapter 3 for details.)

If you've decided to give up tea and black coffee or smoking, this is an inexpensive substitute.

Water improves circulation as it makes the veins and blood vessels more elastic. Alternate 2 times between hot and cold water concluding with cold. The hot should be just warm enough for the skin to become red. Cold is 38°C.

Stand in hot shower with a hand-regulated shower head. Start on the calves of your legs and move up the back. Turn sideways and do the side of the leg and up. Have your arm elevated, then turn to other leg and repeat the process. They spray the front of your body, beginning at your feet and work your way up.

- Cold—Do soles of each foot one at a time to brace the body for the shock, then work up the extremities as before.
- Hot—same as before.
- Cold—then wrap in a warm blanket and rest for 28 minutes.

## FAST DAY AT HOME

If you really want to attain maximum weight-loss while fasting, spend one day in bed. It has been my experience and that of many other spa-goers that one day of bed-fasting will result in a weight loss of about 1 kilo, which is 2.2 pounds.

To start your day, set the mental stage with the attitude that this is a special reprieve day. Rest, relax, enjoy it, and consider what a gift you are giving yourself in terms of renewed energy.

Next set the physical stage. Perhaps you will want to put some fresh cut flowers by your bed and turn on soothing music.

Plan to drink freshly-squeezed juice. If you have a juicer, fresh carrot and spinach juice is a good energizer plus an excellent source of vitamin A, which is good for the skin.

To make the juice seem like it goes further, sip it from a spoon. The process will take longer and you will be able to savor each drop.

Keep on hand several bottles of mineral water. Usually in the course of a one-day fast, you will consume about 2 quarts of liquid. Mountain Spring, Vichy, Poland and Pellagrino are all waters I would recommend. Perrier, the ever popular, has a considerable amount of sodium, which causes the body tissues to retain liquid, so I would not recommend it for a one-day fast, although it is good for a social drink at a party.

At midday, plan to have a vegetable bouillon.

Take several of your favorite reading materials or letters you have been wanting to write and catch up on correspondence.

Plan to nap at midday.

In the evening have a fruit drink, e.g., combination of apricot, peach and orange, or strawberry-apple.

You will find that the investment you make from such a one-day vacation will pay off in renewed energy.

## SWEATING/WATER THERAPY

Sweating can be the most vigorous activity you've had all day. The heat produces an artifical "fever" and urges every body organ into action. While outwardly relaxed, your inner organs are as active as though you were jogging or mowing the lawn. At the same time you are being cleansed from inside out by the skin, your body's largest organ, by sweat, its excretion.

## HOW TO USE A HOT TUB FOR SWEATING

If you suffer from a serious illness or have an acute heart, circulatory or respiratory problem, consult a physician prior to hot tubbing.

1. Eating immediately before bathing puts a strain on the circulatory system. As before swimming, wait an hour after a large meal before taking the plunge. Also, it is best not to bathe on an empty stomach. Overheated bodies, like during any exercise, use energy, and some people in a depleted condition may experience nausea or even fainting. If you are physically exhausted or have had a long illness, consult your doctor prior to submerging in the water.

   —Mental exhaustion is not included in the precaution.

2. Remove jewelry and glasses before taking to the water.
   —Metal gets burning hot and heat causes capillaries and skin to swell, making rings and tight bracelets constricting.
   —Contact lenses may dry and provoke eye irritation—pop them out first.
3. Don't drink alcohol while bathing. One stiff drink when you're in hot water can make you feel drunk since heat stimulates the metabolism. With arteries, veins and capillaries expanded and the heart beating rapidly, alcohol rushes through your system. The "morning after" can be relieved by hot tubbing. The bath's heat speeds the metabolism and hastens the elimination of additives in the alcohol which causes hangovers.
4. For the common headache—usually caused by the constriction of the capillaries in the head, hot tubbing or sweat-baths dilate the vessels, relax the body, and bring relief.
5. Use *after vigorous sports:* keeps the blood circulating and continues the body's natural process of purging fatigue waste, such as lactic acid, without adding strain to the muscles.
6. Use *before yoga or massage* to loosen and prepare the muscles for twisting and turning.
7. Body responses to heat: let your body tell you when it wants out. People not accustomed to heat may feel nausea or faint, and nose-bleeds or other injury to blood vessels may occur. If treated properly, there is little danger. Nausea is induced by a lack of blood to the parasympathetic nervous system and is a sign of impending unconsciousness. This can result from bathing on an empty stomach when your blood sugar is low.
   —Injury to blood vessels sometimes occurs when the sudden dilation of weak vein walls. If this happens, stop the bleeding with a cold compress.
8. During menstruation, the sauna hot tub or other type of sweat bath can alleviate some of the cramps by relaxation and the removal of excessive water caused by sodium retention. For the same reason, sweat-bathing is generally beneficial for healthy pregnant women. However, during cases of toxemia or complicated pregnancy, a physician should be consulted before sweat-bathing.
9. Sauna as delivery room during childbirth. Sweat-baths fulfill many of the requirements of the increasingly popular childbirth methods that is, "soft birth" or birth without violence. These techniques, often practiced at home under the supervision of a midwife or physician, require a warm ambient temperature and

subdued lighting inherent in most sweat-baths. Heat relaxes the woman and smooths delivery, and the child being born is spared the sock of harsh lights. A dip in warm water replaces the hard slap on the newborn's behind and both the woman and the child enjoy the unclinical atmosphere of the earthy sweat-room.

—Sweat-bathing after childbirth releves aching muscles, cleanses the body and gives the new mother needed privacy.
—Until she has recuperated from the ordeal of childbirth, the sweat-bath should be kept at a low temperature.

10. Menopause can be eased by sweat-bathing, which helps to stimulate the autonomic nervous system, the pituitary gland, the adrenal glands and the ovaries. Many medical people consider menopause an elimination crisis which makes sweat-bathing even more useful. The theory is that menstruation is more than just an elimination of the uterine lining: it is an elimination cycle for the entire body. Upon cessation of the woman's reproductive cycle, the body must find other ways of ridding itself of toxic accumulations, and while this adjustment is going on, uncomfortable menopausal symptoms are felt. Sweat-bathing acting as a general toxic eliminator, reduces some of the distress.

## TAKE A BREATH-BREAK IN YOUR HOME SPA

Doctors call it "aerobics," yoga proponents and spa enthusiasts call it inhalation therapy, and the average person says it's breathing. All are talking about rhythmic breathing, an easy way to cleanse your lungs and respiratory system while refreshing your body and mind at home or anywhere.

Why breathe rhythmically? There are many benefits to it. With each complete inhalation and exhalation, carbon dioxide is burned and waste materials are eliminated from the blood. This helps purify the bloodstream as well as supply the blood with oxygen which is needed by all body cells. The entire body is rewarded with a feeling of new vitality when dark blood is changed into fresh red blood. While sitting or reclining, and wearing loose clothes, breathe in deeply, hold for 5 seconds, and then breathe out.

Repeat this exercise 10 times in the morning and evening. It can help you feel refreshed and glowing with health.

1. Upon awakening in the morning, breathe deep exhaled breaths.
2. Repeat in the evening prior to bed to assure a sound sleep.

3. During times of tension do a series of expulsions or lion's postures in yoga.
4. Alternate nostril breaths are good to do if you are having difficult resting.

## HOW TO INJECT MORE VITALITY AND OVERCOME FATIGUE WITH REST

People who habitually put in long hours of work usually need no more sleep than those who sit around doing next to nothing. Fatigue is not a condition exclusive to people who have been working too hard.

1. Do you allow time to rest? Do you take time for a mini-vacation to work on autogenic training during the day? Do you understand your body clock?
2. Do you exercise enough? There is a correlation between exercise and mental alertness. One way to perk up your brain and relieve boredom is to go out and take a brisk walk in the bracing air.

We don't get enough outdoor exercise and activity as our ancestors did. When five o'clock fatigue hits, exercise is usually the best aid. Swimming, mild jogging, mild aerobics and skipping rope will increase the circulation of the blood to the brain and make you feel more alive.

3. Try walking home from work. Brisk walking is a good conditioner, bringing every muscle into play as well as burning up calories.
4. Those who find athletics unappealing or impractical can devise ways for making the office a place of exercise. Bend, stoop, squat, reach and stretch at every possible opportunity. Walk upstairs and avoid the elevator.
5. Eat properly. Have fruits and vegetables and avoid Danish rolls and coffee.
6. Are you depressed? Fatigue often masks depression—a predisposition of perpetual gloomy outlook that develops during childhood when a person first acquires attitudes about himself. Lowered self-esteem also contributes to it.
7. Is noise pollution affecting your energy? Scientists relate noise to hearing loss, nervous disorders, irritability, inefficiency and fatigue. How much noise is too much? Doctors have discovered that noise pollution is as much a threat to certain susceptible people as air pollution is to emphysema or asthma sufferers.

Several studies indicate that either prolonged exposure to noise or sudden sharp noises will produce involuntary responses by the vascular, digestive and nervous systems.

Sound is measured in decibels, with one decibel representing the smallest change in loudness that the normal human ear can detect between two sounds. Conversation in a relatively quiet setting measures about 60 dbs., while the traffic noise or the noise of a machine shop is likely to make it an uncomfortable 80.

Sounds which reach the dangerous levels are: jet plane takeoffs: 150, subway trains screeching along the track: 95, power lawnmower: 96, food blender: 85.

Oversleeping can have as adverse an effect on the performance of daily duties as sleeping too little. Oversleepers feel sluggish because their basal metabolism has dropped too low.

## EXERCISE AND FITNESS

Everything physical requires mental effort. If you want to be healthy, then flex your brain as well as your muscles.

Basic principle: It's not so much what kind of exercise that you do, but that you enjoy it and do it! Don't expect an instant change in your figure and health. Since it has taken time to get flabby and de-energized, it will take an equal amount of time to rev-up your system again. Be patient with progress. Give yourself a couple of months and then see how you look and feel. Make exercise a life-long habit. Choose a favorite activity and do it every day of your life.

Be aware of your mood changes when exercising. Psychologically, exercise is a mood elevator. When you feel tense or overtly aggressive, go out for a walk, jump rope or do something physical.

Are you bored and want to overeat? Stop! Don't head for the kitchen, run outside. When hunger gets you, get away and become occupied with a physical activity (include bioenergetic exercise).

Refer to Chapter 8, on Exercise.

1) Do stretches upon awakening.
2) Walk or run in the morning prior to work or school.
3) Jump rope for a 10 minute break instead of snacking.
4) On weekends, go for long walks, hike or take an all day bike trip.
5) Study a new exercise, such as judo, yoga, racquetball, tennis or bioenergetics.
6) Stand up tall and be aware of your posture, which affects breathing and total body function. Be aware of how you stand and walk

when you pass a mirror. To align your posture, put your feet up against a baseboard and slide down till the small of the back touches wall. Hold your head forward but don't stretch the neck up since this produces a strain on the thyroid gland.

## STRESS AND JOB TENSION— LIFE STYLE AS WELL

Learning to be relaxed is a direct road to being honest with yourself. Many people believe that their business produces their tension. Such people fail to realize that their daily pursuits and hobbies are not forced upon them but are their own voluntary choices.

How to deal with stress:

1. First understand the workings of stress (what made you ill, etc.).
2. Establish a philosophy of life and style of living which allows you to adjust more readily to the inevitable situations of stress that go along with being alive.
3. *Relaxation* is the essence of reducing stress. Dr. Sheely points out that "most illnesses have their outlet within 18 months of an emotional trauma. Since all these diseases can be caused by emotional distress, by controlling emotional excess you can learn to mentally control most symptoms and most disease processes. It's important to put the whole body, mind, emotions and spirit in tune."

Become self-regulated towards health to influence your:

1. Attitude
2. Ability to Relax
3. Physical exercise
4. Mental exercise
5. Habit
6. Faith and beliefs
7. Sanitation
8. Light
9. Diet

True health results from an integrated mind, body and spirit. Relaxation is the antidote to disease. Your ability to relax may eventually be the determining factor in preventing disease or death.

To relax, achieve a fixed concentration: focus your attention upon a specific mental activity so that distracting thoughts and emotions don't interfere.

Tell yourself to relax by beginning to close your eyes and take a deep breath. Refer to Autogenic Training in Chapter 6.

## HOW TO CREATE YOUR OWN BAD OR SPA ATMOSPHERE

### Atmosphere

Come to your senses.

Montaigne, the French essayist, thought that the medical world could promote the cause of health by greater use of scents. Odors, he said, contain qualities to change one's attitudes and spirits.

*Smell:*

The surroundings in a Bad atmosphere, whether in Europe or your home, can appeal to your senses. Herbal blends of peppermint, cloves, and chamomile can contribute a delightful fragrance to your home, and the aroma of fresh flowers, cooking soup or bread baking add a welcoming atmosphere to your abode.

What kind of innovative fragrances can you create? Try blending various spices—cinnamon, nutmeg and allspice; crush mint leaves and place them in an open bowl for a soothing scent: mix herb leaves of linden, peppermint, rose hips and chamomile; blend dried rose petals with cloves, dried, grated lemon and orange peels. Keep the mixture in an open bowl for a month, then put it in a closed jar for a month to enhance its potency. Take it out the next month and smell the fragrant aromas.

*Sound:*

Although classical music touches the soul to create some moods, silence is revitalizing after a tension-filled day. Lie down in a darkened room, close your eyes and listen to the lack of sound. It can be a source of new energy. Save your favorite music for exercising or creating specific moods.

*Sight:*

Your own spa or Bad atmosphere can be one that is calming, refreshing and energizing. How does your home look? Have you tried using freshly cut flowers or dried plant arrangements to heighten the aesthetics? Hanging green plants of Swedish, Baltic or English ivy add feeling to your spa. Consider ferns, aloe veras or splurge and buy an orange tree. Theses touches of nature will contribute to your own sense of naturalness as you work, rest and have fun in your own spa.

Create order around you. If you have a habit of casually throwing things around, take the time to put them away. Organize books, last month's magazines, clothes, etc. You will be surprised at the sense of internal order that results from viewing tidiness around you. Often we become so accustomed to rooms looking like urban renewal projects that we forget how calming it is to view neatness.

### Have a Chaos Day

If you are the type who is an inveterate dropper of anything and everything as you enter the door, allow yourself one day to live in confusion. Sunday might be a good time to throw the *New York Times* all over the living room. Have a picnic on the floor. Discard your shoes momentarily. Allow yourself one day of reprieve, then . . . Clean up the mess. You will be surprised at the sense of relief when you have put order back into your atmosphere. Order and rhythm are innate to the spa atmosphere and you can change the state of your health by changing your habits.

## BAD IN THE BATHROOM

Here is the locale of your own healing spa. Does it have a sense of aesthetics? Do you like the way it looks? How do you feel being in the room? Would you like to change the color, appearance or mood? This special room can be redecorated very inexpensively to appeal to your senses.

In European Bads, the decor varies from ornate pillars, statuary, sea nymphs and Roman graffitti to an antiseptic white. You can adorn your bath with hanging plants, assorted foliage, apothecary jars of potions and salts, or colorful paint or wallpaper. A friend of mine purchased inexpensive colored sheets at a January white sale. She stapled them to the walls and created a tent-like ceiling. The effect was dramatic. The feeling was that of entering a gypsy tent for a clandestine rendezvous. I, however, prefer to have vivid red wallpaper of Moucha sketches as my decor, but to each his or her own.

You have many choices for your Bad decor. Decide what is aesthetically appealing to you and do it.

### Bath Items Needed:

*Loofah sponge or mitt.* This is used for a dry brush massage to scrub away the dead skin cells.

*Sea Salt.* It's very inexpensive, about 39¢ per pound, so buy about five pounds. Keep it in colorful apothecary jars to add to your atmosphere. On wintery days when others are shoveling snow from the walks, put 2 cups of sea salt in your tub, get in, and imagine that you are basking in the sea in a tropical climate.

*Epsom Salts.* Like sea salt it is inexpensive. Keep a generous supply on hand for medical as well as bath purposes. It is great for soaking tired feet, sprained wrists or fatigued bodies.

*Bran.* Either keep a container of this potent solution or make bran bags.

*Lotion.* This is to the body what icing is to cake. Choose a lotion that enhances your body-texture. Vegetable oils that are used in food preparations are excellent. Safflower, soya or corn oil are very good. I particularly like olive oil mixed with equal parts of water, which is nourishing for dry skin. If you are more inclined to buy a lotion, consider one of a papaya, almond or aloe vera.

*Hand-shower attachment.* This can be purchased at a hardware store for about $4.99. If you prefer a more elaborate variety, you can get a more expensive type from a plumbing supply house. The hand-shower is attached to the faucet, and is great for the Faucher douche spraying of the extremities.

*Friction towel.* Yes, velour is much smoother; however, the coarseness of this thick cotton towel with its rough nap of uncut loops increases circulation.

*Herbs.* Consider rose petals, chamomile, linden flowers or peppermint leaves left in a container for an extra special scented bath.

Scents for all seasons: In spring, put fresh daffodils in your bathroom, in summer, use fresh, cut lemons or flowers, in autumn, use leaves, color turned branches, and dried grasses, and in winter, use pine branches with bits of holly.

These are the daily bath items. However, if you would like to really splurge, try some luxury items. Buy a redwood tub for the ultimate luxury, or consider a Jacuzzi whirlpool, home sauna or steam bath. These can be ordered through a plumbing supply house.

Many people familiar with the European Bads are now creating their own home spas. Diane von Furstenburg remodeled the barn on her Vermont home to have it converted into a spa. Some bath devotees are investing in redwood tubs for individual bathing and group celebrations.

## HERBAL TEAS FOR HOME SPA

| NAME | PART | MEDICINAL ACTION |
|---|---|---|
| ANISE<br>Pimpinella anism<br>anise, sweet cumin | root and/or seeds | Aromatic, carminative, diaphoretic pectoral relaxant, stimulant, stomachic, tonic. |
| BAYBERRY<br>bayberry wax<br>tree, wax-myrtle<br>candleberry<br>tallow shrub | bark | Astringent, diaphoretic, emetic (large doses) increases circulation, stimulant, tonic. |
| CHAMOMILE<br>Anthemis nobilis<br>ground apple<br>whig plant | flowers and/or upper half of plant | Appetite stimulant, anodyne, anti-spasmodic, carminative, stomachic, tonic. Affects: bladder, kidneys, spleen. |
| COMFREY<br>Symphytum officinale<br>knitbone, gum plant<br>slippery root | leaves and/or root | Astringent, antiseptic, demulcent, expectorant, mucilaginous, nutritive styptic, vulnerary. Affects: lungs, stomach, bones. |
| DANDELION<br>Taraxacum densleonis<br>Taraxacum officinale<br>priest's crown<br>swine's snout | leaves and/or root | Laxative, depurative, diuretic, hepatic stimulant, stomachic, tonic. Affects: kidneys, liver, bladder, spleen, urinary organs. |

| | | |
|---|---|---|
| blowball<br>cankerwort<br>lion's tooth<br>white endive<br>golden suns | | |
| ELDER<br>Sambucus nigra<br>elderberry | bark and/or leaves, flowers and/or fruit | Bark: catharic, emetic. Flowers: alterative, discutient, diuretic, diaphoretic, emollient, exanthematous, increases circulation. |
| FENNEL<br>Foeniculm vulgare<br>sweet fennel, finkel<br>hinojo, fenkel, wild fennel | leaves and/or seeds | Aromatic, carminative, diaphoretic, diuretic, pectoral stimulant, stomachin. Affects: internal organs (stimulation), brain (poor memory), eyes (strengthening). |
| FENUGREEK<br>Trigonella foenumgraecum<br>bird's foot<br>greek hay seed | seed | Farinaceous, mucilaginous. Affects: intestines, lubricates bowels. |
| GINSENG<br>Panax quinquefolla<br>five fingers<br>red berry<br>man's health | root | Disease preventative, demulcient, diaphoretic stimulant (mild), stomachic, tonic. Affects: stomach, nerves, lungs. |
| GOLDEN SEAL<br>Hydrastis canadensis<br>Indian paint<br>turmetic root | root | Antiperiodic, antiseptic, alternative aperient, deobstruent, detergent diuretic, laxative, opthalmicum, stomachic, tonic. Affects: eyes, liver, mucous membranes, stomach. |

| NAME | PART | MEDICINAL ACTION |
|---|---|---|
| GOLDEN SEAL (Cont'd)<br>wild curcuma<br>yellow root | | |
| GOTO KOLA<br>Hydsrocotyle asiatica<br>Indian pennywort<br>march penny<br>white root | leaves | Diuretic, aperient, alternative, stimulant (small doses), narcotic (large doses). |
| HOREHOUND<br>Marrubium vulgare<br>white horsehound<br>marvel | flowering tops and/or leaves | Aromatic, diaphoretic, diuretic, expectorant, hepatic, laxative (large doses), pectoral, tonic, stimulant. |
| HORSETAIL<br>Equisetum<br>hyemale<br>shave grass<br>scouring rush<br>bottlebrush<br>paddock pipes | barren stems | Anthelmintic, astringent, depurative, diuretic, detergent, decongestant, hepatic, nervine, pectoral, stomachic. Affects: kidneys, bladder. |
| HYSSOP<br>Hyssopus | whole plant | Antiseptic, aromatic, aperient, anthelmintic, carminative, diaphoretic, expectorant, febrifuge, rubifacient, |

| | | |
|---|---|---|
| officinalis<br>holy herb | | laxative, sudorific, stimulant. Affects: bladder, kidkeys, spleen, mucous lining (stomach bowels). |
| JUNIPER<br>Juniperus communis<br>juniper bush<br>juniper bark | berries | Carminative, diuretic, stomachic. Affects: kidneys, bladder. |
| LINDEN<br>Tilia platyphyllos<br>linden flowers<br>common lime, lime flowers | flowers | Expectorant, dicphoretic, nervine, stimulant. Affects: mucous membranes, digestive and nervous system. |
| LOBELIA<br>Lobelia inflata<br>emetic weed<br>washma weed<br>wild tobacco<br>indian or wild tobacco<br>pukeweed, gagroot | plant and/or seed | Antispasmodic, emetic, expectorant, diaphoretic, nervine, relaxant (large doses), stimulant (small doses). |
| MARSHMALLOW<br>Althea officinalis<br>althea, sweet weed<br>mortification root<br>wymote | leaves and/or root | Demulcent, diuretic, emollient, mucilaginous. Affects: kidneys. |

# GLOSSARY

Alterative ................ Blood purifier, corrects symptoms of minor functional disorders
Anodyne ................ Relieves pain
Anthelmintic ............ Expels worms
Antiperiodic ............ Arrests morbid periodical movements
Antispasmodic ........... Relieves or prevents spasms
Antiseptic ................ Opposed to putrification
Aperient .................. Gentle laxative
Aromatic .................. Mildly stimulant or pleasing odor
Astringent ............... Draws tissues together checking discharges
Carminative .............. Expels gas from bowels, stomach, intestines
Cathartic .................. Strong laxative
Cephalic .................. Used in diseases of head
Cholagugue .............. Increases bile flow
Demulcent ............... Soothing relieves inflammation
Deobstruent .............. Removes obstructions from organs
Depurative ............... Removes waste from body (purifies blood)
Diaphoretic .............. Increases perspiration
Discutient ................ Dissolves and removes tumors
Diuretic ................... Increases urine flow
Emetic .................... Produces vomiting
Emmemagogue ........... Promotes menstruation
Emollient ................ Softening and soothing to inflamed parts
Exanthematous ........... Remedy for skin eruptions and diseases
Expectorant .............. Facilitates expulsion of mucus from respiratory tract

Febrifuge ................ Reduces fevers
Hepatic .................. Remedy for Liver Diseases
Laxative ................. Promotes bowel action and/or corrects constipation
Mucilaginous ............. Soothing to inflammed parts
Nervine .................. Quiets nervous irritation
Parturient ............... Promotes labor at childbirth
Pectoral ................. Relieves chest affections
Refrigerant .............. Cooling or relieves thirst
Resolvent ................ Dissolves or removes tumors
Relaxant ................. Relieves strain or tension
Rebifacient .............. Increases circulation
Sedative ................. Allays nervous irritability, soothing or quieting to nervous system
Stomachic ................ Strengthens or tones stomach, promotes appetite, aids digestion
Styptic .................. Stops hemorrhaging or bleeding
Vermifuge ................ Expels worms
Vulnerary ................ Heals wounds

# DIRECTORY OF EUROPEAN BADS AND SPAS

When I decided to go to the Bads I initially wrote to the national tourist office of each country. Within three weeks, a packet of spa and bad information was mailed. You can do the same. For more detailed information regarding costs and specific programs, write to the individual spas or bads.

## Austria

Contact: Austrian National Tourist Office
545 Fifth Avenue, New York, NY 10017
(212) 697-0651

*Bad vie Wien,* located in the Weinerwald, Vienna Woods; a half hour from Vienna. From early Roman times to the present, the creme de la creme have congregated here. Beethoven completed his 9th Symphony here. A medical diagnostic center, underwater therapy treatments, fango (mud packs) and varied water therapies are available. In addition, sports like skiing, biking, golf, riding and swimming are but a few of the possibilities for the athletically minded.

*Bad Gastein-Bad Hofgastein,* these spas are located about 12 miles from one another. I prefer the old world elegance of Bad Gastein over the newer Bad Hofgastein complex. Both places are quiet and offer the usual water treatments and sporting activities. A special treatment is radon heat from a cave. The indoor pool offers man-made waves so you can feel like you are by the sea. As a side trip, you can be in Zagreb, Yoguslavia in about 45 minutes from Bad Hofgastein.

*Salzburg Therapeutic Center* provides a variety of thermal water treatments.

## Belgium

Contact: Belgian National Tourist Office
720 5th Avenue
New York, NY 10019
(212) 582-1750

## Bulgaria

Contact: Bulgarian Tourist Office
50 East 42nd Street
New York, New York 10017

## Czechoslovakia

Contact: CEDOK
10 East 40th Street
New York, New York 10016
(212) MU9-9720

*Marienbad and Karlovy Vary (Carlsbad)* are the prime Bads to visit. Pavilions, fashionable promenades and the elegance of another era abound there. Strauss, Chopin, Beethoven, Ibsen, and Goethe are only some of the former visitors to these renown spas.

## Denmark, Finland, Sweden, Norway

Contact: Scandinavian National Tourist Office
505 Fifth Avenue
New York, New York 10017
(212) 582-2802

## France

Contact: French National Tourist Office
610 Fifth Avenue
New York, New York 10020
(212) 757-1125

*Vichy*, of mineral water fame, is possibly the best known spa in France. Its water is considered very good for digestive problems, liver and gall bladder difficulties and children's diseases. A casino, horse races, water sports and cultural events are some of the other attractions.

## Germany

Contact: German National Tourist Office
630 Fifth Avenue
New York, New York 10036
(212) 757-8570

Germany is the home of the Bads. Kurort spas, are everywhere. At last count there were 250 treatment centers in existence. Of note are Bad Homberg, Bad Pyrmont, Bad Neuenahr, Badenweiler, and Bad Wiessee.

*Baden-Baden* is the ultimate for spa goers. The Brenner's Park hotel offers an adjoining Klinik Stephanie which has an outstanding anti-stress program. Besides the best in Bad treatment, you can experience an elegant life here. The casino, horse races, tennis, golf, hiking in the nearby Black Forest, swimming, and treatments in the Augustabad and Friedrichs Bad are unique in Europe. The fango mudpacks, underwater massages and Roman-Irish steam baths cannot be rivaled. The Kurpath and kurgarden and a stroll along the romantic River Oas are all musts when you visit this international spa.

*Wiesbaden* If you find yourself in Frankfurt, consider staying in Wiesbaden. Trains leave the lower level of the Frankfurt air terminal about every 18 minutes for this spa. Wiesbaden offers traditional spa activity: a variety of thermal waters for drinking and bathing, mud baths, gymastics, theaters, concerts and twenty-six brine springs. Many charter flights arrive at Frankfurt.

## Great Britain

Contact: British Tourist Authority
680 Fifth Avenue
New York, New York 10022

Bath, Forest Mere, Enton Hall, Cheltenham are a few of the British spas available.

## Greece

Contact: Greek National Tourist Organization
645 Fifth Avenue
New York, New York 10022
(212) 421-5777

Loutraki and Kammena Vourla are spas located near gulfs, and are excellent for swimming or bathing. In Athens, you can swim in the Mediterranean and take spa treatments nearby. Consider sightseeing at the many archeological sites.

## Hungary

Contact: Hungarian Mission to the U.N.
10 East 75th Street
New York, New York 10021

Budapest is virtually a spa city. However, the stifling atmosphere in the city can be oppressive. Be sure and get a visa several days in advance. You can either write to the Hungarian embassy in Washington, D.C., or apply to an IBEZ office in Vienna several days in advance.

## Ireland

Contact: Irish Tourist Board
590 Fifth Avenue
New York, New York 10036
(212) 246-7400

## Israel

Contact: Israel Government Tourist Office
488 Madison Avenue
New York, New York 10022
(212) 754-0140

Tiberias Hot Springs and the Dead Sea are two viable spas in Israel. Tiberias is known for the treatment of eye problems, rheumatism and diseases of the joints, cancer, and female disorders. The Tiberias springs are located in the Galilee area which is naturally beautiful. These springs are probably the oldest in the world, mentioned in Joshua (19:35) and later named by a Roman emperor. The Dead Sea is a marvelous place to float, but does not offer the extensive medical treatments of Tiberias.

## Italy

Contact: Italian Government Tourist Office
630 Fifth Avenue
New York, New York 10020
(212) 245-4822

Spas abound in this country. Montecatini, Merano, and Fiuggi are some of the popular thermal establishments. Flowing fountains, Baroque architecture and verdant gardens are some of the attractions.

## Luxembourg

Contact: Luxembourg Information Office
Dag Hammerskjold Plaza
200 East 42nd Street
New York, New York 10017
(212) 751-9650

## Netherlands

Contact: National Tourist Office
576 Fifth Avenue
New York, New York 10036
(212) 245-5320

## Poland

Contact: Polish Travel Office, ORBIS
500 Fifth Avenue
New York, New York, 10036

Thirty-six health spas can be found in Poland.

## Portugal

Contact: Portuguese Tourist and Information Office
548 Fifth Avenue
New York, New York 10036
(212) 354-1487

Mineral springs containing deposits of radium, flouride, sulfur, sodium and chloride offer thermal treatments to spa goers.

## Romania

Contact: The Romanian Tourist Office
543 Third Avenue
New York, New York 10036
(212) 697-6971

The Black Sea provides the setting and climate for spa enthusiasts. Over one hundred-fifty health resorts have treatments for digestive ailments, allergies and cardiovascular diseases. Many Romanian spas offer the Gerovital treatment developed by Dr. Ana Aslan to prevent aging.

## Spain

Contact: Spanish National Tourist Office
665 Fifth Avenue
New York, New York 10017

Seascapes, two hundred spas and lovely scenery are available to spa-seekers in Spain.

## Switzerland

Contact: Swiss National Tourist Office
250 Stockton Street
San Francisco, California 94108
(415) 362-2260

Be sure and write for the Swiss pocket guide to Climatic health resorts. It has complete information about the numerous spas available in Switzerland.

Baden, St. Moritz, Bex, les Bains, Bad Ragaz and Vals are some of the outstanding spas. Thermal pools and baths, assorted water therapies, golfing, tennis, swimming, riding, fishing, skiing, and mountain hikes are some of the attractions.

## Yugoslavia

Contact: Yugoslav State Tourist Office
630 Fifth Avenue
New York, New York 10020
(212) 757-2801

# Index

**Y**

# Coal Production and Processing Technology

# Coal Production and Processing Technology

*Editor*

Ombir Kumar

scitus
academics

**Coal Production and Processing Technology**
Edited by **Ombir Kumar**

ISBN: 978-1-68117-679-6
Library of Congress Control Number: 2016958830

© 2018 by
SCITUS Academics LLC,
616, Corporate Way, Suite 2, 4766,
Valley Cottage, NY 10989

www.scitusacademics.com

This book contains information obtained from highly regarded resources. Copyright for individual articles remains with the authors as indicated. All chapters are distributed under the terms of the Creative Commons Attribution License, which permits unrestricted use, distribution, and reproduction in any medium, provided the original author and source are credited.

**Notice**

Reasonable efforts have been made to publish reliable data and views articulated in the chapters are those of the individual contributors, and not necessarily those of the editors or publishers. Editors or publishers are not responsible for the accuracy of the information in the published chapters or consequences of their use. The publisher believes no responsibility for any damage or grievance to the persons or property arising out of the use of any materials, instructions, methods or thoughts in the book. The editors and the publisher have attempted to trace the copyright holders of all material reproduced in this publication and apologize to copyright holders if permission has not been obtained. If any copyright holder has not been acknowledged, please write to us so we may rectify.

Printed in United States of America on Acid Free Paper

# Preface

Coal is one of the cheapest and most reliable sources of energy, and as demand soars new technology will be crucial. With global demand for coal widely expected to rise over the next 20 years. Modern mining methods allow us to easily reach most of our coal reserves. Due to growth in surface mining and improved mining technology, the amount of coal produced by one miner in one hour has more than tripled since 1978. Surface mining is used to produce most of the coal because of less expensive than underground mining. Surface mining can be used when the coal is buried less than 200 feet underground. In surface mining, giant machines remove the top-soil and layers of rock to expose large beds of coal. Once the mining is finished, the dirt and rock are returned to the pit, the topsoil is replaced, and the area is replanted. The land can then be used for croplands, wildlife habitats, recreation, or offices or stores. Underground mining, sometimes called deep mining, is used when the coal is buried several hundred feet below the surface. Some underground mines are 1,000 feet deep. To remove coal in these underground mines, miners ride elevators down deep mine shafts where they run machines that dig out the coal. After coal comes out of the ground, it typically goes on a conveyor belt to a preparation plant that is located at the mining site. The plant cleans and processes coal to remove dirt, rock, ash, sulfur, and other unwanted materials, increasing the heating value of the coal.

*Coal Production and Processing Technology* delivers exclusively comprehensive analysis of the state-of-the-art coal technologies used in everything from mining to greenhouse gas mitigation.

# Table of Contents

# Chapter 1

# Theory and Practice of Integrated Coal Production and Gas Extraction

**Liang Yuan**[1]

*State Key Laboratory of Deep Coal Mining & Environment Protection, Huainan Mining Group Co., Ltd., Huainan 232001, China*

## ABSTRACT

The integrated extraction of coal and gas combines coal mining with gas capture. Taking into account the gas deposition and flow conditions in the Chinese coal basins, this paper describes the status of the theory and key technologies of this integrated extraction system, and presents its application and practice in the Shaqu, Zhongxing, Fenghuangshan and Pingmei mines. Areas for further improvements in future studies are discussed, focusing in particular on the fundamentals of the extraction system to make it greener, more scientific, and more advanced in both the exploitation and utilization of coal and the gas in coal.

**Keywords:** Integrated coal production Gas extraction De-stress mining Pillarless mining Circular overlying zone

## 1 INTRODUCTION

Most coal mines in China extract coal from seams with low permeability and high gas content. Gas control in such mining seams is a worldwide problem and the associated techniques are not completely optimized. Gas outburst accidents frequently occur during mining of these seams, therefore the productivity is lower, and it is very difficult to achieve safe and efficient mining. The Huainan mining area is a typical example of these conditions, having low permeability, high gas content, and complex geological conditions. Since 2004, the mining depth in Huainan coal mines has reached 700–1000 m, all 15 mines are classified as being outburst-prone, and the coal seams are characterized by low permeability (0.001 mD), high gas content (12–36 $m^3$/t), and high gas pressures (up to 6 MPa). Mining of these seams by conventional methods generates many problems, including coal pillars left in the panels, high abutment stress in the protected seams, the risk of outbursts, high gas emissions from the first-mined seam, gas accumulation at the upper corner of the longwall working face, a large amount of roadway excavation in rocks and at great depths, and the high cost of gas control.

Integrated coal and gas production combines coal mining with gas capture. This is a typical model for the development of dual resources (coal and gas in coal mine). Mining activity leads to desorption and flow of gas in the coal and creates favorable conditions for gas drainage. Furthermore, coal mining and its associated ventilation systems provide operating space for gas extraction. Efficient drainage of gas reduces the gas concentration and amount at the working face, which can effectively prevent gas explosions and eliminate coal and gas outbursts, thereby promoting safer and more efficient coal mining (Fields 1973; Garcia and Cervik 1985; Hargraves and Martin 1993; Creedy et al. 2001; Cheng et al. 2004, 2006). In recent years, integrated coal production and gas extraction has been developed and promoted rapidly in China, Australia, and other coal-mining countries, and has been demonstrated to be an effective method for safe and efficient mining of coal seams with high gas content and low permeability (Xie et al. 2006; Yuan 2008a).

This paper summarizes the fundamental theory and key technologies of integrated coal production and gas extraction in an effort to promote its wider application. Applications to four coal mines in China are also presented to showcase its applicability and effectiveness.

## 2 RESEARCH STATUS

Integrated coal production and gas extraction must be considered as a system which involves the exploration and measurement of stress field redistribution, deformation and failure of coal and rock, gas pressure and permeability, and gas desorption and migration during the process of coal mining.

## 2.1 Fundamental theory

### 2.1.1 Deformation and failure of overlying roof strata and overburden pressure

Theories of a natural equilibrium arch, pressure arch, cantilever beam, prefabricated fissures, articulated rock, elastic foundation beam, and many other well-known hypotheses have been proposed. In China, the masonry-beam structure model, passing-stress rock beam structure model, and key-layer theory have been proposed (Qian and Liu 1984; Song 1988; Qian and Shi2003).

### 2.1.2 Crack distribution in the overlying strata

To optimize the design of the bore for drainage of pressure-relieved gas from a mining area, detailed fracture distribution behaviors generated by mining have been developed by Chinese scholars. For example, the O-ring fracture (Qian and Xu 1998), the elliptical parabolic band (Li et al. 1999), and the annular ring fracture distributions (Yuan 2008b) have been investigated and proven.

### 2.1.3 Gas relief caused by mining flow patterns

Based on empirical data, two models of relieved gas emissions have been established in Germany (Noack 1998), as shown in Fig. 1. One model the relationship between the extent of gas emission and different roof and floor heights, while the other relates gas pressure to different heights of the roof and floor. Both models have been widely applied to forecast gas emission volumes from adjacent layers and evaluate gas drainage technologies. In addition, empirical models of gas emissions from adjacent layers in the typical high-gas mining areas of Yangquan and Huainan coal mines have been established (Cheng et al. 2004, 2006).

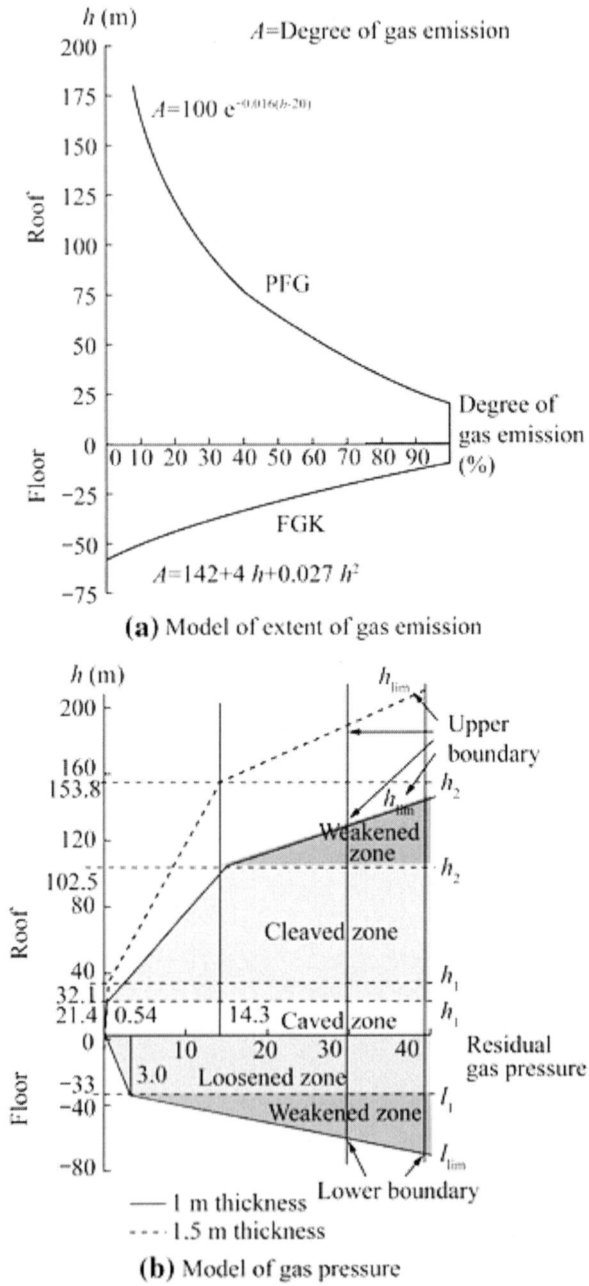


**Figure 1.** Model of mining gas desorption emissions (Noack 1998). *PFG* curve of degree of roof gas emissions; *FGK* curve of degree of bottom gas emissions

### 2.1.4 Variation of permeability and flow of relieved gas

The relationship between stress distribution and permeability in the front of the working face and the surrounding goaf rock was analyzed. The permeability coefficient reduces as a function of the abutment pressure of the working face, while the permeability sharply increases in the gob with the transfer of mining-induced stress and then reduces again as the mining stress is removed. However, the permeability in the surrounding rock after compaction is still much larger than the original permeability. Variation of rock permeability was also studied by Palchik (2005), Unver and Yasitli (2005), and Usanov et al. (2014). Permeability distribution of the overlying relief gob seam along the advancing direction of the working face was analyzed by dividing it into three stages: initially increasing permeability and flow by pressure relief, followed by high permeability and flow by continued relief, and then reducing permeability and flow by pressure recovery (Yu 1984).

## 2.2 Technical practice

Gas extraction can be carried out before, during, and after mining. In countries such as the US or Australia, coal seams have higher permeability and occur at shallower depths (Fields 1973; Hargraves and Martin 1993; Steven et al. 2007). The main methods of gas extraction include pre-extraction by vertical wells (Garcia and Cervik 1985) and long ground directional drilling or bedding drilling. In recent years, coal bed methane development has gradually achieved a certain economy of scale. Gas extraction during and after mining is generally applied to low permeability coal seams by methods such as drilling through the coal seam, horizontal roof drilling, gob area wells, and special gas extraction tunnels (Noack et al. 1995; USEPA 1998,1999). Drilling through coal seams and horizontal roof drilling are widely used in China and other countries, and gob area wells are widely used in countries with shallower coal depths, such as the US and Australia (Creedy et al. 2001; Michael 2007). In recent years, long ground directional drilling has become a new trend, and has been successfully applied in the US and Australia (Fig. 2). Coal mine methane extraction by directional drilling from the ground into the coal seam has been applied in Australia, and advanced navigation systems for directional drilling have been developed. In China, techniques for gas extraction have been developed for conditions when pressure relief has been extended at a coal mine, such as in the Huainan, Yangquan, and Huaibei groups. Simultaneous extraction coal and gas by roadway retention and borehole drilling has been successfully implemented at Huainan coal mines.

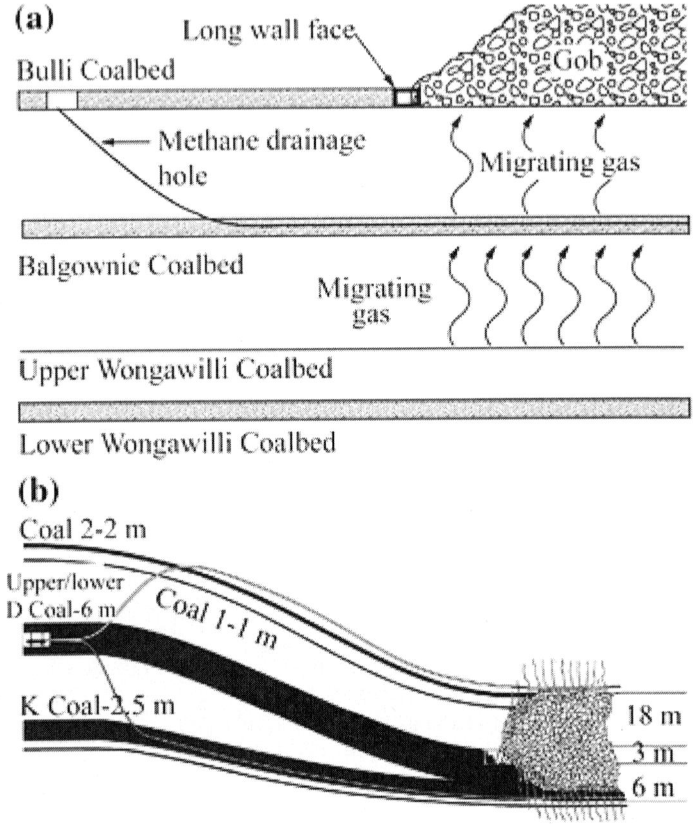


**Figure 2.** Gas extraction by long ground directional drilling in the US and Australia

# 3 TECHNIQUE OF INTEGRATED COAL PRODUCTION AND GAS EXTRACTION

## 3.1 Principles

The principle of integrated coal production and gas extraction follows a sequence of phenomena. Following mining-induced failure and the consequent movement of surrounding rocks, the gas desorbs from the broken coal seams and becomes free-flowing, and is thereby able to move into fractures and accumulate in the coal and rock strata. This accumulated gas is extracted by gas drainage boreholes and/or tunnels concurrently with the mining of the coal seams. Figure 3 illustrates this principle.

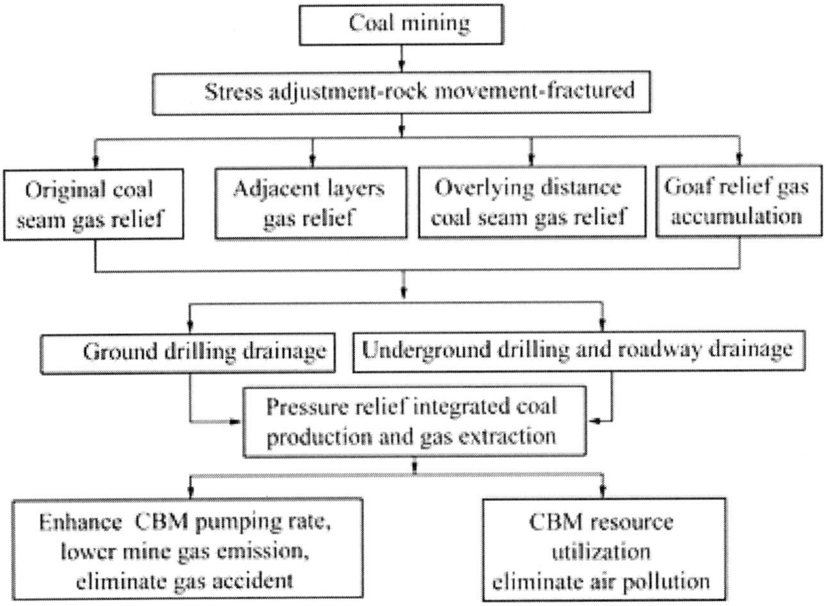


**Figure 3.**Principle of integrated coal production and gas extraction

By integrating coal production with gas extraction, coal seam gas becomes a useful resource. Advantage is taken of the effect of strata movement on gas pressure-relief and flow during the coal mining process to establish a single production system for simultaneous coal and gas extraction. By including gas drainage as part of the regular coal mining process, the traditional single coal resource mining pattern is transformed into an integrated production facility for both coal and gas.

## 3.2 Theoretical foundations

### 3.2.1 The annular-shaped overlying zone theory

The "annular-shaped overlying zone" theory has been proposed. The stress-relief coefficient of the overlying strata is obtained from numerical simulation results (Yuan et al. 2011a). The overlying zone can be considered an "annular-shaped fractured zone", which is located at a certain height above the goaf and has a particular width and extends upward at a particular angle. The zone has the following characteristics: (i) it can be divided into three sections along the strike, i.e., front, center, and rear. The front section is adjacent to the working face and runs through the working face in the direction of dip, and is the main region where gas desorption and emission occur. The central section connects the front and rear sections along two mining boundaries, and forms channels between these sections to allow large-scale gas flow. The rear section is near the cut and is smaller than the front section in size; (ii) the overlying annular-shaped fracture zone extends upward at a certain angle in the dip section, and the extension angles of the outward and inward boundaries are different; (iii) the overlying annular-shaped fracture zone is located in the strike section above the goaf at particular intervals and extends upward at a particular angle. The front range is larger than the rear range.

### 3.2.2 Three-band structure in stress-relief layer

The distribution and evolution of three bands in the stress-relief layers due to mining of the first seam have been clearly identified. These provide for the occurrence of desorption and formation of flow channels of gas in gas-enriched regions. In the process of mining a working face without a pillar, the front abutment stress region is located 0–30 m ahead of the working face and the concentration factor is about 2–3. The stable stress-relief region is located 300–500 m ahead of the working face in the advancing direction, the fracture development area is 0–50 m behind the working face of the first-mined seam, the active strata movement region is some 50–500 m behind the working face, and the attenuation region is more than 500 m behind the working face developed toward the goaf in the form of a wedge (Yuan 2008a).

### 3.2.3 Gas drainage by stress relief

Technical principles for enhancing gas drainage by stress relief have been proposed. Mining-induced stress, gas pressure and permeability, strata movement, and fracture evolution behavior have been investigated. A linear relationship between gas pressure and stress and a negative exponential relationship between permeability and stress have been demonstrated. Additionally, mining of the first seam can induce expansionary deformation, stress relief, and permeability enhancement of neighboring coal seams (Yuan 2008b).

## 3.3 Key Technologies

### 3.3.1 Excavation of a special roadway for gas drainage

A special roadway should be excavated in the de-stressed and fractured region formed in the first or protective seam for gas drainage. This technology has been developed to target the gas-rich zones in this region.

This gas-rich region, which has a width of 0–30 m and height of 8–25 m, is located in the annular-shaped fractured zone above the two roadways of the working face (Yuan 2008c).

This technology has been further developed to extract desorbed gas from overlying de-stressed coal seams that are spaced some distance from the first-mined seam. Once the first (protective) seam is mined, the range of the de-stressed region develops upward at a strike fracture angle of 80°–85° and the de-stressed layer is located 10–150 m above the protective seam (Yuan 2009a).

This technology has also been applied to extract desorbed gas from the underlying de-stressed protected coal seams. After the first seam is mined, the de-stressed range develops downward at strike and dip fracture angles of 99°–100° and 102°–110°, respectively, and the de-stressed layer is located 15–100 m below the protective seam (Yuan 2009b).

Ground well technology for gas drainage from de-stressed regions has been developed. This includes well construction and operating procedures. Technologies for controlling deformation of the surrounding roadway rocks in soft coal seams have also been developed. These include bolt-grouting support of soft rock roadways with high stress and controlled pre-stressing of fractured roofs with obviously inclined separation.

### 3.3.2 Roadway controlling technologies in pillarless mining

Technologies for roadways include support with strengthened bolting, meshing, and grout injection, a self-moving shield for reinforced support in mining-perturbed roadways, and building of packing walls for retaining gob-side roadways. Other key technologies include the development of materials capable of withstanding high loading for the packing walls, a modular shield for constructing the packing walls, and pre-fracturing of the working face roof for de-stressing. The initial and periodic caving intervals can be reduced by weakening the roof strength using advanced deep-hole pre-splitting blasting. An initiative for support roofing with high stiffness has been proposed, which emphasizes the “three high” bolting system, i.e., high strength, high pretension, and high stiffness of bolts (Yuan et al. 2011a, b).

### 3.3.3 Gas drainage by boreholes drilled in the retained roadway

A new concept for safe and efficient gas extraction has been proposed based on pillarless mining with a Y-shaped ventilation system. Boreholes in the retained roadways are drilled into the de-stressed and gas-rich zones in the overlying and underlying regions to extract gas (Yuan 2010).

# 4 MAIN ACHIEVEMENTS

## 4.1 Overlying annular fractured zone

Three-dimensional computational fluid dynamics modeling of a typical mining panel has revealed the existence of an overlying annular-shaped fractured zone in which gas-rich sections are located. The basic geometric features for highly efficient gas drainage are fully understood. A zone with a certain width locates at a particular height above the goaf and extends along the vertical direction at a particular angle, as shown in Fig. 4.

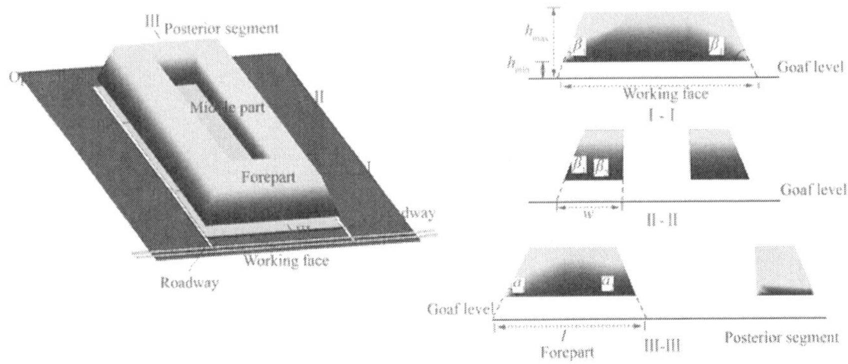


**Figure 4.** Annular-shaped overlying zone

The basic criteria for identifying this zone in multiple coal seams with low permeability are as follows:

(1)High gas desorption rate: Based on specific coal seam conditions, the effective stress reduction factors can be determined when gas desorbs significantly, and the zones in which high gas desorption occurs are identified according to the overlying strata stress-relief model.

(2)High permeability: High permeability is used to identify zones where mining-induced fractures are highly developed and compaction starts to occur. Regions with high permeability are determined using the overlying permeability distribution model. The upper boundary of the range for effective gas drainage does not exceed the upper boundary of the horizontal high permeability zone.

(3)High concentration of gas extracted: The minimum purity requirement of the gas extracted is determined and the range of gas purities is determined by applying the basic laws of gas dynamic flow.

Based on the above, the regions of highly efficient gas extraction from multiple coal seams can be determined.

## 4.2 De-stressed extraction of coal and gas

Gas drainage is implemented by placing roadways and/or boreholes in the de-stressed and/or fractured zones formed by mining of the first (protective) seam in multiple coal seams. A sketch of the gas drainage system is shown in Fig. 5.

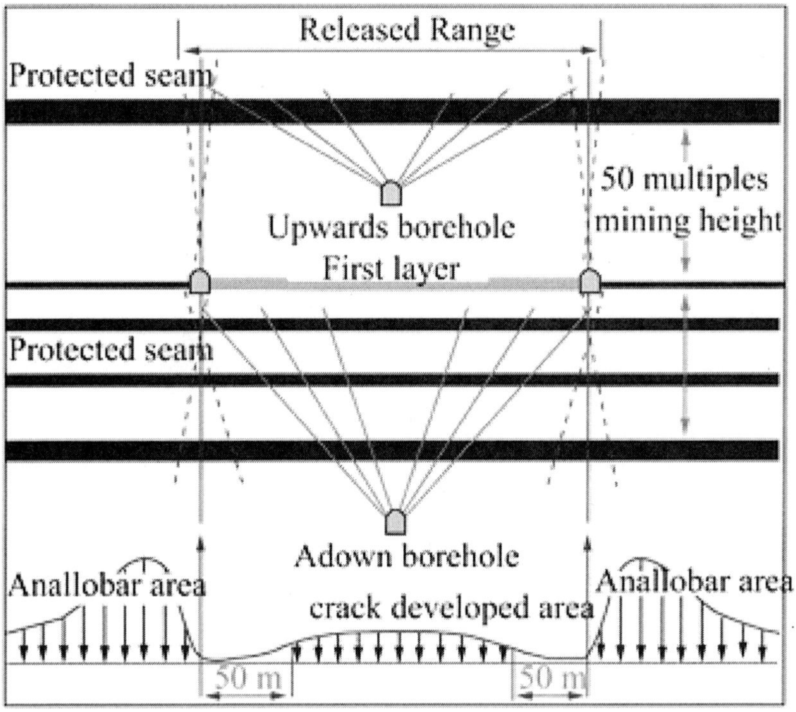


**Figure 5.** De-stressed gas drainage system

## 4.3 Pillarless extraction of coal and gas

With the use of a Y-type ventilation system, the coal in front of the working face in the first seam is mined, while gas from both the protective and protected seams is extracted through boreholes drilled in the retained roadways. In this way, integrated coal production and gas extraction is achieved. The extracted gas is separated into high- and low-purity components, and transported to the surface for use in electric power plants and domestic cooking and heating, respectively.

Depending on the location of the gas-rich zones, boreholes in the retained roadway can be drilled up- and/or downward to target the gas-rich zones in both overlying and underlying strata. The pillarless extraction of coal and gas is schematically shown in Fig. 6.

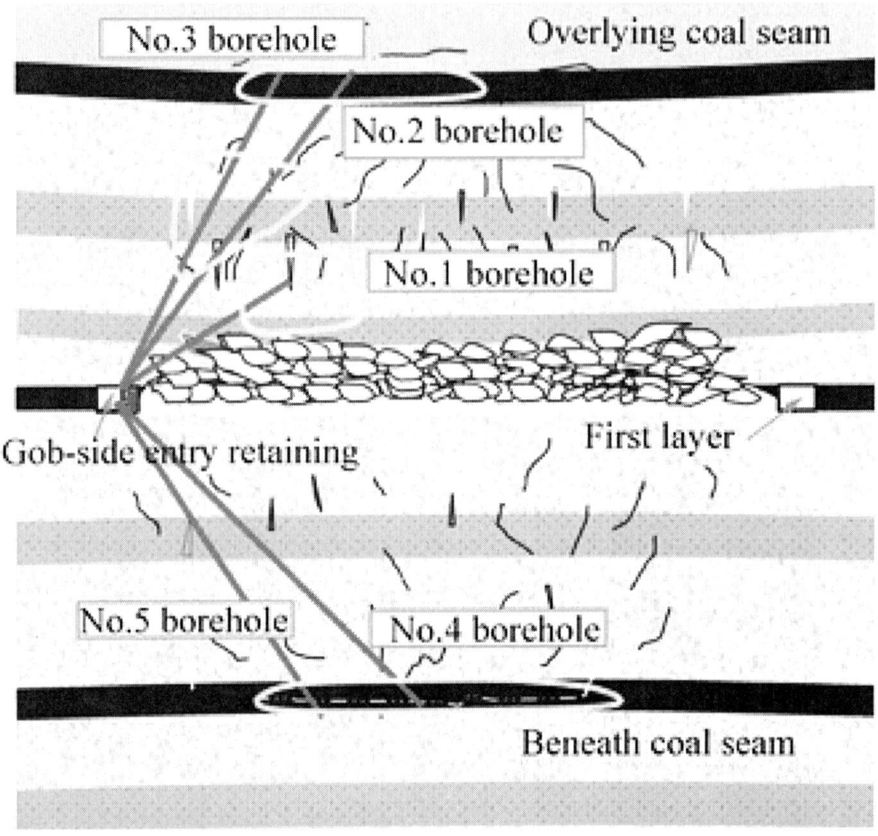


**Figure 6.**Pillarless extraction of coal and gas

## 4.4 Innovative research methods

A large-scale physical model has been developed for fundamental research into integrated coal production and gas extraction, as shown in Fig. 7. The main components of the model include an outburst simulation instrument, an excavation system, a data monitoring and recording system, a dynamic data-analyzing system, and a virtual early-warning system. The geometric dimensions of the model are 3000 mm × 3500 mm × 2000 mm (length × width × height) and it can be easily transported. Large-scale geomechanical tests can be implemented with advanced monitoring systems to study integrated coal and gas production in seams with low permeability. Development and evolution of the stress and fracture zones in a retained roadway and in overlying or underlying seams with pillarless mining can be investigated under various stress, geological, and excavation conditions.

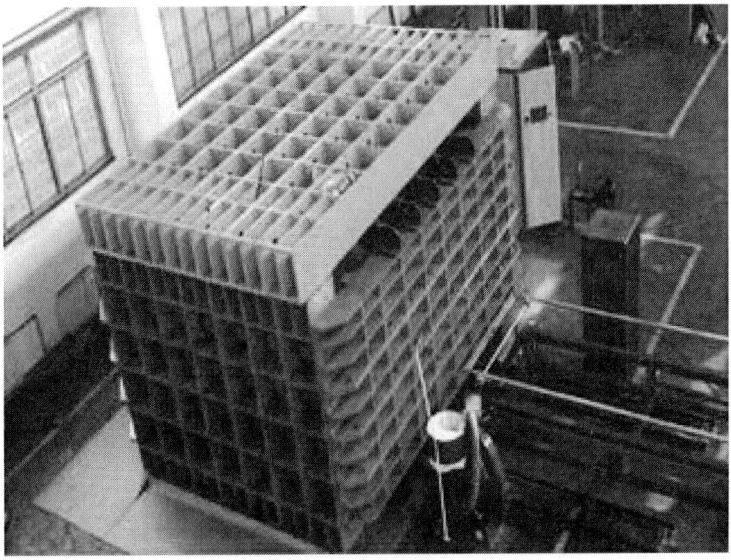

(a) 3D model

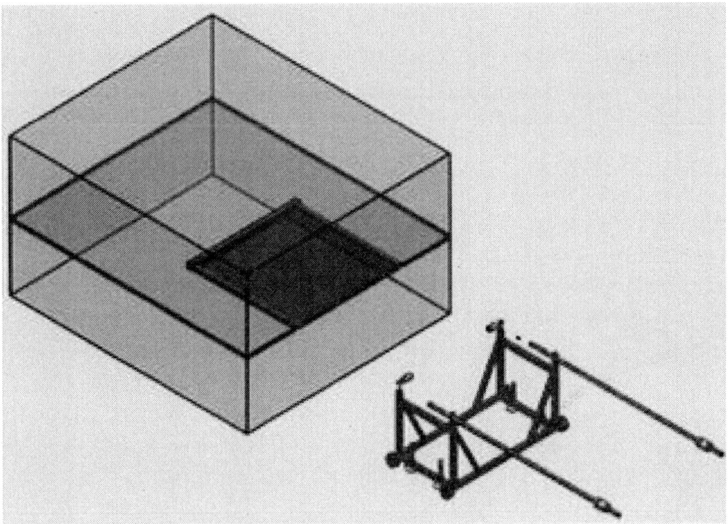

(b) Excavation system

**Figure 7.** Large-scale physical model for simulation of coal and gas extraction

# 5 OPERATING PRACTICE

The core ideas relating to the integrated extraction of coal and gas are consistent with scientific, efficient, and practical engineering principles. Coal resources in China differ vastly in the nature of their deposition; the theoretical and technological innovations with respect to integrated extraction of coal and gas take different deposition conditions and different mining methods into account.

Integrated extraction of coal and gas originated in the Huainan coal mining group. Huainan was once one of the areas with the most serious gas outburst and explosion hazards in the Chinese coal industry. Because of the high gas content and low permeability of coal seams in Huainan, innovative methods were developed to enhance seam permeability to resolve these issues. Coal permeability is improved by mining-induced de-stressing, thereby enabling the integrated extraction of coal and gas. These technological developments have completely prevented the reoccurrence of gas explosion accidents and greatly improved coal productivity and gas extraction efficiency. All coal mines in Huainan now simultaneously extract coal and gas. Annual gas extraction from the mines is about 500 $Mm^3$.

The successful demonstration of this technology in Huainan played an important role in resolving gas control in other gas-containing Chinese coal mines. It has been applied in Shanxi, Henan, Shanxi, Heilongjiang, Hebei, Xinjiang, and other major coal-producing provinces. Coal production from mines using this technology is some 21 billion tons.

As a first example, the geological conditions of the Shaqu coal mine in Shanxi province are very complex and it is one of the highest gas-emitting mines in China. The gas content is 29 $m^3/t$, the pressure is up to 2.4 MPa, and the absolute gas gushing quantity is 473 $m^3/min$. In 2008, the gas concentration exceeded the statutory limit in 3635 incidents, in each incident exceeding a concentration of 2.5 % (Yuan 2008c). In the 6 years prior to 2012, coal production was about 200 Mt (design capacity was 300 Mt), and production capacity was seriously restricted by this gas problem. Integrated extraction of coal and gas was implemented in 2011, with comprehensive gas-control measures, such as protective mining, progressive drainage, Y-type ventilation, expansion of the gas extraction system, underground gas drainage from retained roadways, surface well drainage, and gas use. By the end of 2012, the number of gas incidents had dropped to five, and none occurred in 2013.

The second example is the successful implementation of integrated coal production and gas extraction with pillarless mining in the 1205 working face of the Zhongxing coal mine, Fenxi Coal Mining Group. This mine comprises typical "three soft" multiple coal seams with close intervals and composite fragmented thick roof conditions. Field observations indicate that the retained roadway (cross-sectional area of 12 $m^2$) is well maintained and its cross-sectional shrinkage is only 11.11 %. The average gas extraction from the working face is 43.17 % and the average gas concentration at the tail entry is 0.33 %, indicating of the effective gas extraction of the mine.

A third example is the successful application of integrated coal production and gas extraction at the working face 154,307 (with thick and hard roof conditions) of the Fenghuangshan coal mine, Jincheng Coal Group. The overlying seam of the mine was outburst-prone and the accumulated gas needed to be drained. Gas drainage is carried out through boreholes in the retained roadway of the working face, arranged in the overlying seam and supplemented by surface drainage wells. Field observations show that the number of gas incidents dropped by 88 % and the risk of outbursts in the overlying seam was eliminated.

As a final example, the mining depth of the working face in the Henan Pingdingshan Coal Group was 1100 m and the retained roadway was under conditions of high stress with a thick, hard roof. The roadway floor seriously heaved, and the abutment stress resulting from sudden breaking of a large area of overhanging roof in the working face was very high. Various measures were taken to resolve these issues. Roof stress was relieved by pre-splitting explosion with roof long boreholes and the "three high and one strong" support technique was used to control roadway stability. In addition, a Y-shaped ventilation system, gas drainage boreholes arranged in the de-stressed seams, development of a new high-strength material for the packing wall, and the use of a mechanized filling technique to build the packing wall were also implemented.

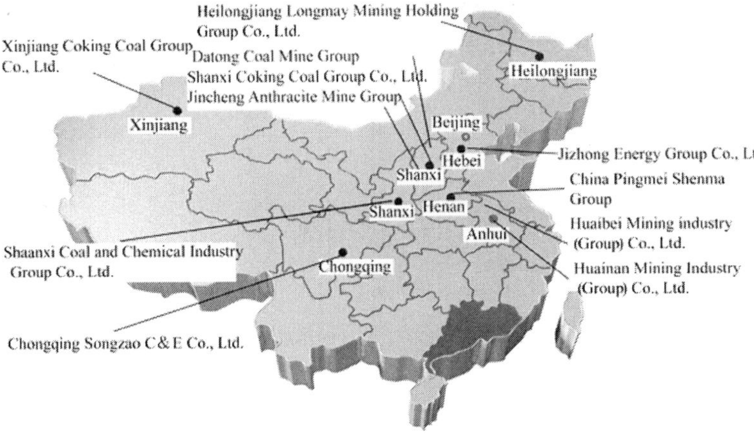


**Figure 8.** Chinese coal mines practicing integrated extraction of coal and gas

These achievements provide robust technical support for the extraction of deep coal and gas resources. Figure 8 shows the Chinese coal mines in which integrated extraction of coal and gas is applied.

# 6 CONCLUSIONS

China has rich coal resources. With increasing energy consumption and a greater demand for a cleaner environment, integrated coal production and gas extraction will play an increasingly important role. As demonstrated over the last 10 years in Huainan and other mines with similar conditions, integrated production of coal and gas is probably the only way to make coal mining greener and more scientific. The main theoretical and technological achievements for this technology are summarized as follows:

(1)Dynamic evolution and distribution of mining-induced stress, fracture, and gas flow fields in mining multiple seams of high gas content and low permeability;

(2)Identification of a circular overlying zone for efficient gas extraction;

(3)Excavation of overlying and underlying gas drainage roadways in de-stressed fractured zones induced by mining the first (protective) seam;

(4)Pillar mining with a retained roadway and Y-type ventilation;

(5)Gas drainage via boreholes drilled in the retained roadway into gas-rich zones in overlying and underlying strata.

Implementation of integrated coal and gas production can not only secure energy supply for sustainable economic development in China, but also enhances the scientific and technological level of China's coal mining industry. Further theoretical and technological research is required to make coal mining greener, more scientific, and more efficient.

# REFERENCES

1. Cheng YP, Yu QX, Yuan L (2004) Experimental research on coal and gas safely and efficiently remote relief exploitation. J China Univ Mining Technol 33(2):132–136
2. Cheng YP, Zhou DY, Yu QX (2006) Research on protection layer relief gas drainage and emission laws. J Mining Saf Eng 23(1):12–18
3. Creedy DP, Garner K, Holloway S et al (2001) A review of the worldwide status of coalbed methane extraction and utilisation. Report No. COAL R210, DTI/Pub URN 01/1040

4. Fields HH (1973) Degasfication through vertical shafts. In: Methane Control in Eastern U.S. oal ines. United States Department of Interior & Bureau of Mines Information Circular IC 8621, 25–38

5. Garcia F, Cervik J (1985) Methane control on longwalls with corss-measure boreholes. Report of Investigations 8985, United States Department of the Interior

6. Hargraves AJ, Martin CH (1993) Australasian coal mining practice. The Australasian Institute of Mining and Metallurgy

7. Li SG, Shi PW, Qian MG (1999) Research on overburden elliptical parabolic crack with dynamic distribution. Ground Press Strata Control 3–4:44–46

8. Michael B (2007) High performance longwall mining in deep and methane rich coal deposits in Germany taking into account methods and technologies for controlling the estimated gas liberation. In: Proceeding of 2007 China (Huainan) international symposium on coal gas control technology, Huainan, China, 57–75

9. Noack K (1998) Control of gas emissions in underground coal mines. Int J Coal Geol 35:57–82

10. Noack K, Koppe U, Kunz E (1995) Control of high gas emissions in underground coal mines. In: International symposium workshop on Management and Control of High Gas Emissions and Outbursts in Underground Coal Mines. 20–24 March, Wollongong, Australia, 16–24

11. Palchik V (2005) Localization of mining-induced horizontal fractures along rock layer interfaces in overburden: field measurements and prediction. Environ Geol 48:68–80

12. Qian MG, Liu XC (1984) Mine pressure and control. China Coal Industry Publishing House, Beijing

13. Qian MG, Shi PW (2003) Mining pressure and strata control. China University of Mining & Technology Press, Xuzhou

14. Qian MG, Xu JL (1998) Research on overburden fracture distribution "O" ring features. J China Coal Soc 23(5):466–469

15. Song ZQ (1988) Practical mine pressure. China University of Mining & Technology Press, Xuzhou

16. Steven S, Bruce A, Crosdale P et al (2007) Coal petrology and coal seam gas contents of the Walloon Subgroup-Surat Basin, Queensland, Australia. Int J Coal Geol 70:209–222

17. Unver B, Yasitli EE (2005) Modelling of strata movement with a special reference to caving mechanism in thick seam coal mining. Int J Coal Geol 66(4):227–252

18. Usanov SV, Mel'nik VV, Zamyatin AL (2014) Monitoring rock mass transformation under induced movements. J Min Sci 49(6):913–918

19. USEPA (1998) Coalbed methane recovery and electric power generation project-opportunity at the Wesola Mine Myslowice, Poland

20. USEPA (1999) White paper: guidebook on coalbed methane drainage for underground coal mines

21. Xie HP, Peng S, He M (2006) Deep mining basic theory and engineering practice. Science Press, Beijing

22. Yu QX (1984) Gas prevention in coalmine. China University of Mining & Technology Press, Xuzhou

23. Yuan L (2008a) Key technique of safe mining in low permeability and methane-rich seam group. Chin J Rock Mech Eng 27(7):1370–1379

24. Yuan L (2008b) Theory and practice of integrated pillarless coal production and methane extraction in multi-seams of low permeability. China Coal Industry Publishing House, Beijing

25. Yuan L (2008c) Gas distribution of the mined-out side and extraction technology of first mined key seam relief-mining in gassy multiseams of low permeability. J China Coal Soc 33(12):1362–1367

26. Yuan L (2009a) Theory of pressure-relieved gas extraction and technique system of integrated coal production and gas extraction. J China Coal Soc 34(1):1–8

27. Yuan L (2009b) Theory and practice of integrated pillarless coal production and methane extraction in multiseams of low permeability. Eng Sci 11(5):72–80

28. Yuan L (2010) Concept of gas control and simultaneous extraction of coal and gas. China Coal 6:5–12

29. Yuan L, Guo H, Shen BT, Qu QB, Xue JH (2011a) Circular overlying zone at longwall panel for efficient methane capture of mutiple coal seams with low permeability. J China Coal Soc 36(3):357–365

30. Yuan L, Xue JH, Liu QS, Liu B (2011b) Surrounding rock stability control theory and support technique in deep rock roadway for coal mine. J China Coal Soc 36(4):535–543

# Chapter 2

# Development and Application of an Efficient Gas Extraction Model for Low-Rank High-Gas Coal Beds

**Baiquan Lin[1,2] • He Li[1,2] • Desheng Yuan[1,2,3] • Ziwen Li[1,2]**

[1] *The State Key Laboratory of Coal Resources and Mine Safety, China University of Mining and Technology, Xuzhou 221008, China*

[2] *Faculty of Safety Engineering, China University of Mining and Technology, Xuzhou 221008, China*

[3] *Shaanxi Binchang Mining Group Co., Ltd., Xianyang 721000, China*

## ABSTRACT

To promote gas extraction in low-rank high-gas coal beds, the pore structure characteristics of the coal and their effect on gas desorption were studied. The results show that micropores are relatively rare in low-rank coal; mesopores are usually semi-open and inkpot-shaped whereas macropores are usually slit-shaped. Gas desorption is relatively easy at high-pressure stages, whereas it is difficult at low-pressure stages because of the 'bottleneck effect' of the semi-open inkpot-shaped mesopores. A 'two-three-two' gas extraction model was established following experimental analysis and engineering practice applied in the Binchang mining area. In this model, gas extraction is divided into three periods: a planning period, a transitional period and a production period. In each period, surface extraction and underground extraction are performed simultaneously, and pressure-relief extraction and conventional extraction are coupled to each other. After applying this model, the gas extraction rate rose to 78.8 %.

**Keywords:** Low-rank coal Pore structure Gas extraction Inkpot-shaped pore

# 1 INTRODUCTION

Underground gas extraction has been a conventional method to guarantee safe production in high-gas coal beds in China (Lin 2010). Since the 1980s, coalbed methane extraction through surface wells has been popular in China, achieving the simultaneous extraction of coal and gas (Li et al. 2014). At present, the exploitation of coalbed methane in China is concentrated in medium- and high-rank coalfields. Research in low-rank coalbed methane extraction is immature (Qiao 2009). Owing to advances in low-rank methane exploitation in the Powder River Basin, Raton Basin and Alberta Basin, the economic value of low-rank coalbed methane increased (Fu et al. 2006; Sun et al. 2009; Ye et al. 2009). In China, coalbed methane resources in low-rank coalfields account for 47 % of the gross amount (Liu and Gao 2014). A typical low-rank coal bed is characterized by multiple layers, large thicknesses, high permeability and low gas content. The huge reserve of coal can be offset by its poor gas content, and thus coalbed methane from low-rank coal has good prospects for future development (Han 1980).

Coalbed methane is a natural gas resource adsorbed within a coal reservoir. Its production must involve a depressurization desorption stage (Qin et al. 2012). In addition, the geological carrier of coalbed methane, coal itself, is an important source of energy. How to break the limitations of the two independent industries involved with surface and underground gas extraction, and how to organically coordinate the safety of coal mining and the high-efficiency exploitation of coalbed methane, are problems of efficient gas extraction in high-gas coal beds.

The Binchang Jurassic coalfield area is located on the southwest margin of the Erdos basin. It is one of the most promising low-rank mining areas in China (Liu et al. 2011; Tian et al. 2012). Coal and gas reserves in the Binchang mining area reach $5.03 \times 10^9$ tons and $9.75 \times 10^9$ $m^3$, respectively. However, as the mining area extends, gas emissions have become a growing problem that seriously restricts coal production. Therefore, coalbed methane must be efficiently extracted. In this paper, the pore structure characteristic of the Jurassic low-rank coal in the Binchang mining area and its effect on gas desorption were studied by means of maceral experiments, vitrinite reflectance experiments, liquid nitrogen and carbon dioxide adsorption experiments and mercury injection experiments. A 'two-three-two' gas extraction model has been proposed by summarizing experimental analysis and engineering practices.

# 2 MICROSTRUCTURAL CHARACTERISTICS OF JURASSIC LOW-RANK COAL

## 2.1 Petrographic characteristics of Jurassic low-rank coal

The microscopic petrographic properties of coal are key parameters that characterize its metamorphic grade. Differences in coal maceral determine the pore size and distribution. Additionally, it also affects the adsorption and desorption of gas (Duan et al. 2009a, b). Six coal samples collected from different coal mines were selected for this experiment. Their maceral and vitrinite reflectance analyses are listed in Table 1.

**Table 1.** Results of the maceral and vitrinite reflectance experiments

| Coal samples | Buried depth (m) | Vitrinite (%) | Inertinite (%) | Exinite (%) | Minerals (%) | $R_{o,max}$ (%) | Coal rank | Metamorphic grade |
|---|---|---|---|---|---|---|---|---|
| Dafosi | 475 | 42.67 | 55.68 | 0 | 1.65 | 0.76 | Bitumite C | Low |
| Yuanzhuang | 490 | 63.68 | 34.29 | 0 | 2.03 | 0.89 | Bitumite C | Low |
| Xinyu | 258 | 77.10 | 22.13 | 0 | 0.77 | 1.36 | Bitumite B | Medium |
| Pingdingshan No. 4 coal | 800 | 80.21 | 11.68 | 6.93 | 1.18 | 1.83 | Bitumite A | Medium |
| Pingdingshan No. 8 coal | 720 | 82.96 | 9.57 | 6.07 | 1.40 | 1.90 | Bitumite A | Medium |
| Guqiao | 956 | 86.80 | 10.67 | 0 | 2.53 | 2.06 | Anthracite C | High |

As listed in Table 1, the vitrinite reflectance of coal samples of the Dafosi Coal Mine and Yuanzhuang Coal Mine is 0.76 and 0.89, respectively, which means the samples are from low-rank coals. The vitrinite reflectance of samples from the Guqiao Coal Mine is 2.06, thus the samples are high-rank coals. The rest of the samples are medium-rank coals. It has been indicated (Qin and Ye 1999) that more vitrinite in coal corresponds to a better adsorption capacity of gas because the vitrinite contains significant numbers of micropores that can provide huge specific surface areas for gas absorption. The vitrinite content of coal samples from the Dafosi Coal Mine is 42.67 %, much lower than that of the medium- and high-rank coal. Thus, the gas adsorption capacity of the low-rank coal is weak.

## 2.2 Pore structure characteristics of Jurassic low-rank coal

The gas adsorption capacity of coal is closely related to its specific surface area, and the specific surface area is dominated by its pore structure characteristics (Li et al. 2014). To assess the pore structure characteristics of Jurassic low-rank coal, gas adsorption experiments and mercury injection experiments were conducted.

Coal samples (0.2–0.25 mm in size) and an ASAP-2000 absorption instrument were selected to conduct low-temperature liquid nitrogen adsorption experiments that aimed to investigate the distribution of micropores and mesopores. The testing temperature was 77 K and the relative pressure was 0.050 to 0.995. As the diffusion of nitrogen molecules in micropores under low temperature conditions is slow, results from micropore distributions are not accurate. Thus, the $CO_2$ adsorption experiments were conducted as a supplement to study the distribution of micropores. In the $CO_2$ adsorption experiments, the AUTOSORB-1 absorption instrument ran at 273 K. The results of the gas adsorption experiments are illustrated in Tables 2 and 3, and the liquid nitrogen adsorption and desorption curves are presented in Fig. 1.

**Table 2.** Results of low-temperature nitrogen adsorption experiments

| Coal samples | Total surface area ($m^2/g$) | Mean pore size (nm) | Pore volume ($\times 10^{-3}$ mL/g) | | | |
|---|---|---|---|---|---|---|
| | | | Total | Micropore | Mesopore | Macropore |
| Dafosi | 4.65 | 11.40 | 8.34 | 0.51 | 4.68 | 3.05 |
| Xinyu | 1.62 | 10.33 | 2.35 | 0.12 | 1.36 | 0.87 |
| Pingdingshan No.8 | 4.46 | 5.75 | 7.92 | 0.38 | 3.96 | 3.58 |
| Guqiao | 3.32 | 4.70 | 6.42 | 0.39 | 3.54 | 2.49 |

**Table 3.** Results of the $CO_2$ adsorption experiments

| Coal samples | Volume ($\times 10^{-3}$ mL/g) | Superficial area ($m^2/g$) | Mean pore size (nm) |
|---|---|---|---|
| Dafosi | 2.39 | 21.84 | 0.60 |
| Xinyu | 2.65 | 26.07 | 0.84 |
| Pingdingshan No. 8 | 3.18 | 39.30 | 0.55 |
| Guqiao | 3.46 | 41.06 | 0.79 |

Table 2 indicates that the pore volume, and especially the mesopore volume, of Jurassic low-rank coal is relatively large, and can thereby provide broad spaces for gas adsorption. However, the surface area of micropores in the Jurassic low-rank coal is relatively small, which impedes gas adsorption in low-pressure stages.

Figure 1 illustrates that the gas adsorption of Jurassic low-rank coal increases slowly under low pressure. Conversely as the pressure increases ($P/P_0 > 0.5$), an adsorption hysteresis loop appears within all samples. The appearance of the adsorption hysteresis loop mainly depends on the capillary condensation that occurs on the solid surface. The adsorption hysteresis loops of different coal samples vary considerably, indicating different pore structure characteristic effects on gas adsorption (Jiang et al. 2011). According to the shape of pores, the adsorption hysteresis loop can be divided into four categories (Kondo et al. 2006). As shown in Fig. 1, the adsorption hysteresis loop for Jurassic low-rank coal emerges under pressures of 0.5–0.8 and

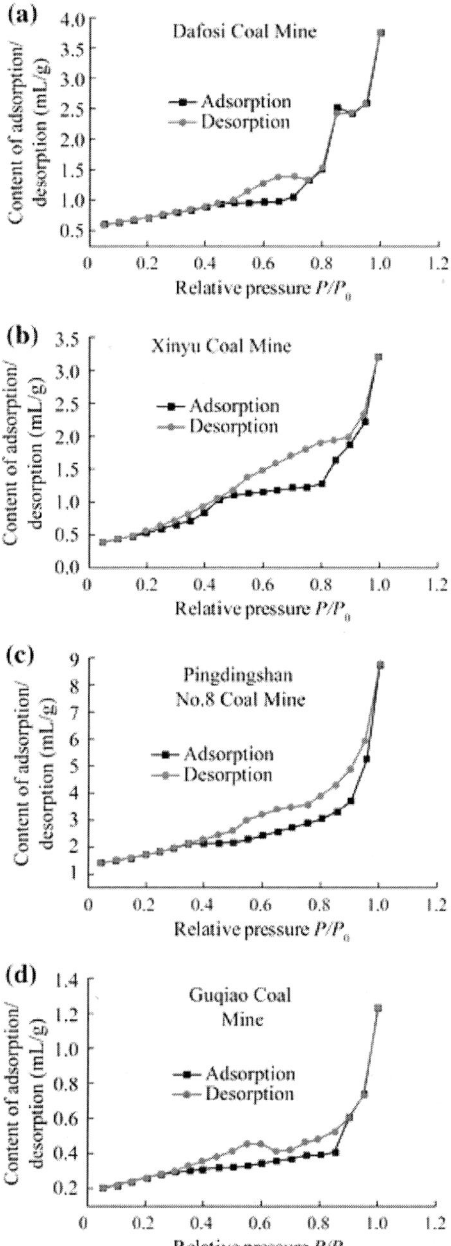


**Figure 1.** Nitrogen adsorption/desorption curves

gradually disappears as the pressure increases. This phenomenon confirms that mesopores in low-rank coal samples usually have semi-open inkpot-shapes and macropores are usually slit-shaped. Curves for medium- and high-rank coal samples indicate that the samples contain numerous wedge-shaped and slit-shaped pores, which contribute greatly to gas desorption.

To assess the distribution of macropores, mercury injection experiments were conducted to obtain the pore size distribution, specific surface area, permeability and porosity of the coal. The experimental results are shown in Table 4, and the pore size distribution is shown in Fig. 2.

**Table 4.** Results of the mercury injection experiments

| Coal samples | Dafosi | Pingdingshan No. 8 coal | Guqiao | Xinyu |
|---|---|---|---|---|
| Pore volume (mL/g) | 0.1194 | 0.0237 | 0.0342 | 0.0435 |
| Specific surface area ($m^2/g$) | 42.317 | 12.668 | 19.178 | 20.205 |
| Mean pore size (nm) | 11.3 | 7.5 | 7.1 | 8.6 |
| Apparent density (g/mL) | 1.1264 | 1.3206 | 1.2008 | 1.1752 |
| Skeletal density (g/mL) | 1.3014 | 1.3633 | 1.2521 | 1.2386 |
| Porosity (%) | 13.4486 | 3.1340 | 4.1017 | 5.1173 |
| Permeability (mD) | 10.3368 | 2.9158 | 5.8122 | 7.6307 |

Figure 2 shows that the pore size of Jurassic low-rank coal is characterized by a bimodal distribution of mesopores and macropores. The peak pore size of the mesopores and macropores is 10 nm and 70 nm, respectively. In contrast, the pore size of medium- and high-rank coal shows a unimodal distribution with smaller magnitude. The mercury injection experiments indicate that the pore volume and specific surface area reach 0.1194 mL/g and 42.317 $m^2/g$, respectively. These properties are significantly higher than those of medium- and high-rank coal samples. Moreover, the permeability and porosity of low-rank coal are relatively high. Larger pore volume and specific surface area are conducive to gas storage and aggregation, whereas higher permeability will promote gas flow in the coal seam.

# 3 EFFECT OF GAS DESORPTION IN JURASSIC LOW-RANK COAL BEDS

The proportion of mesopores and macropores in coal samples, as shown in Fig. 3, can be obtained from the gas adsorption experiments and mercury injection experiments.

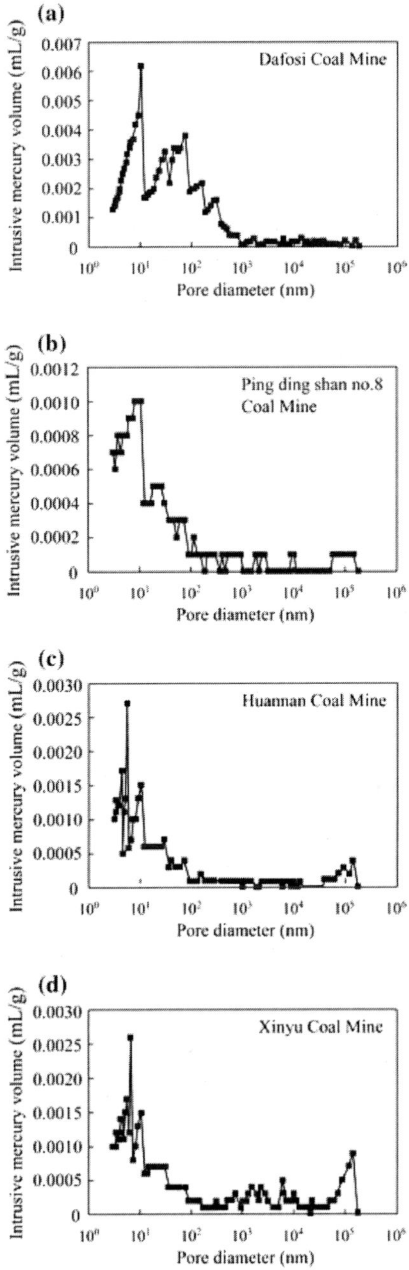


**Figure 2.** Pore size distribution of coal samples

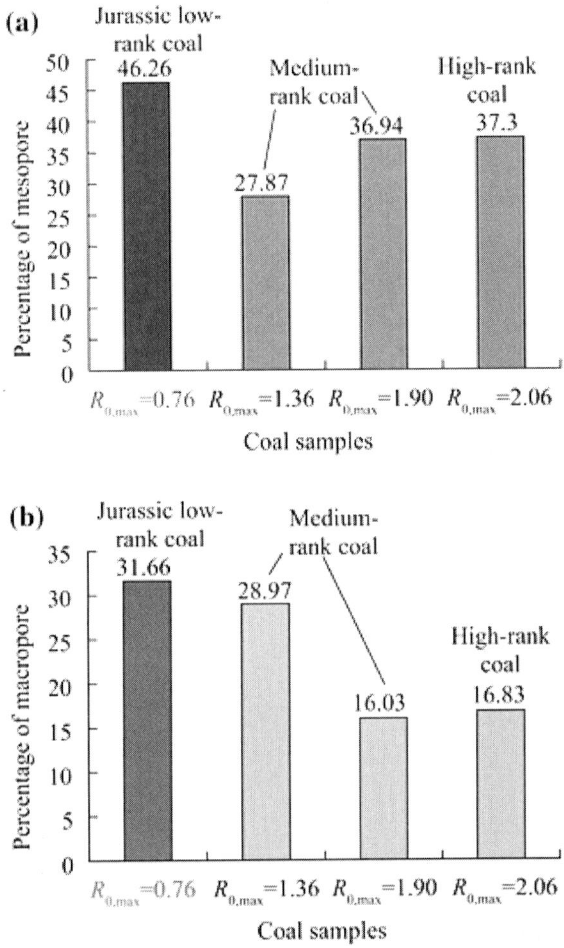


**Figure 3.** Proportion of mesopores and macropores in coal samples

Figure 3a illustrates that the proportion of the slit-shaped macropores in Jurassic low-rank coal reaches 31.66 % and the permeability of macropores reaches 10.34 mD, which promotes gas flow in high-pressure stages. However, the percentage of the slit-shaped macropores in medium- and high-rank coals is relatively small. Figure 3b illustrates that semi-open inkpot-shaped mesopores in Jurassic low-rank coal account for 46.26 % of the total, which is significantly higher than that of the medium- and high-rank coal samples. Gas desorption at low-pressure stages is restricted by the ‘bottleneck effect’ of the semi-open inkpot-shaped mesopores and further weakens gas extraction.

Micropores are rarely developed in low-rank coal; mesopores are dominated by semi-open inkpot shapes whereas macropores are usually slit-shaped. The special pore structure of Jurassic low-rank coal results in a 'multi-stage controlling effect' on gas desorption. Gas desorption at high-pressure stages is mainly dominated by the slit-shaped macropores; gas can be rapidly released with large flow rates and high concentrations. Because gas desorption at low-pressure stages is mainly dominated by semi-open inkpot-shaped mesopores, gas desorption is severely limited; the flow rate and concentration decay rapidly with abrupt mutations. Such uneven extraction would lead to a large amount of remanent gas, greatly restricting the simultaneous extraction of coal and gas. Therefore, it is essential to establish an efficient gas extraction model to realize the stepped exploitation of gas.

## 4 GAS EXTRACTION MODEL FOR LOW-RANK HIGH-GAS COAL BEDS

### 4.1 'Two-three-two' gas extraction model

On the basis of the special pore structure of Jurassic low-rank coal and the space–time replacement law for coal production, a 'two-three-two' gas extraction model was proposed (Fig. 4). In this model, gas extraction is divided into three periods: a planning period, a transitional period and a production period. In each period, surface extraction and underground extraction are performed simultaneously, and pressure-relief and conventional extraction are coupled to each other. Using this model, surface well gas extraction was first applied in the Dafosi Coal Mine in December 2009. Gas extraction maintained high efficiency in the early period of the engineering project, and the highest daily output of an individual well reached 16 582.3 $m^3$. However, as time went on, the coal bed entered a low-pressure stage. Gas desorption becomes more and more difficult and the gas extraction quantity rapidly decays. Thus, underground extraction is extremely urgent to debase the gas content of the coal seam.

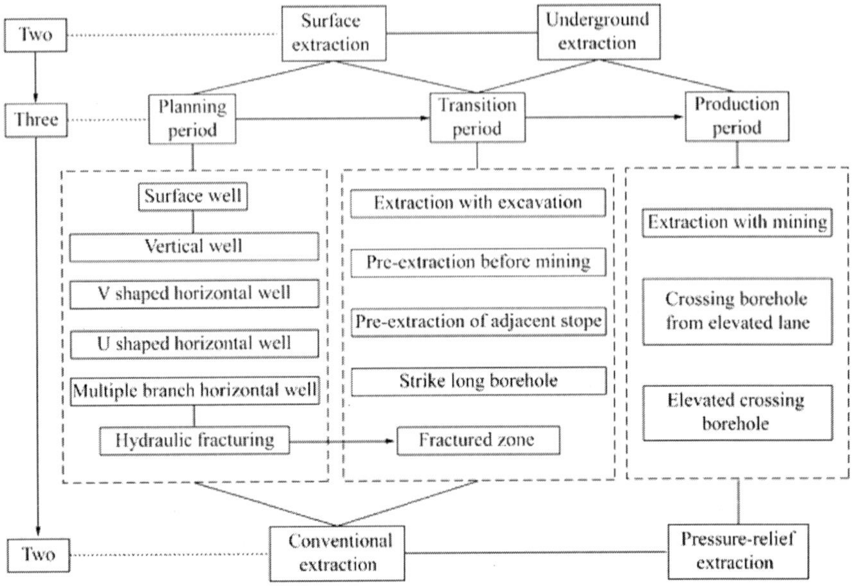


**Figure 4.** The 'two-three-two' model of gas extraction in low-rank high-gas coal beds

The planning period corresponds to the 5–10 years prior to the underground exploitation of the coal mine. In this period, large quantities of surface wells would be arranged to pre-extract the coalbed methane. The arrangement of the surface wells (type, orientation and density) should coordinate with factors of geology, geography and resource. Well densification or multiple-branch horizontal wells should be applied in gas-rich area. At the meantime, the relative location of surface wells and underground roadways should also be taken into consideration to avoid any adverse effects on coal production. After the well drilling has been completed, hydraulic fracturing would be adopted to form a fractured zone in the coal seam. At high-pressure stages, large quantities of gas were desorbed and extracted through the fractured zone and the wells. When the decay of the gas-extraction quantity occurs, the gas extraction enters the transitional period.

The transitional period corresponds to the underground exploitation period, when roadways are gradually constructed while coal mining is not being carried out. As the pre-extraction area is full of the original coal mass that has not been induced by mining, fractures are gradually closed under in situ stress and, as a result, gas flow is hampered. At this point, long horizontally striking boreholes should be drilled from roadways along the coal seam to intersect the fractured zone, forming a local stripped pressure-relief zone.

The surface wells together with long boreholes jointly extract gas. In addition, extraction by excavation, pre-extraction before mining and pre-extraction of adjacent panels should also be carried out to eliminate blank areas of gas extraction.

The formation of the mining face marks the beginning of the production period, when the decrease of gas-extraction in surface wells and long boreholes runs counter to the urgent demands of production. During the planning and transitional periods, the geostress is relatively high and fracture development is weak. Limited effects of gas extraction can be achieved. Therefore, the pressure-relief effects induced by mining should be taken advantage of in the production period. Additionally, crossing boreholes from elevated lanes should be undertaken to avoid gas overrunning at the mining face.

## 4.2 Staged division of gas extraction

To assess the efficiency of gas extraction over different periods, a mathematical model of the permissive coal-bed gas content for safe coal mining was established considering factors such as coal-bed gas geology, coal mining activity and mine ventilation (Qin et al. 2007):

$$C = C_{\mathrm{ic}}(1 - R) + \beta\varepsilon \frac{M_{\mathrm{c}} S_{\mathrm{h}} v_{\mathrm{h}}}{nP}, \qquad (1)$$

where $C_{ic}$ is the original gas content of the coal bed ($m^3$/t); $R$ is the gas desorption ratio (%); $\beta$ is the recovery ratio of coal resource (%); $\varepsilon$ is a combined influence factor; $M_c$ is the permitted volume fraction of gas in the ventilation roadway (%); $S_h$ is the sectional area of the ventilation roadway ($m^2$); $v_h$ is the permitted air speed in the ventilation roadway (m/s); $n$ is the ratio of the affected distance in front of the excavation face to the excavation speed; and $P$ is the coal production (t/s).

After substitution of the relevant parameters from the Dafosi Coal Mine into Eq. (1), a division criterion for gas extraction can be obtained (Fig. 5). According to the gas extraction rate of the Dafosi Coal Mine (73.2 %), the proportion of gas extraction periods can be calculated: 3.2 %–6.6 % for the planning period (with an average of 4.9 %), 17.3 %–22.3 % for the transitional period (with an average of 19.8 %), and 47.8 %–49.3 % for the production period (average of 48.5 %). The proportions of gas extraction in the Dafosi Coal Mine are shown in Fig. 6. Note that the production can be dynamically adjusted by the mining deployment and geological conditions. Therefore, we can form a flexible and efficient gas extraction system.

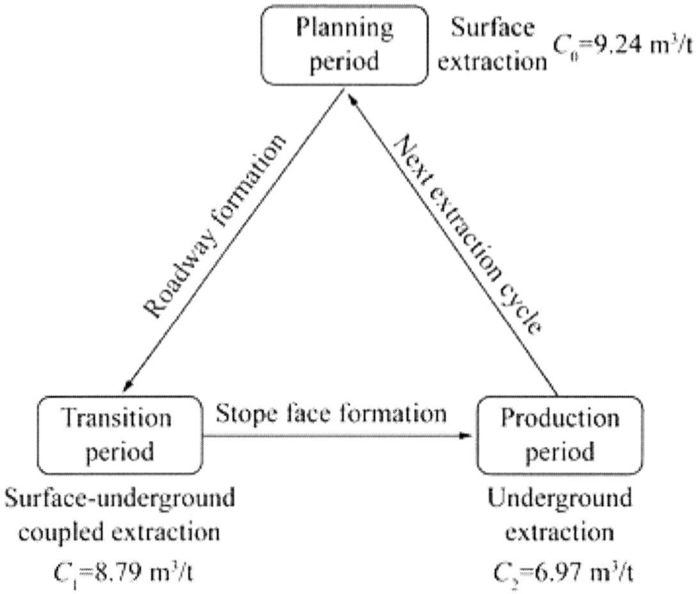


**Figure 5.** Staged division of gas extraction in the Dafosi Coal Mine

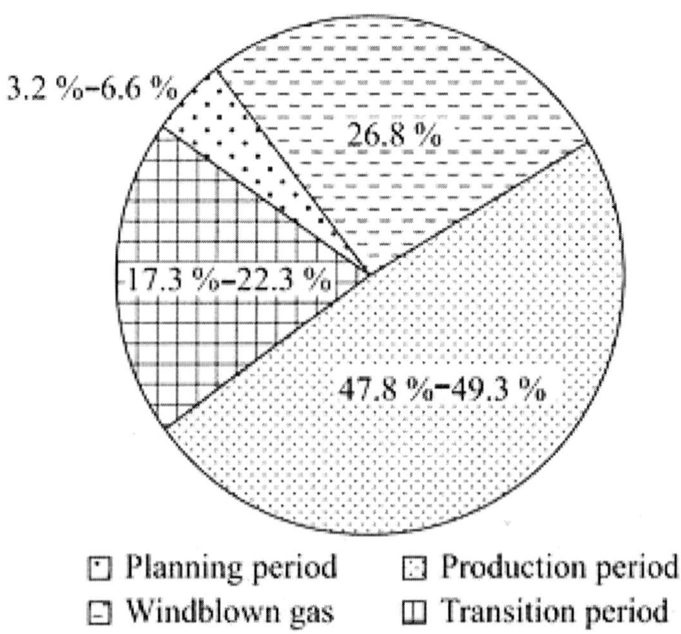


**Figure 6.** Proportions of gas extraction in the Dafosi Coal Mine

# 5 APPLICATIONS

In this section, the gas extraction effect of the 'two-three-two' gas extraction model is investigated, taking panel 40110 from the Dafosi Coal Mine as an example. The exploitable reserves, original gas content and total gas content of panel 40110 are 3.55 × $10^6$ tons, 9.2 $m^3/t$ and 32.66 × $10^6$ $m^3$, respectively. The roadway layout for panel 40110 is illustrated in Fig. 7.

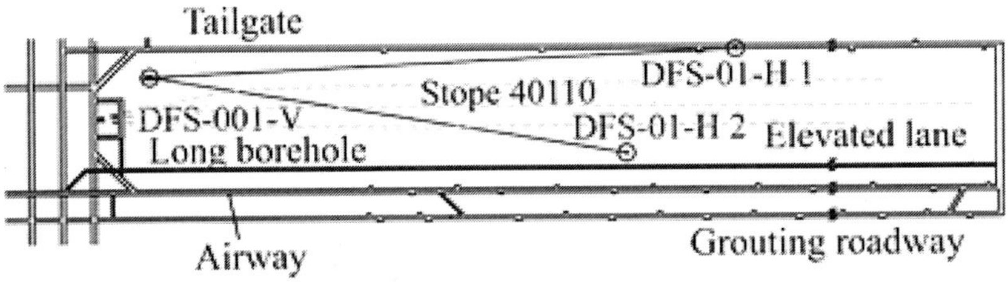


**Figure 7.** Roadway layout of the panel 40110 in the Dafosi Coal Mine

The planning period: DFS-01 surface well covers panel 40110. Gas extraction from this well commenced on 4 July 2009 and ended on 12 March 2011 (a total of 617 days) induced by the mining activities at panel 40108. The cumulative gas production during this period was 416 × $10^3$ $m^3$.

The transitional period: gas extraction during the transitional period consists of the combined extraction from the DFS-01 surface well and the underground long boreholes, the extraction with excavation of the tailgate, airway and grouting roadway of panel and pre-extraction of panel 40110. The total gas production was up to 807 × $10^6$ $m^3$.

The production period: gas extraction during the production period consists of mining panel 40110 and the area of the crossing boreholes from the elevated lane and the grouting roadway. The total gas production was up to 17.23 × $10^6$ $m^3$.

After applying the 'two-three-two' gas extraction model, the gas extraction rate for panel 40110 reached 78.8 %, which exceeds the original rate (73.2 %). The proportion of gas extraction from panel 40110 over the three periods is presented in Fig. 8. Compared with Fig. 6, the proportion of gas extracted in the planning period (1.6 %) is lower than the theoretical value (3.2 %–6.6 %), resulting in an increase in gas extraction rates for the transitional and production periods. The lack of surface extraction may put greater pressure on underground mining. Therefore, we suggest that the surface extraction in this area should be extended or densified.

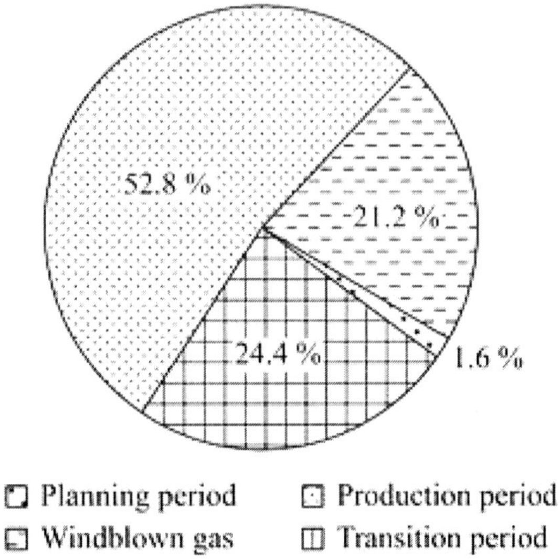


**Figure 8.**Proportions of gas extracted from panel 40110 in the Dafosi Coal Mine

We will investigate the extraction situation for the DFS-02-V surface well in the following section. Coal and gas storage capabilities in the area around this well are $12 \times 10^6$ tons and $110.49 \times 10^6$ $m^3$, respectively. Up to 30 August 2013, the cumulative gas production of this well was $841.63 \times 10^6$ $m^3$. The proportion of gas extracted during the planning period (10.4 %) is higher than the theoretical value (3.2 %–6.6 %). Thus the extraction in the planning period has already risen to the standard quality, and can be attributed to the transitional period. Owing to the large proportion extracted in the planning period, the transitional and production periods can be reduced, appropriately. The quantity of boreholes should be reduced and the extraction duration shortened to affect rapid production.

# 6 CONCLUSIONS

(1)Micropores are relatively rare in low-rank coal; mesopores usually have semi-open inkpot shapes whereas macropores are usually slit-shaped. At high-pressure stages, gas desorption is mainly dominated by the slit-shaped macropores. Gas can be rapidly released with high flow rates and concentrations. In contrast, during low-pressure stages, gas desorption is mainly dominated by the semi-open inkpot-shaped mesopores. Gas desorption is severely limited. Both the flow rate and concentration decay rapidly with abrupt mutations.

(2)A 'two-three-two' gas extraction model was developed based on the combination of experimental analysis and engineering practice in the Binchang mining area. In this model, gas extraction is divided into three periods: a planning period, a transitional period and a production period. In each period, surface and underground extraction are undertaken simultaneously. In addition, pressure-relief and conventional extraction are coupled to each other.

(3)Based on gas extraction rates at the Dafosi Coal Mine, the proportions of gas extraction periods were calculated. After applying the 'two-three-two' gas extraction model, the gas extraction rate for panel 40110 reached 78.8 %. Production can be dynamically adjusted by mining deployments and geological conditions so that a flexible and efficient gas extraction system can be formed.

## ACKNOWLEDGMENTS

The research was supported by the National Basic Research Programme of China (973 Project) (2011CB201205), National Natural Science Foundation of China (51474211), and the National Key Technology R&D Program (2012BAK04B07).

## REFERENCES

1. Duan XQ, Qu JW, Wang ZN (2009a) Pore structure of macerals from a low rank bituminous. J China Univ Min Technol 38(2):224–228
2. Duan XQ, Qu JW, Wang ZN (2009b) Wettability of macerals from low rank bituminous. J China Coal Soc 34(2):243–246
3. Fu XK, Huo YZ, Hu AM, Fan ZQ (2006) Exploration and development of low rank seam coal bed methane in America. China Coal 5:75–76
4. Han DX (1980) Coalfield geology in China, Beijing
5. Jiang WP, Song XZ, Zhong LW (2011) Research on the pore properties of different coal body structure coals and the effects on gas outburst based on the low-temperature nitrogen adsorption method. J China Coal Soc 36(4):609–614
6. Kondo JY, Ishikawa DX, Abe YF (2006) Adsorption Science, Beijing
7. Li ZW, Lin BQ, Hao ZY, Gao YB (2013) Characteristics of pore size distribution of coal and its impacts on gas adsorption. J China Univ Min Technol 6:1047–1053

8. Li GF, Li B, Jiao HB, Liu X (2014) Three-region integrated CBM stereo-extraction in Jincheng mining area. China Coalbed Methane 11(1):3–7

9. Lin BQ (2010) Theory and techniques of coal mine gas control. Xuzhou, China University of Mining and Technology Press

10. Liu Y, Gao XK (2014) Reservoir forming characters of low-rank CBM in Binchang block, Ordos basin. Reserv Eval Dev 4(2):70–75

11. Liu HB, Hu SB, Yin RS, Cao J, Wang F (2011) Occurrence features of coalbed methane of Binchang mining area in Ordos basin. Coal Geol Explor 39(4):20–23

12. Qiao JW (2009) Research on the low rank coal of pore characteristics and desorption laws, Xi'an University of Science and Technology

13. Qin Y, Ye JP (1999) Characteristics and mechanism of gas controlling in the factor of rock physics in China coal reservoir. J China Univ Min Technol 28(1):14–19

14. Qin Y, Wu CF, Hu AM, Yang ZB, Fan ZQ, Ye JP (2007) Mathematical model of permissive coalbed-gas content for safe coal-mining. J China Coal Soc 32(10):1009–1013

15. Qin Y, Yuan L, Hu QT, Ye JP, Hu AM, Shen BH, Cheng YP, He XQ, Zhang SA, Li GF, Zhang Q (2012) Status and development orientation of coal bed methane exploration and development technology in China. Coal Sci Technol 10:1–6

16. Sun P, Wang B, Sun FJ, Zheng GQ, Li GZ, Wang HY, Liu HL, Deng Z (2009) Research on reservoir patterns of low-rank coal-bed methane in China. Acta Petrolei Sin 30(5):648–653

17. Tian C, Tang DZ, Zhou ZJ, Tao S, Chen XZ, Song CL (2012) Hydrogeological characteristics and their control on coalbed methane in Binchang mining area. Coal Geol Explor 40(1):43–46

18. Ye X, Chen CF, Jiang WL, Deng HC, Xu CH (2009) Geological characteristics and new development progress of low rank seam coalbed methane in China. Coal Sci Technol 8:111–115

# Chapter 3

# Comprehensive Technical Support for High-Quality Anthracite Production: A Case Study in the Xinqiao Coal Mine, Yongxia Mining Area, China

**Wei Zhang [1,2], Dongsheng Zhang [3,*], Hongzhi Wang [3] and Jixin Cheng [3]**

[1]*IoT Perception Mine Research Center, China University of Mining & Technology, Xuzhou 221008, China*

[2]*The National and Local Joint Engineering Laboratory of Internet Application Technology on Mine, China University of Mining & Technology, Xuzhou 221008, China*

[3]*School of Mines, China University of Mining & Technology, Xuzhou 221116, China*

## ABSTRACT

The effective production of high-quality anthracite has attracted increasing global attention. Based on the coal occurrence in Yongxia Mining Area and mining conditions of a coalface in Xinqiao Coal Mine, we proposed a systematic study on the technical support for the production of high-quality anthracite. Six key steps were explored, including coal falling at the coalface, transport, underground bunker storage, main shaft hoisting, coal preparation on the ground, and railway wagon loading. The study resulted in optimized running parameters for the shearers, and the rotating patterns of the shearer drums was altered (one-way cutting was employed). Mining height and roof supporting intensity were reduced. Besides, loose presplitting millisecond blasting and mechanized mining were applied to upgrade the coal quantity and the lump coal production rate. Additionally, the coalface end transloading, coalface crush, transport systems, underground storage, and main shaft skip unloading processes were improved, and fragmentation-prevention techniques were used in the washing and railway wagon loading processes. As a result, the lump coal production rate was maintained at a high level and fragmentation was significantly reduced. Because of using the parameters and techniques determined in this research, high-quality coal production and increased profits were achieved. The research results could provide theoretical guidance and methodology for other anthracite production bases.

**Keywords:** coal mining; high-quality anthracite; lump coal production rate; fragmentation-prevention; mining optimization

# 1. INTRODUCTION

As one of six approved domestic anthracite production bases, Yongxia Mining Area (YMA) of Henan Province in China has an intended capacity of 10 million tons yearly. The quantity of anthracite is about 20% of all coal produced, but contributes 45% of total coal income. Despite the poor performance of the coal market over the past three years, anthracite sales have not been plagued with overstocking and sluggish demand. Therefore, it is significant to provide a series of customized technical supports for producing high-quality anthracite.

The Lump coal production rate (LCPR) is a key index of anthracite's quality. Among the various factors affecting the LCPR, physical properties and occurrence conditions of the coal seam are the most important ones [1,2,3]. The LCPR of anthracite has been intensively studied over the past few decades and various reports have been published, all of which can be categorized into the following five aspects:

(1) Reformations of shearer drums [4,5,6,7,8]. Since 1972, attempts have been made to increase the LCPR by enlarging the chipping areas of cutting picks, optimizing their arrangements and improving drum parts in Poland, Russia and China.

(2) Improvements in blasting methods [9,10,11,12,13]. The Cardox blasting technique (CBT) has been widely applied to increase LCPR in Turkey and Colombia. Also, based on the controlled blasting principle, loose control blasting, uncoupled water medium millisecond blasting, and high-pressure gas millisecond blasting have been developed to improve the blasting effect.

(3) Adjustments in mining techniques. Zhao *et al.* [14] proposed a method that combines the blasting mining workface and fully mechanized workface to achieve enhanced LCPR. Song *et al.* [15] proposed a technique involving low cutting depth and fast traction two-way cutting using an AM-500 Shearer (TMM Group, Taiyuan, China), and achieved to enhance LCPR from raw coal. Zhang *et al.* [16] introduced a coal planer (DBT Company, Lünen, Germany) used in the mining of thin coal seam with a thickness of 1 m. The LCPR was increased using effective mining of workface obviously.

(4) Optimizations of transport and storage. Li *et al.* [17] reported a stretchable mini-sized bin to mitigate the high drop damage on coal in the bunker. As a result, lump coal losses were reduced by 6%. Kozan *et al.* [18] proposed a demand-responsive decision support system by integrating the operations of coal shipment, coal stockpiles and coal railing within a whole system. A generic and flexible scheduling optimization method is developed to identify, represent, model, solve and analyze the coal transport problem in a standard and convenient way. Zhang *et al.* [19] reported the air-supported membrane shed as a new building structure for storing coal. Wang *et al.* [20] reported wave-like coal drops with horizontally attached transloading points and spiral coal drops with vertically attached transloading points based on the *in situ* analysis of underground conditions. As a result, the fragmentation of mined anthracite was reduced. Lv *et al.* [21] introduced a massive vertical bunker on-wall buffer system with a unique structure and fixing patterns. Compared with conventional column coal drops placed in the bunker center, this buffer system effectively prevented coal from fragmenting during its dropping process, thus lessening lump coal loss. Liu *et al.* [22] reported an innovative methodology for optimizing the coal train scheduling problem. To construct feasible train schedules, an innovative constructive algorithm called the SLEK algorithm is proposed. To optimise the train schedule, a three-stage hybrid algorithm called the SLEK-BIH-TS algorithm is developed based on the definition of a sophisticated neighbourhood structure under the mechanism of the Best-Insertion-Heuristic algorithm and Tabu Search metaheuristic algorithm. Singh *et al.* [23] described a MILP (Mixed Integer Linear Programming) model for determining the capacity requirements, and the most cost effective capacity improvement initiatives, to meet demand while minimizing the total cost of infrastructure and demurrage. Then, they presented results of computational experiments on the model's performance along with a comparison of the model's output with detailed analyses from the coal chain analysts and planners.

(5) Innovations in coal preparation plants. Wang *et al.* [24] reported that an ultrasonic wave sensor was placed on top of the lump coal buffer bunker, and the work site was equipped with coal level alarms. The dropping height was maintained between 2–3.8 m, and in this way, both the LCPR and safety

were enhanced. Xie *et al.* [25] introduced a sizing crusher (FP5012, ZGME Company, Zhengzhou, China) was used to increase the size uniformity of crushed particles and decrease the over-crushing rate. Chen *et al.* [26] introduced attempts made to adjust the unloading opening size, optimize the separating density, and perform separate storage of filtrated coal. As a result, the LCPR of anthracite has been increased by 4.5%.

In summary, despite great achievements made in producing high-quality anthracite, previous reports focus on only one key step, and few attempts have been made to investigate the entire production process in an integrated way. As we know, underground mining in itself is a complicated process, which is easily affected by several determining factors (e.g., geological conditions, mining techniques, and production systems). Therefore, a significant improvement in the quality of mined anthracite is a systematic undertaking that can only be achieved by modifications in all relevant production links. In other words, overall product quality is determined by the poorest performance of individual processes (Cannikin Law). Based on the occurrence of the coal seam in YMA and the mining conditions of a coalface in Xinqiao Coal Mine (XCM), we proposed a systematic study on the technical supports for the production of high-quality anthracite in this paper (the remaining sections includes mine conditions and mining techniques, techniques for increased LCPR of raw coal, fragmentation-prevention techniques for lump coal, and economic benefits). It should be pointed out that the proposed coal mining methods are only used for underground mining. The results of this study have been widely adopted for high-quality anthracite production in other coal mines, YMA.

## 2. MINE CONDITIONS AND MINING TECHNIQUES

As shown in Figure 1, XCM is located in the southwest part of Yongcheng City, Henan Province, China. Its terrestrial coordinates are 116°13′34″–116°18′07″ East longitudes, 33°47′21″–33°53′58″ North latitudes. With a length of 14 km (North to South) and a width of 1.6–4 km (East to West), the mine has a total area of 36 $km^2$. As one of the largest coal mines managed by Yongcheng Coal & Power Company Limited (YCPLC), XCM has been designed with a capacity of 1.2 million tons each year and a service life of 56.6 years. A pair of shafts was established in a uni-vertical up and down pattern and with a horizontal elevation of −550 m. Mining is executed in a bottom up fashion; the bottom coal seam (#$2_2$) is mined before mining the top coal seam. In addition, horizontal mining occurs in a forward pattern.

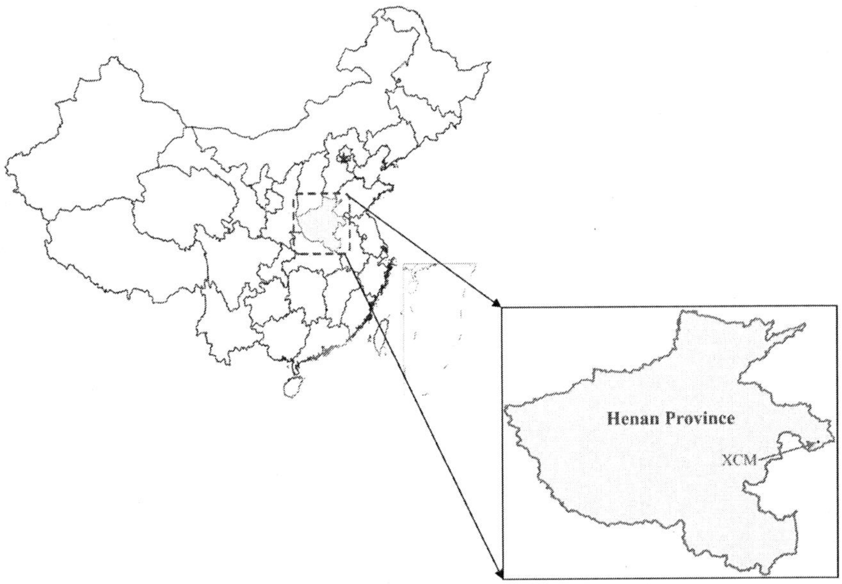


**Figure 1.** The geographical location of XCM.

The #$2_2$ coal seam of the North Second Panel (NSP) was mined first. The generalized column of the NSP is presented inFigure 2. The geological structure and occurrence conditions of this field are favorable for mining; the coal seam thickness ranges from 1.69 to 4.34 m and the average thickness is 3.33 m. The dip angle ranges from 10° to 16° and the average angle is 13°. The roof of the #$2_2$ coal seam is made up of fine sandstone and sandy mudstone, with magmatic rock in some local regions. The base of the #$2_2$ coal seam is made up of mudstone and siltstone. In this area, strike longwall fully mechanized mining (FMM) (mining height is equal to 2.85 m) and roof caving (for mined-out areas) were employed.

## 3. TECHNIQUES FOR INCREASED LCPR OF RAW COAL

In coal mining, the LCPR is positively related to the unit price of the product and decrease of pulverized coal rate. Mostly, raw coal mining is the key stage of lump coal formation. Moreover, the parameters (running parameters and drum parameters) of the shearer and the mining methods play a key role in the formation of lump coal.

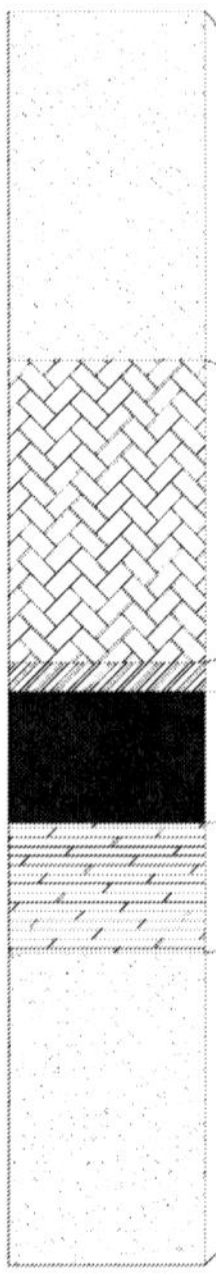

| Number | Lithology | Thickness | Remarks |
|---|---|---|---|
| 1 | Siltstone | 8.26 m | / |
| 2 | Fine sandstone | 8.61 m | Main roof |
| 3 | Sandy mudstone | 0.22 m | Immediate roof |
| 4 | Coal | 3.33 m | #$2_2$coal seam |
| 5 | Mudstone | 2.85 m | Immediate floor |
| 6 | Siltstone | 9.46 m | Main floor |

**Figure 2.** The generalized column of the NSP.

## 3.1. Optimization of Shearer's Parameters

### 3.1.1. Mathematical Description of Shearer's Cutting Thickness

The cutting thickness of a shearer refers to the thickness cut by each pick in one rotation of the drum. This parameter is not an intrinsic one; instead, it is a condition parameter that is determined by the arrangement of cutting picks, the rotating speed of the drum, and traction speed of the shearer [27,28]. Due to the effects of the drum rotation and shearer traction used for this study, arc-shape cutting was generated and the cutting shape was a crescent [29] (Figure 3).

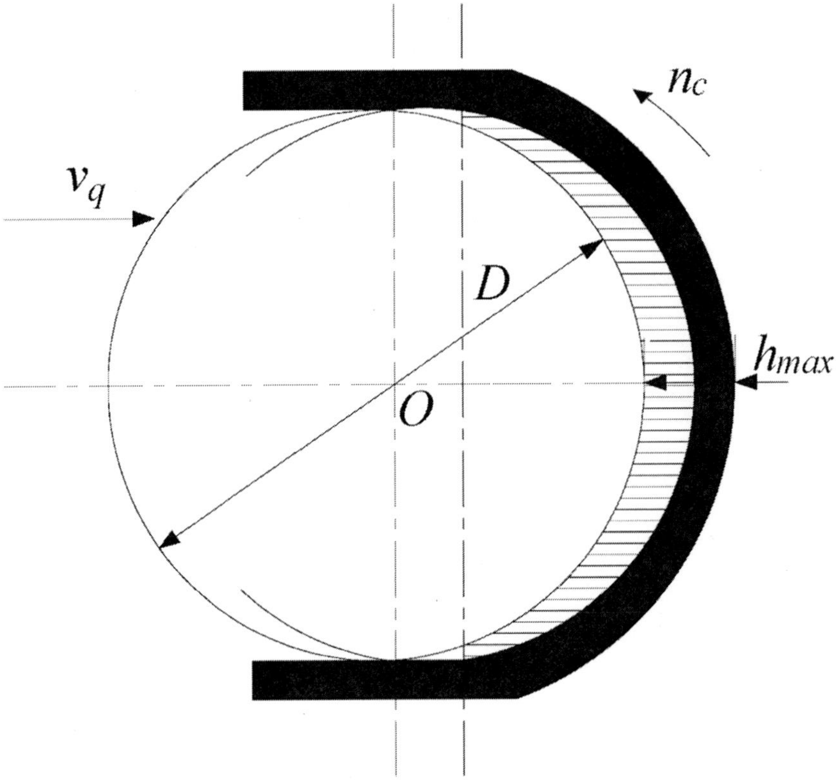


**Figure 3.** The ranges of drum cutting thickness.

The cutting thickness along the traction direction in one rotation can be expressed as [30]:

$$h_{\max} = \frac{1000 v_q}{z_1 n_c} \tag{1}$$

$$\bar{h} = \frac{2}{\pi} h_{\max} \tag{2}$$

where: $v_q$ is the traction speed of the shearer, m/min; $z_1$ is the number of picks in a transversal (determined by the picks arrangement and the number of helical blades); $n_c$ is the rotating speed of the drum, r/min; $h_{max}$ and h¯ are the maximum and minimum cutting thickness, respectively.

According to Equations (1) and (2), cutting thickness is also determined by the picks arrangement and the number of helical blades.

### 3.1.2. Optimization of Running Parameters

According to the relationship between traction/rotating speeds and cutting thickness, the ratio of traction speed and rotating speed must be optimized to improve the LCPR. For instance, the traction speed/rotating speed ratio is decreased for hard coal while increased for soft coal. Previous studies have revealed that traction speed/rotating speed ratio should be kept within 0.0762–0.1524 [31,32]. The parameters of the double-drum shearers (MG200/500-QWD, TST Company, Beijing, China) currently used in XCM are as follows: traction speed is 0–6 m/min, drum diameter is 1600 mm, cutting depth is 630 mm, and designed drum rotating speed is 42 r/min. With consideration to the situation in this study, traction and rotating speeds were adjusted to 4–5 m/min and 35 r/min, respectively, so that the ratio remained at 0.11–0.14. As a result, the LCPR was enhanced by 3.8%.

### 3.1.3. Optimization of Cutting Pick Parameters

In theory, the LCPR can be enhanced by either increasing the pick length or decreasing the pick density. Nevertheless, both measures lead to increasing shearer vibrations, thus lessening the service life of the shearer. To counter this, a novel shearer drum with unique picks (Figure 4) was used in XCM. As shown in Figure 4a, the cutting blades presented large cutting depth and digging capabilities. Each drum had three blades and each transversal had three cutting picks; the distances between transversals could be 100, 122, 142, or 162 mm. The cutting cross-section of kerfs is shown in Figure 4b. Herein, $A_1$–$A_4$, $B_1$–$B_4$, and $C_1$–$C_4$ sketch the cross-sections of picks No. 1 to No. 4 on the blades.

The 18 cutting picks on the plate were maintained, while the picks on the blade were reduced from six to four. Three cutting picks were installed on each transversal and the inter-transversal distance was increased from 80 to 162 mm. To mitigate the increased cutting resistance, a more powerful drum (Kennametal Company, Fort Mill, SC, USA) was employed. Meanwhile, high-strength point-attack picks (U92 and U94) were used in different situations: extended U92 picks (from 92 to 125 mm) were used for completed cutting cases, and U94 picks were used for coal seams with small structures. Since then, compared to the production using conventional drums, the LCPR was enhanced by 5.1%.

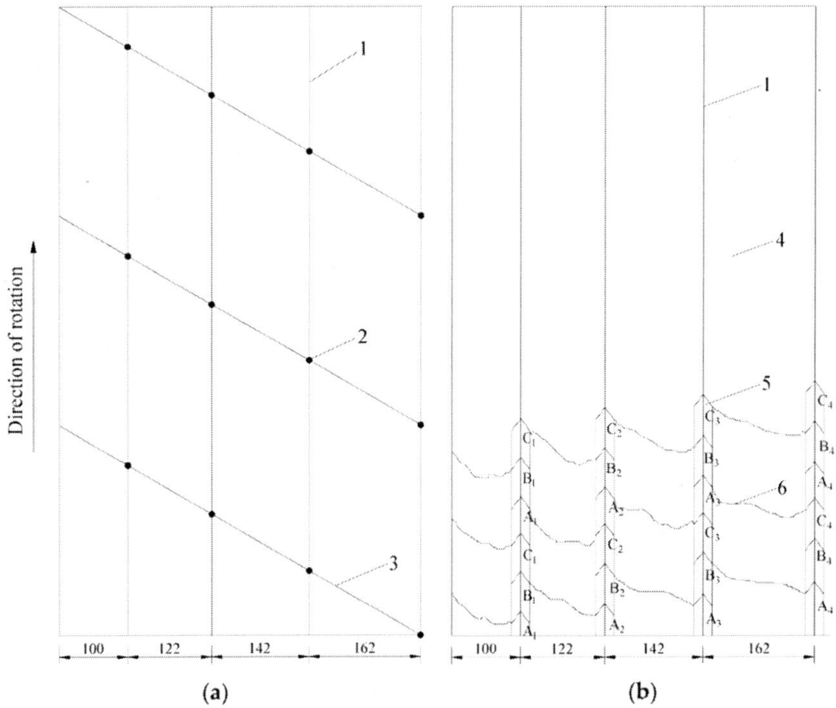


**Figure 4.** A novel shearer drum with large cutting depth and digging capabilities: (**a**) arrangement of cutting picks on blades; (**b**) cutting cross-section of kerfs; 1, transversals; 2, cutting picks; 3, blades; 4, anthracite; 5, kerfs; 6, cracks.

## 3.2. Allocation of Reasonable Mining Techniques

### 3.2.1. Selection of Rotating Direction of the Drums and Cutting Approach

To improve the stability of the shearer, the two drums rotated in opposite directions (front/rear equals clockwise/anti-clockwise or anti-clockwise/clockwise, as shown in Figure 5). Therefore, the cutting resistances on the different drums worked in opposite directions. Usually, a clockwise/anti-clockwise pattern was employed. This can be attributed to the fact that the specific power consumption was minimized when the front and rear drums were responsible for cutting and loading, respectively. Additionally, the floating dust was also reduced. Nevertheless, the anti-clockwise/clockwise pattern was used in XCM. In this case, the fragmentation of lump coal was reduced by 4.9%, as loading of both drums did not involve the rocker arm.

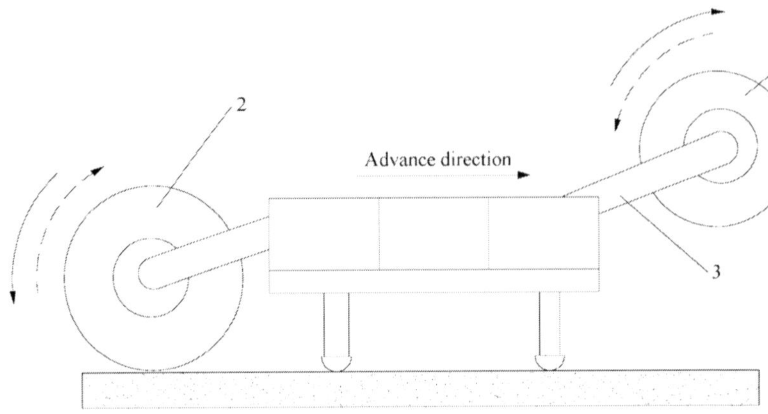


**Figure 5.** Clockwise/anti-clockwise or anti-clockwise/clockwise patterns of front and rear drums: 1, front drum; 2, rear drum; 3, rocker arm.

Currently, two-way and one-way cutting approaches are both widely used in the mining industry. Theoretically, two-way cutting approaches are more effective than one-way cutting. However, two-way approaches are limited by various issues in practice. For instance, the height of the shearer body is limited by the thickness of the coal seam, and low underneath clearance may be met. The maximum underneath clearance of the shearer was 468 mm in this study, and coal cut by the front drum would accumulate at the front end of the shearer in front-rear cutting, which could result in undesired fragmentation. On the other hand, one-way cutting approaches showed reasonable efficiency, and the LCPR could be enhanced by using this method. Therefore, in this study, a rear-front one-way cutting approach was used and the coal was kept away from the bracket. Using one-way cutting approach, the NSP has an average yield of 100,000 tons each month, with the highest monthly yield of 180,000 tons.

### 3.2.2. Reduction of Mining Height and Roof Supporting Intensity

In cases of strong coal walls and roof, mining height and roof supporting intensity would be reduced accordingly to allow spontaneous caving of the top coal upon cutting (Figure 6). In this way, massive coal cubes can be gained at a relatively low drum rotating speed. At the same time, cutting resistance on the unit area is lessened. Mining height of the NSP was designed to 2.85 m and a dual-column shield hydraulic support (ZY4000/17.5/38, ZMJ Company, Zhengzhou, China, supporting height is 1.75–3.8 m and initial support is 3077 kN) was used. For practical purposes, the mining height was reduced from 2.85 to 2.80 m, and the initial support was lowered from 3077 to 2800 kN. As a result, the LCPR was enhanced by 3.7%.

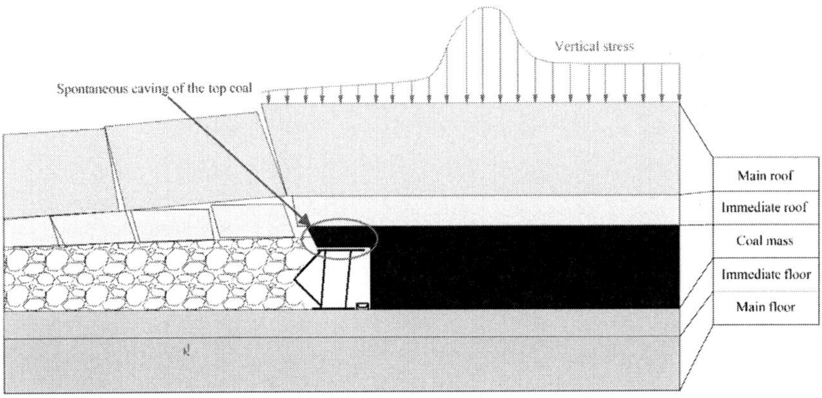


**Figure 6.** Schematic illustration of the coalface mining process.

### 3.2.3. Implementation of LPMB on Coal Mass

In mining, many specific situations arise. For instance, some mines are located in geological crack zones, while others have issues of parting bands. Without additional measures, the LCPR of the product could be extremely low. Previous studies reported positive effects on the LCPR using blasting. In accordance with that, LPMB was executed on the coal body based on the variation of the coal seam thickness. More specifically, a loose blast was conducted once a day so that the presplitting depth met the need during working progress. Blasting was carried out while mine maintenance was conducted.*In situ* measurements revealed that the LCPR was increased by 12.37% (Table 1) with LPMB and FMM.

**Table 1.** LCPR comparison of two different mining techniques.

| Mining Technique | Total Output (t) | Lump Quantity (t) | LCPR (%) | | Cutting Way |
|---|---|---|---|---|---|
| LPMB + FMM | 1st: 390 | 186.5 | 47.82 | Average: 46.47 | One-way |
| | 2nd: 390 | 174.3 | 44.69 | | |
| | 3rd: 390 | 182.9 | 46.90 | | |
| FMM | 1st: 390 | 134.5 | 34.49 | Average: 34.10 | One-way |
| | 2nd: 390 | 131.9 | 33.82 | | |
| | 3rd: 390 | 132.6 | 34.00 | | |

# 4. FRAGMENTATION-PREVENTION TECHNIQUES FOR LUMP COAL

As it will undergo long transport routes (including coalface end transloading, transport through headgate, panel, and main roadway), lump coal mined from the coalface by the shearer is stored in an underground bunker and hoisted to the surface. Raw coal will be also washed and sieved in a series of processes that involve repetitive squeezing, colliding and abrading (as well as secondary crushing of massive cubes), which results in reduction of LCPR. Indeed, a large amount of coal is pulverized into powder, causing a severe decline in the quality of anthracite. In this section, we proposed a study of fragmentation-prevention techniques for lump coal in view of the whole coal flow system.

## 4.1. Principles of Coal Fragmentation

Fragmentation refers to the process in which large lumps are crushed into smaller ones. The collision of coal cubes against one another is believed to be the main cause of fragmentation [33,34]. It is generally believed that the LCPR of the final product is positively related to the percentage of large lumps in the raw coal. However, the LCPR of the final product is also affected by various reasons from the transport and transloading systems. Particularly, collision is regarded as a main reason for the LCPR of the final product. Despite the limited understanding of lump coal fragmentation principles, the collisions can be generally described by the following equation (Momentum Theorem) [35]:

$$F = \frac{m(v_t - v_o)}{t} \tag{3}$$

where: *F* is the force experienced by the cube during collisions; *m* is the mass of the cube; *t* is the collision time; vo and vtare the velocities before $(v_o = \sqrt{2gh})$ and after collisions, respectively.

According to Equation (3), the collision force experienced by the lumps is determined by the collision time *t*, lump mass*m*, and velocities before and after collisions (vo and vt). In most cases, vt is negligible, as lumps after collision are static. According to classical physics, vo is positively related to the falling height $(v_o = \sqrt{2gh})$.As the inner surface (made of concrete) of bunker is rigid, the collision time is extremely short. As a result, the collision force is large and the lumps are easily fragmented. Additionally, the force on each lump increases with its mass. Therefore, the LCPR is reduced as the average lump mass increases.

## 4.2. Reconstructions of Coalface End Transloading

Because of the large height difference (1.2–1.5 m) between the transloader end and the extensible belt conveyer, lumps falling from the transloader gain a large amount of speed causing violent collisions between the lumps and the conveyer surface. As a result, the overall LCPR is reduced in this process. To solve this, an additional buffer unit was installed at the transloader exit to lessen the collisions between the lumps and the conveyer, so as to reduce lump fragmentation by 4.7%.

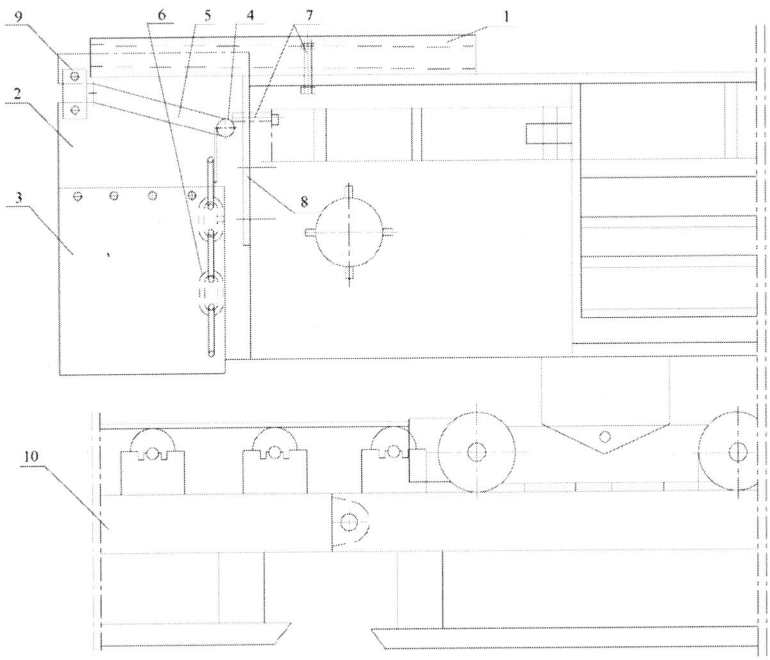


**Figure 7.** Basic configuration of the buffer unit: 1, fixed flange beam; 2, fixed side protecting plate; 3, movable side protecting plate; 4, buffer axis; 5, guide slot; 6, buffer chain; 7, fixed bolt; 8, connection plate; 9, damper; 10, extensible belt conveyor.

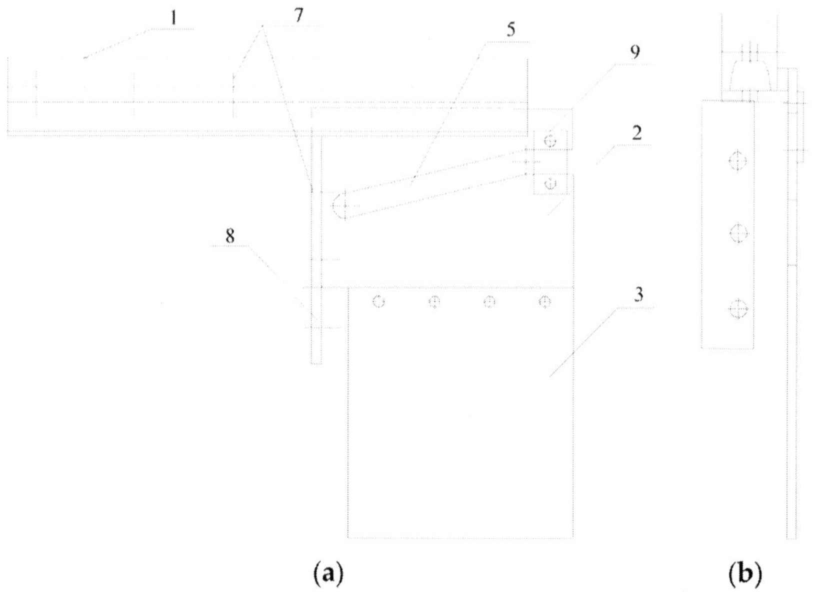


**Figure 8.** Schematic illustration of a side protecting plate: (**a**) front view; (**b**) side view.

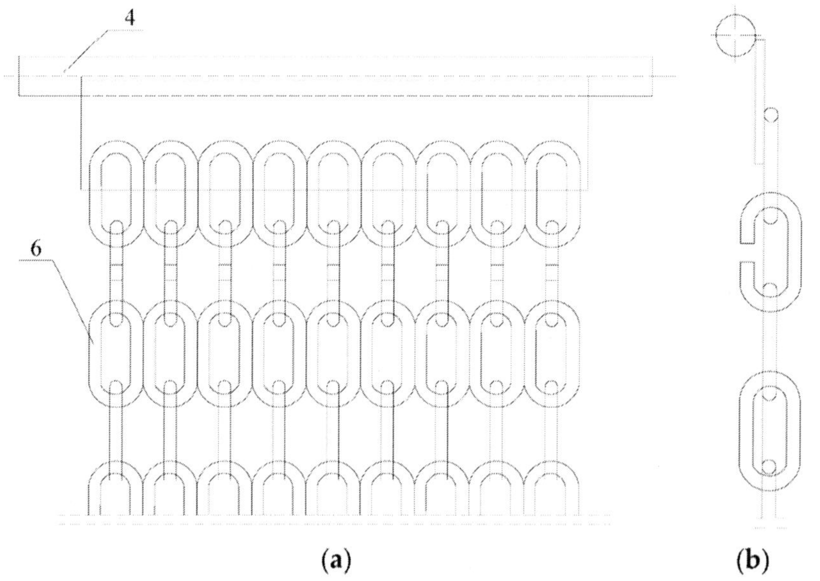


**Figure 9.** Schematic illustration of a buffer axis: (**a**) front view; (**b**) side view.

The basic configurations of the buffer unit are shown in Figure 7. As viewed, the buffer unit mainly consists of side protecting plate components (Figure 8) and buffer axis components (Figure 9). Symmetrical side protecting plates were attached to the spill plates at the sides of the transloader. Components of the side protecting plate included a fixed flange beam, fixed side protecting plate, movable side protecting plate, fixed bolt, connection plate, and damper. The components of the buffer axis included a buffer axis, connection plate, buffer chain, and split ring.

The buffer axis and chains were placed at the exit of the transloader to set up a semi-confined space with the side protecting plates. As a result, the lumps were converged in the center part of the conveyer belt and decelerated, which result in reduced collisions with the conveyer belt. In case of a sudden increase in impacts on the buffer axis, it moved upwards along the guide grooves on the fixed side protecting plates to avoid severe damage to the unit's components. Once the impacts were balanced by gravity, the buffer axis stayed in place. Unlike buffer teeth, the buffer axis actively responded to varying impacts and the lump speeds were kept without severe damage to the buffer unit. A fixed protecting plate and movable protecting plate replaced the transloader folding plate so that the plate length could be adjusted according to variations in the roadway floor.

## 4.3. Applications of Wheel Crusher

In practical situations, large anthracite lumps mined from the coalface are pulverized by a coalface crusher connected to the transloader. In this process, conventional crushers (e.g., jaw crushers and hammer crushers) rely on compressive forces to crush the lumps. Nevertheless, cracks are formed in the lumps as the loading area of lumps is large. Meanwhile, their mechanical strengths degrade after compression. As a result, the lumps become extremely small and may be pulverized into powder in consecutive processes, and then reduce the LCPR of the anthracite. To avoid it, a Wheel Crusher (PLM 1000, ZMJ Company, Zhengzhou, China) that works well with the coalface end transloader is applied in XCM.

Specifically designed for domestic coal mines, this wheel crusher consists of a pulley, crushing chamber, unloading chamber, crushing axis components, and dust curtains (Figure 10) [36]. The crusher is connected to the transloader at both ends by connection holes. An additional joint is designed at its loading end so that a rigid connection between the crusher and the transloader could be established.

Conventionally, coal shows an average lump size below 100 mm after crushing, with 84% having a diameter no larger than 100 mm and 30% being of fine grade. As a result of crushing, the overall LCPR is reduced by 5%. By using the wheel crusher proposed in this study, the LCPR loss was reduced by only 2%. According to market surveys and customer feedback, this was achieved by optimizing the gear and crusher exit diameter (200–400 mm).

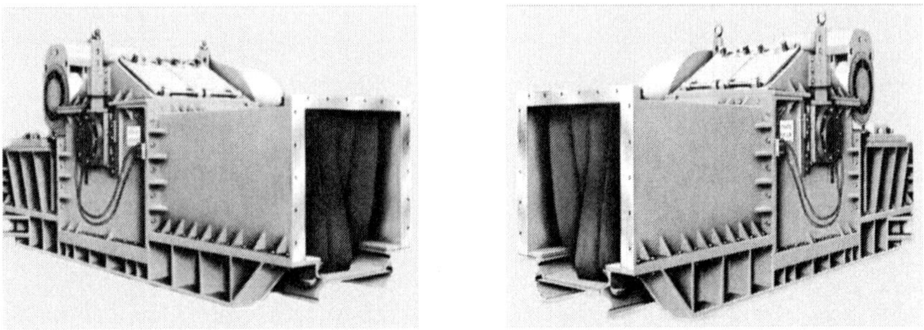

(a) (b)

**Figure 10.** PLM 1000 Wheel Crusher: (**a**) left front view; (**b**) right front view.

## 4.4. Adjustments in Transport Systems

Before being stored in underground bunkers, crushed raw coal is transported over a long distance and transloaded several times. Because of the long transport distance and the height differences in overlapping sections, the lumps fall a large distance at transloading points, resulting in lump fragmentation and reduced LCPR. The LCPR loss at each transloading point is estimated to be 0.5%. To mitigate this loss, the following adjustments were made to optimize the transport systems: (1) The roadway layout was improved so that the number of transloading points and height differences was lessened; (2) the height of overlapping sections of transloading points was reduced so that the falling heights of the lumps would be less than 0.5 m; (3) the steel wire mesh and flakes were replaced with a buffer device at transloading points (Figure 11).

## 4.5. Optimizations of Underground Storage

As a key component of the coal production system, underground bunkers show significantly varying stock levels, resulting in unpredictable falling heights of the lumps. Collisions in the falling process caused great losses of lumps. Statistics revealed that the losses of LCPR in this process were as high as 6%–12% [37,38]. Therefore, it was essential and urgent to reduce the lump coal loss by improving the design of underground bunkers.

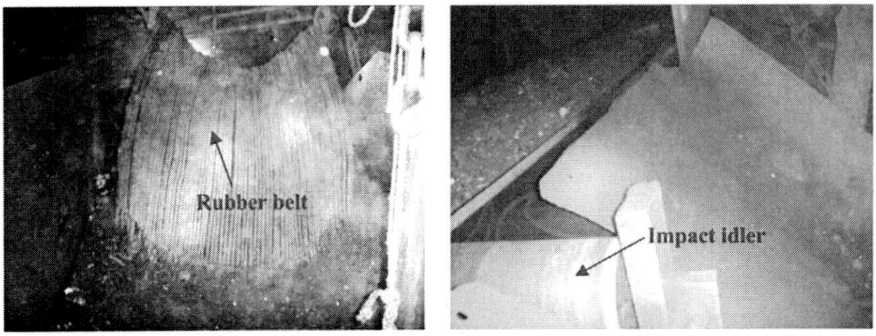


(a) (b)

**Figure 11.** Buffer device: (**a**) rubber belt; (**b**) impact idler.

Designed bunker height of XCM was 28 m, which exceeded the optimized value for bunker bottom protection and lump preservation. To mitigate this issue, spiral bunkers are sometimes used. However, because construction and maintenance of spiral bunkers require significantly increasing costs and time, a novel bunker design was proposed. Specifically, the cross-section of the bunker was designed to be circular and permanently supported with anchor rod/anchor mesh/concrete (concrete support thickness is 0.4 m). Hanging spiral chutes were installed on the outside wall of the bunker and the junctions of these chutes were processed to strengthen its resistance to corrosion, rust, and wear. As a result, the final speed of the lumps was reduced and their collisions with the bunker were lessened, indicating that the LCPR was enhanced and damages to the bunker were reduced. Additionally, bunker blockings were also lessened. Practical applications revealed that the LCPR of bunkers equipped with spiral chutes increased by 30%.

The application of hanging spiral chutes had a significant effect on the LCPR. However, in the coal dumping process, it is difficult for operators to make reasonable decisions based purely on visual observations, resulting in over-dumping. As a result, the LCPR is reduced to a higher extent than expected in this process. To mitigate this issue, a stock level monitoring system (Figure 12) was installed at the bunker opening to promote the dumping process. In this way, both underground and ground operators can accurately control the bunker level. Additionally, an alarm is triggered once the stock level is below a prescribed value (17 m in this case) so that over-dumping would be prevented.

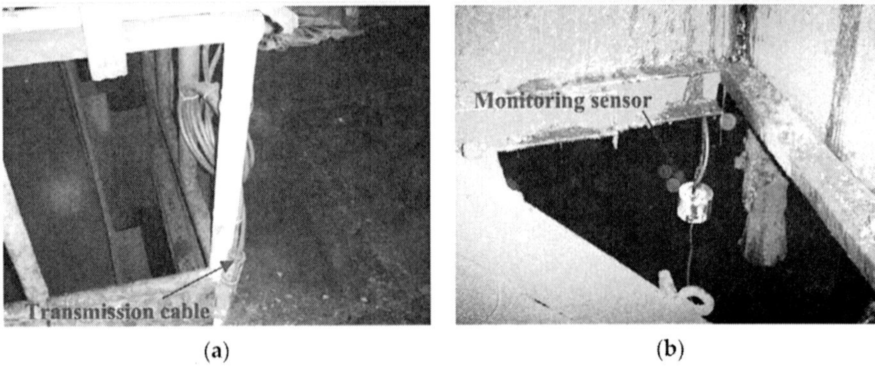


**Figure 12.** Bunker stock level monitoring system: (**a**) bunker opening; (**b**) sensor layout.

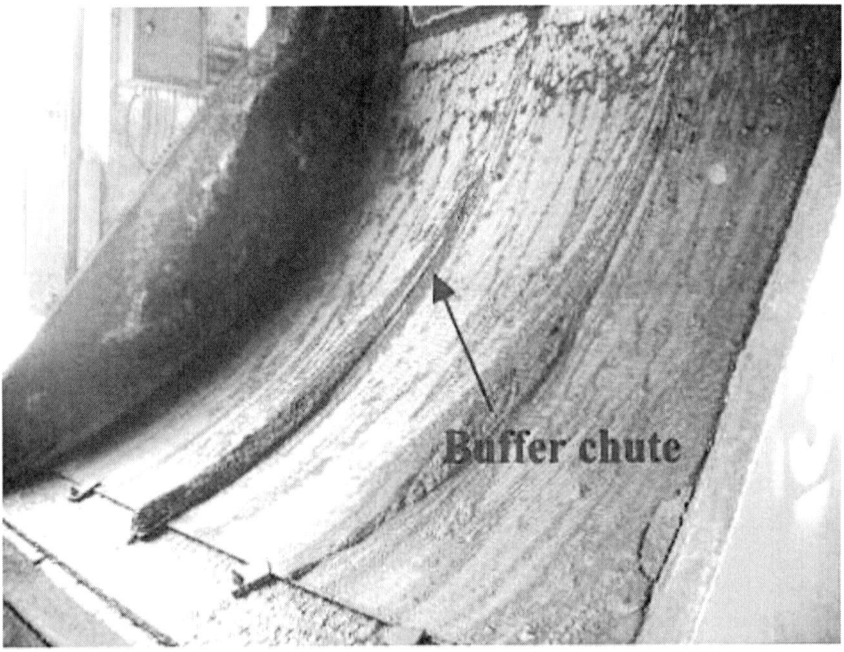


**Figure 13.** Buffer chute.

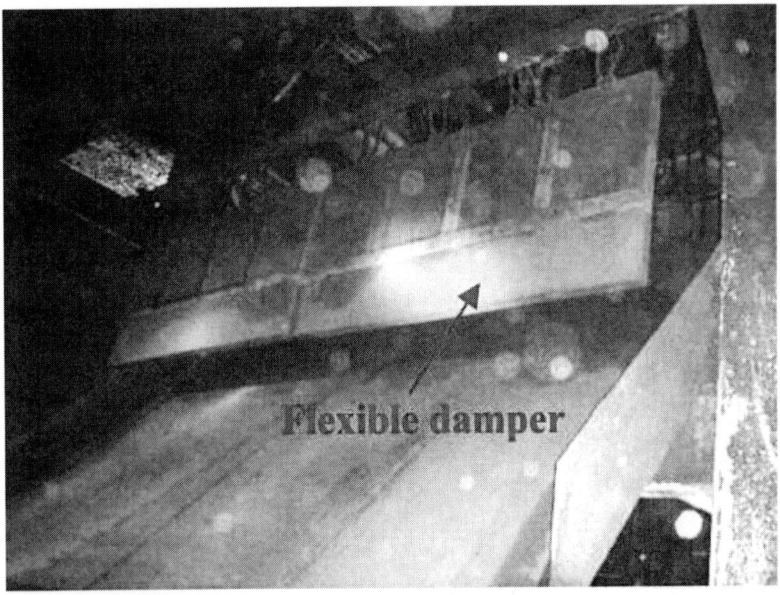


**Figure 14.** Flexible damper.

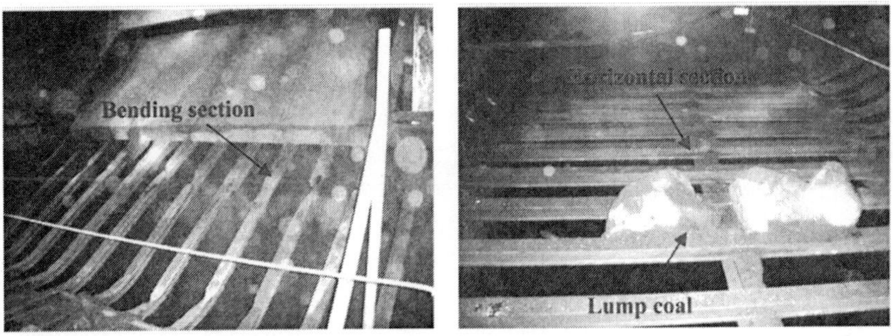


(a) (b)

**Figure 15.** Interval blocking units: (**a**) bending section; (**b**) horizontal section.

## 4.6. Improvements to the Main Shaft Skip Unloading Processes

The main shaft is regarded as the core of a coal mine production system. In large and medium-sized mines, coal lifting is carried out at the main shaft with a skip. The raw coal is then lifted to the ground by the shaft skip and transloaded to the conveyer on the ground. Because of production rate needs, transloading rates are kept at a high level [39,40], resulting in violent collisions between the lumps and wellhead bunker walls. Therefore, a buffer chute (Figure 13), a flexible damper (Figure 14) and interval blocking units (Figure 15) were installed at the transloading sections to relieve the collisions and reduce lump loss of about 15%.

## 4.7. Fragmentation-Prevention in Washing Processes

According to previous studies, fragmentation in washing process contributes significantly to the overall lump loss [41,42]. To improve the washing process and overall LCPR, measures such as process flow optimization, screening, transloading modifications, and storage adjustments were used.

In cases where the screening plant is under maintenance, raw coal from the shaft is immediately transloaded to the storage. To avoid this, a heavy media separator for lumps is commonly used. In XCM, a +25 mm heavy media bevel wheel for lumps, a 0.5–25 mm heavy media cyclone for fines, and a −0.5 mm flotation slime unit was integrated and used. However, lump fragmentations resulting from high-speed rotation in the pumps, squeezing in the pipes, and collisions in heavy media cyclones were observed. Therefore, the sieve size was reduced from 25 to 13 mm so that lumps over 13 mm were injected into the heavy media bevel wheel separator. In this way, the LCPR was increased by 5.4%.

In the washing, and particularly the screening and transloading processes, lumps gain much energy while being relatively brittle. As a result, significant lump fragmentation occurs. To mitigate this issue, several measures were adopted: (1) A cushion was placed on the feeding chute of the sizing sieve to decelerate fast-moving lumps entering the sieve and reduce lump loss about 5.8%. (2) The front end chute of the medium-removing sieve was adapted to decelerate the falling lumps. Specifically, the chute angle was optimized and buffer plates were placed inside the chute. In this way, the traveling times of lumps in the chute were increased, resulting in a collection of coal. (3) Height differences at various transloading points were reduced. For those with height differences larger than 500 mm, buffer systems (rubber and plastic strips) were installed to reduce lump fragmentation as shown in Figure 16.

A fragmentation-prevention system (LKK-1, Figure 17) was installed in the bunker to mitigate lump fragmentation in the storage process. The coal lumps dropped into the chute after being processed through the sizing screens. The impeller coal feeder at the coal chute exit monitored and properly adjusted the fall of the screened lumps into the surge bunker so that the stock level of the bunker was kept at suitable levels.

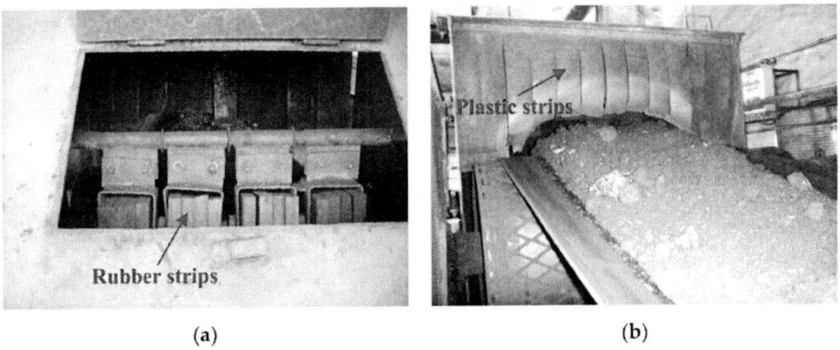


**Figure 16.** The buffer systems at transloading points: (**a**) rubber strips; (**b**) plastic strips.

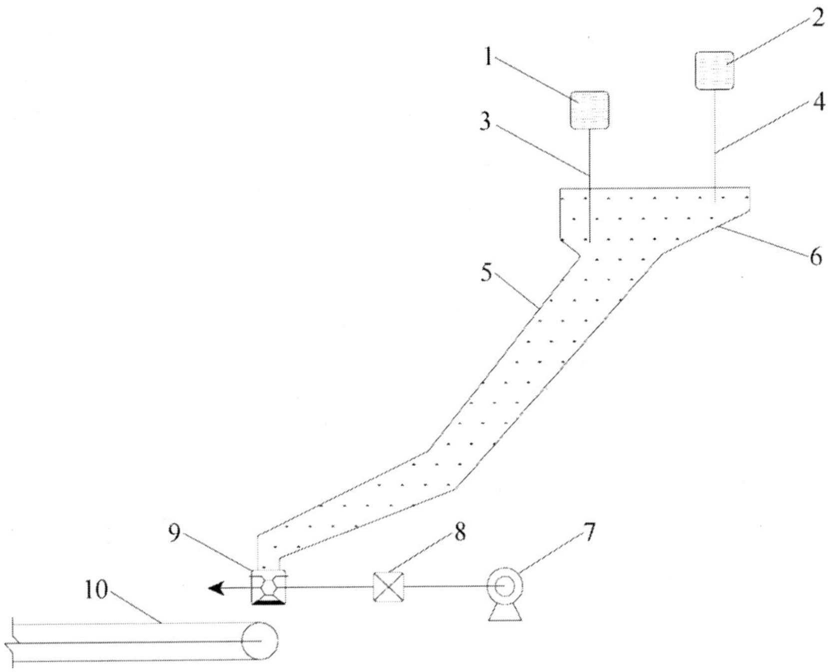


**Figure 17.** LKK-1 fragmentation-prevention system: 1, signal relay of low stock level; 2, signal relay of high stock level; 3, electrode of low stock level; 4, electrode of high stock level; 5, coal chute; 6, surge bunker; 7, electromotor; 8, gearbox; 9, impeller coal feeder; 10, main conveyor.

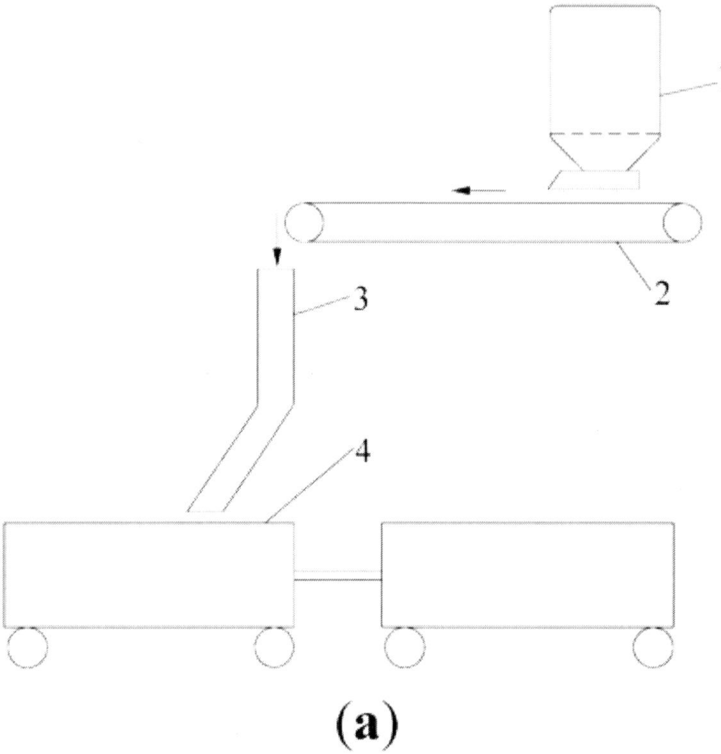


**Figure 18.** Railway wagon loading processes: (**a**) conventional loading system; (**b**) fragmentation-prevention loading system; 1, feeder; 2, belt conveyor; 3, chute; 4, railway wagon; 5, display of stock level; 6, sensor of stock level; 7, storage hopper; 8, winch; 9, valve.

## 4.8. Fragmentation-Prevention in Railway Wagon Loading Processes

To overcome the limits of the conventional wagon loading processes, a novel fragmentation-prevention system was designed (Figure 18). This system consisted of a feeder, belt conveyer, and a chute stock level control unit. The feeder was placed on top of the belt conveyer and a storage hopper between the conveyer and the chute was incorporated. A stock level control unit consisting of a sensor and display was installed at the hopper entrance. The hopper exit was connected with the buffer chute and a gravity-controlling valve was installed at the chute exit, which was on top of the railway wagon. This fragmentation-prevention system presented distinct advantages. First, the hopper acted as a buffer unit and the falling heights of the lumps were kept within a suitable range by controlling the valve.

Consequently, both noise and lump loss was reduced by 9.2%. This system is also expected to adapt coal lumps of various sizes, demonstrating great potential for industrial applications. Another noteworthy benefit of this system is that it is highly automatic and few operators are needed, which can greatly reduce working costs.

## 5. ECONOMIC BENEFITS

The application of the techniques and optimization processes developed in this study significantly improved the quality of the coal products and increased the anthracite yield, and finally increase profits of the coal mine. As shown in Table 2, an increase of 12 million CNY (113,851,993 × 10.54% = 12,000,000) per year was viewed from the increased LCPR alone.

**Table 2.** Quantity and quality situation of coal products in 2009.

| Months \ Contents | | Raw Coal Quantity (t) | LCPR (%) | Ash Content (%) | Moisture Content (%) | Calorific Value (kcal·kg$^{-1}$) | Incomes (CNY) |
|---|---|---|---|---|---|---|---|
| 2009 | January | 155,736 | 20.65 | 10.10 | 4.9 | 6399 | - |
| | February | 151,808 | 22.21 | 9.85 | 5.1 | 6449 | - |
| | March | 171,138 | 21.08 | 9.90 | 4.9 | 6369 | - |
| | April | 168,369 | 19.22 | 10.21 | 4.8 | 6193 | - |
| | May | 168,631 | 23.05 | 9.79 | 5.4 | 5960 | - |
| | June | 162,735 | 21.74 | 12.11 | 5.2 | 6072 | - |
| | July | 160,838 | 19.31 | 11.10 | 4.8 | 6131 | - |
| | August | 159,737 | 19.19 | 10.26 | 5.2 | 5820 | - |
| | September | 167,610 | 20.87 | 10.64 | 5.3 | 5651 | - |
| | October | 157,847 | 22.34 | 9.89 | 4.9 | 6057 | - |
| | November | 153,856 | 19.98 | 9.71 | 5.2 | 5848 | - |
| | December | 177,511 | 23.69 | 10.36 | 5.4 | 5943 | - |
| Indexes of 2009 | | 1,955,816 | 21.11 | 10.33 | 5.09 | 6074 | 586,744,800 |
| Indexes of 2008 | | 1,681,680 | 10.57 | 19.46 | 6.05 | 5876 | 472,892,807 |
| Difference values | | 274,136 | 10.54 | −9.13 | −0.96 | 198 | 113,851,993 |

## 6. CONCLUSIONS

**(1)**Based on the analysis of the cutting thickness of the shearer drums, the influence factors have been understood, including traction speed, drum rotating speed, arrangement of cutting picks, and the number of helical blades.

**(2)**For optimized shearer performance in XCM, the following parameters should be employed: traction speed of 4–5 m/min, drum rotating speed of 35 r/min (initial design speed is 42 r/min), and 30 cutting picks (initial design number is 36). Additionally, the pick length was increased while the pick density was decreased. Moreover, a rear-front one-way cutting approach was used in the mining process, and the mining height and roof supporting intensity were reduced accordingly. A combination of LPMB and FMM was also applied.

**(3)**Based on the principles of lump fragmentation, the coalface end transloading, coalface crushing, transport systems, underground storage, and main shaft skip unloading processes were all improved. Fragmentation-prevention techniques were also applied in the washing and wagon loading processes. As a result, fragmentation of the lump coal was obviously reduced. The LCPR was maintained at a high level, and a great increase in annual profits was achieved.

**(4)**In order to widely and confidently use the parameters and techniques determined in this study, some research directions should be required in future studies such as more on-site measurements of LCPR, laboratory analysis of mechanical mechanisms for coal fragmentation, and techniques for high-quality anthracite production of open-pit mining.

## ACKNOWLEDGMENTS

The research is financially supported by the National Basic Research Program of China (No. 2015CB251600), the National Natural Science Foundation of China (No. 51404254), the China Postdoctoral Science Foundation (Nos. 2014M560465 and 2015T80604), the Jiangsu Planned Projects for Postdoctoral Research Funds (No. 1302050B) and the Fundamental Research Funds for the Central Universities (No. 2013QNB24). We wish to thank the XCM for supporting to conduct this important study, as well as Rong Zhou from YCPLC for the assistance of data collection. Special thanks are given to Jie-qing Yu from the China University of Mining & Technology, for his assistance with making illustrations, and Cheng-guo Zhang from the University of New South Wales, Australia, for his language assistance. The authors are also grateful to the two anonymous reviewers for their constructive comments and helpful recommendations.

## AUTHOR CONTRIBUTIONS

All the authors contributed to publishing this paper. Wei Zhang performed the technological development and prepared and edited the manuscript. Dong-sheng Zhang revised and reviewed the manuscript. Hong-zhi Wang and Ji-xin Cheng partially participated in the literature research and data processing during the research process.

## CONFLICTS OF INTEREST

The authors declare no conflict of interest.

## REFERENCES


1. Guo, J.Q.; Kang, T.H.; Kang, J.T.; Zhao, G.F.; Huang, Z.M. Effect of the lump size on methane desorption from anthracite. J. Nat. Gas Sci. Eng. 2014, 20, 337–346.
2. Huang, B.X.; Wang, Y.Z.; Cao, S.G. Cavability control by hydraulic fracturing for top coal caving in hard thick coal seams. Int. J. Rock Mech. Min. Sci. 2015, 74, 45–57.
3. Yarushina, V.M.; Bercovici, D.; Oristaglio, M.L. Rock deformation models and fluid leak-off in hydraulic fracturing.Geophys. J. Int. 2013, 194, 1514–1526.
4. Pang, L.; Hosseini, A.; Hussein, H.M.; Deiab, I.; Kishawy, H.A. Application of a new thick zone model to the cutting mechanics during end-milling. Int. J. Mech. Sci. 2015, 96–97, 91–100.
5. Somanchi, S.; Kecojevic, V.J.; Bise, C.J. Analysis of force variance for a continuous miner drum using the Design of Experiments method. Int. J. Min. Reclam. Environ. 2006, 20, 111–126.
6. Liu, X.H.; Liu, S.Y.; Tang, P. Coal fragment size model in cutting process. Powder Technol. 2015, 272, 282–289.
7. Jiang, H.X.; Du, C.L.; Liu, S.Y.; Gao, K.D. Nonlinear dynamic characteristics of load time series in rock cutting. J. Vibroeng. 2014, 16, 292–302.
8. Saurabh, D.; Somnath, C.; Sergej, H. Investigation into coal fragmentation analysis by using conical pick. Procedia Mater. Sci. 2014, 5, 2411–2417.
9. Vidanovic, N.; Ognjanovic, S.; Ilincic, N.; Ilic, N.; Tokalic, R. Application of unconventional methods of underground premises construction in coal mines. Tech. Technol. Educ. Manag. 2011, 6, 861–865.
10. Lai, X.P.; Shan, P.F.; Cao, J.T.; Sun, H.; Suo, Z.Y.; Cui, F. Hybrid assessment of pre-blasting weakening to horizontal section top coal caving (HSTCC) in steep and thick seams. Int. J. Min. Sci. Technol. 2014, 24, 31–37.
11. Reddy, S.K.; Sastry, V.R. Gallery monitoring in blasting gallery panel during depillaring—A case study. J. Mines Metals Fuels 2013, 61, 257–260.
12. Satyanarayana, I.; Budi, G.; Deb, D. Strata behaviour during depillaring in Blasting Gallery panel by field instrumentation and numerical study. Arab. J. Geosci. 2015, 8, 6931–6947.

13. Wang, F.T.; Tu, S.H.; Yuan, Y.; Feng, Y.F.; Chen, F.; Tu, H.S. Deep-hole pre-split blasting mechanism and its application for controlled roof caving in shallow depth seams. Int. J. Rock Mech. Min. Sci. 2013, 64, 112–121.

14. Zhao, T.B.; Zhang, Z.Y.; Tan, Y.L.; Shi, C.Z.; Wei, P.; Li, Q. An innovative approach to thin coal seam mining of complex geological conditions by pressure regulation. Int. J. Rock Mech. Min. Sci. 2014, 71, 51–52.

15. Song, J.; Lian, Q.W. The relation between coal lump rate and cutting method of miner. Shanxi Coal 2003, 23, 20–21. (In Chinese).

16. Zhang, L.M. The current situation and developing trend of extremely thin coal seam mining of China. Appl. Mech. Mater. 2013, 295, 2918–2923.

17. Li, Z.Q.; Oyediran, I.A.; Tang, C.; Hu, R.L.; Zhou, Y.X. FEM application to loess slope excavation and support: Case study of Dong Loutian coal bunker, Shuozhou, China. Bull. Eng. Geol. Environ. 2014, 73, 1013–1023.

18. Kozan, E.; Liu, S.Q. A demand-responsive decision support system for coal transportation. Decis. Support Syst. 2012,54, 665–680.

19. Zhang, L.; Zhu, G.Q.; Zhang, G.W.; Han, R.S. Performance-based fire design of air-supported membrane coal storage shed. Procedia Eng. 2013, 52, 593–601.

20. Wang, X.W.; Qin, Y.; Tian, Y.K.; Yang, X.Y.; Yang, Z.J. Analysis on flow features of bulk coal during coal unloading period based on EDEM. Coal Sci. Technol. 2015, 43, 130–134. (In Chinese).

21. Lv, H.L.; Ma, Y.; Zhou, S.C.; Liu, K. Case study on the deterioration and collapse mechanism and curing technique of RC coal bunkers. Procedia Earth Planet. Sci. 2009, 1, 606–611.

22. Liu, S.Q.; Kozan, E. Optimising a coal rail network under capacity constraints. Flex. Serv. Manuf. J. 2011, 23, 90–110.

23. Singh, G.; Sier, D.; Ernst, A.T.; Gavriliouk, O.; Oyston, R.; Giles, T.; Welgama, P. Mixed integer programming model for long term capacity expansion planning: A case study from The Hunter Valley Coal Chain. Eur. J. Oper. Res. 2012,220, 210–224.

24. Wang, Y. Using the limiting transferring device to increase the lump coal rate of anthracite. Coal Process. Compr. Util.2008, 3, 10–12. (In Chinese).

25. Xie, W.N.; He, Y.Q.; Zhu, X.N.; Ge, L.H.; Huang, Y.J.; Wang, H.F. Liberation characteristics of coal middlings comminuted by jaw crusher and ball mill. Int. J. Min. Sci. Technol. 2013, 23, 669–674.

26. Chen, J.; Chu, K.W.; Zou, R.P.; Yu, A.B.; Vince, A. Prediction of the performance of dense medium cyclones in coal preparation. Miner. Eng. 2012, 31, 59–70.

27. Zeng, R.; Du, C.L.; Chen, R.J.; Wang, W.J. Reasonable location parameters of pick and nozzle in combined cutting system. J. Cent. South Univ. 2014, 21, 1067–1076.

28. Reid, A.W.; McAree, P.R.; Meehan, P.A.; Gurgenci, H. Longwall shearer cutting force estimation. J. Dyn. Syst. Meas. Control 2014, 136, 1–9.

29. Gao, H.B.; Yang, Z.J. Fluctuation analysis of thickness about roller shearer. Coal Mine Mach. 2013, 34, 106–108. (In Chinese).

30. Mazurkiewicz, D. Empirical and analytical models of cutting process of rocks. J. Min. Sci. 2000, 36, 481–486.

31. Liao, X.; Zhang, J.; Feng, T.; Li, P. Intensity nonlinear analysis of central groove of coal shearer under limiting conditions. J. Southeast Univ. 2014, 44, 531–537. (In Chinese).

32. Bilgin, N.; Balci, C.; Copur, H.; Tumac, D.; Avunduk, E. Cuttability of coal from the Soma coalfield in Turkey. Int. J. Rock Mech. Min. Sci. 2015, 73, 123–129.

33. Senneca, O.; Urciuolo, M.; Chirone, R. A semidetailed model of primary fragmentation of coal. Fuel 2013, 104, 253–261.

34. Zhou, Y.D.; Liu, Y.L.; Tang, X.W.; Cao, S.Q.; Chi, C.J. Numerical investigation into the fragmentation efficiency of one coal prism in a roller pulveriser: Homogeneous approach. Miner. Eng. 2014, 63, 25–34.

35. Thorpe, J.F. On the momentum theorem for a continuous system of variable mass. Am. J. Phys. 1962, 30, 637–640.

36. Hao, Q.S. Increase setting in use of middle digging coalface by modifying crusher and optimizing coal drift.Northwest Coal 2008, 6, 56–57. (In Chinese).

37. Yu, T.F. Design and application of spiral chute in preventing lump coal crushing. Coal Mine Mach. 2014, 35, 207–209. (In Chinese).

38. Deng, J.J.; Huang, J.Y.; Kuang, Y.L. Design of integrated manufacturing system of coal preparation plant based on multi-agent. Procedia Earth Planet. Sci. 2009, 1, 713–717.

39. Kou, B.F.; Liu, Q.Z.; Liu, C.Y.; Liang, Q. Characteristic research on the transverse vibrations of wire rope during the operation of mine flexible hoisting system. J. China Coal Soc. 2015, 40, 1194–1198. (In Chinese).

40. Peterka, P.; Kresak, J.; Kropuch, S.; Fedorko, G.; Molnar, V.; Vojtko, M. Failure analysis of hoisting steel wire rope.Eng. Fail. Anal. 2014, 45, 96–105.

41. Wang, Z.G.; Kuang, Y.L.; Deng, J.J.; Wang, G.H.; Ji, L. Research on the intelligent control of the dense medium separation process in coal preparation plant. Int. J. Miner. Process. 2015, 142, 46–50.

42. Noble, A.; Luttrell, G.H. A review of state-of-the-art processing operations in coal preparation. Eng. Fail. Anal. 2015,25, 511–521.

# Chapter 4

# Key Technologies and Equipment for a Fully Mechanized Top-Coal Caving Operation with a Large Mining Height at Ultra-Thick Coal Seams

**Jinhua Wang[1], Bin Yu[2], Hongpu Kang[1], Guofa Wang[1], Debing Mao[1], Yuntao Liang[3], Pengfei Jiang[1]**

[1] *China Coal Technology & Engineering Group, Beijing 100013, China*

[2] *Datong Coal Mine Group Co., Ltd., Datong 037003, China*

[3] *CCTEG Shenyang Research Institute, Shenyang 110016, China*

## ABSTRACT

Thick and ultra-thick coal seams are main coal seams for high production rate and high efficiency in Chinese coal mines, which accounts for 44 % of the total minable coal reserve. A fully mechanized top-coal caving mining method is a main underground coal extraction method for ultra-thick coal seams. The coal extraction technologies for coal seams less than 14 m thick were extensively used in China. However, for coal seams with thickness greater than 14 m, there have been no reported cases in the world for underground mechanical extraction with safe performance, high efficiency and high coal recovery ratio. To deal with this case, China Coal Technology & Engineering Group, Datong Coal Mine Group, and other 15 organizations in China launched a fundamental and big project to develop coal mining technologies and equipment for coal seams with thicknesses greater than 14 m. After the completion of the project, a coal extraction method was developed for top-coal caving with a large mining height, as well as a ground control theory for ultra-thick coal seams. In addition, the mining technology for top-coal caving with a large mining height, the ground support technology for roadway in coal seams with a large cross-section, and the prevention and control technology for gas and fire hazards were developed and applied. Furthermore, a hydraulic support with a mining height of 5.2 m, a shearer with high reliability, and auxiliary equipment were developed and manufactured. Practical implication on the technologies and equipment developed was successfully completed at the No. 8105 coal face in the Tashan coal mine, Datong, China. The major achievements of the project are summarized as follows: 1. A top-coal caving method for ultra-thick coal seams is proposed with a cutting height of 5 m and a top-coal caving height of 15 m. A structural mechanical model of overlying strata called cantilever beam-articulated rock beam is established. Based on the model, the load resistance of the hydraulic support with a large mining height for top-coal caving method is determined. With the analysis, the movement characteristics of the top coal and above strata are evaluated during top-coal caving operation at the coal face with a large mining height. Furthermore, there is successful development of comprehensive technologies for preventing and controlling spalling of the coal wall, and the top-coal caving technology with high efficiency and high recovery at the top-coal caving face with a large mining height. This means that the technologies developed have overcome the difficulties in strata control, top-coal caving with high efficiency and high coal recovery, and enabled to achieve a production rate of more than 10 Mtpa at a single top-coal caving face with a large mining height in ultra-thick coal seams; 2. A hydraulic support with 5.2 m supporting height and anti-rockburst capacity, a shearer with high reliability, a scraper conveyor with a large power at the back of face, and a large load and long distance headgate belt conveyor have been successfully developed for a top-coal caving face with large mining height. The study has developed the key technologies for improving the reliability of equipment at the coal face and has overcome the challenges in equipping the top-coal caving face with a large mining height in ultra-thick coal seams; 3. The deformation characteristics of a large cross-section roadway in ultra-thick coal seams are discovered. Based on the findings above, a series of bolt materials with a high yielding strength of 500–830 MPa and a high extension ratio, and cable bolt material with a 1 × 19 structure, large tonnage and high extension ratio are developed. In addition, in order to achieve a safe roadway and a fast face advance, installation equipment for high pre-tension bolt is developed to solve the problems with the support of roadway in coal seams for top-coal caving operation with a large mining height; 4. The characteristics of gas distribution and uneven emission at top-coal caving face with large mining height in ultra-thick coal seams are evaluated. With the application of the technologies of gas drainage in the roof, the difficulties in gas control for high intensive top-coal caving mining operations, known as "low gas content, high gas emission", are solved. In addition, large flow-rate underground mobile equipment for making nitrogen are developed to solve the problems with fire prevention and safe mining at a top-coal caving face with large mining height and production rate of more than 10 Mtpa. A case study to apply the developed technologies has been conducted at the No. 8105 face, the Tashan coal mine in Datong, China. The case study demonstrates that the three units of equipment, i.e., the support, shearer and scraper conveyor, are rationally equipped. Average equipment usage at the coal face is 92.1 %. The coal recovery ratio at the coal face is up to 88.9 %. In 2011, the coal production at the No. 8105 face reached 10.849 Mtpa, exceeding the target of 10 Mtpa for a top-coal caving operation with large mining height performed by Chinese-made mining equipment. The technologies and equipment developed provide a way for extracting ultra-thick coal seams. Currently, the technologies and equipment are used in 13 mining areas in China including Datong, Pingshuo, Shendong and Xinjiang. With the exploitation of coal resources in Western China, there is great potential for the application of the technologies and equipment developed.

**Keywords:** Ultra-thick coal seams Top-coal caving mining Large mining height Mining method Mining equipment Roadway support Safety guarantee

## 1 INTRODUCTION

In China, there is approximately 1341 Bt of proven coal resource, including 279.58 Bt of basic coal resource for coal mine construction. Among them, coal resource in thick coal seams accounts for 44 % of the total available. The annual underground coal production from thick coal seams exceeds 45 % of total coal production. Since the Eighties in the last century, there have been many research projects focusing on mechanical coal extraction from thick coal seams. The mining technologies and systems for thick and ultra-thick coal seams have been gradually developed in China. Until recently, there have been three major mechanical mining methods for thick coal seams, i.e., a fully mechanized longwall top-coal caving mining method (thereafter LTCC mining method), a fully mechanized sub-level coal mining method, and a fully mechanized mining with a large mining height method. There are some limitations with the fully mechanized sub-level coal mining method, including the thickness variation of coal seams, spontaneous combustion, unit mining cost and efficiency. Due to the low production efficiency (Qian and Shi 2003; Wang 2005; 2006a; Mao and Yao 2010; Wang 2010a), the fully mechanized sub-level coal mining method is currently replaced by the other two mining methods. Compared with the fully mechanized sub-level coal mining method, the fully mechanized coal mining with a large mining height method can reduce the amount of roadway development, mitigate the tension between mining and development, and simplify the mining process. With the progress of mining technologies and equipment in China, the fully mechanized coal mining with a large mining height method has seen widely used (Yan and Yin 2008; Yan 2009; Yan et al. 2011), and has achieved significant mining profit and coal recovery. The method is only applicable to the coal seams of low dip, relative stable, and good roof conditions, and is also limited by the shearer's cutting height and coal wall spalling. For this reason, the mining height for one mining pass is 7.0 m (Wang et al. 2012), and cannot meet the requirement for safe and efficient mining in ultra-thick coal seams above 7 m. In terms of ultra-thick coal seams above 7 m, the top-coal caving mining method is the first choice. For coal seams with thicknesses ranging from 7 to 14 m, the top-coal caving mining method can be applied as the technologies and the equipment are well established and manufactured. In order to achieve safe and efficient coal extraction in ultra-thick coal seams with thicknesses ranging from 14 to 20 m, the authors propose a fully mechanized large mining height longwall top-coal caving mining method (thereafter LLTCC mining method), developed a full range of technologies and equipment for a LLTCC mining operation. The technologies and equipment developed have been successfully applied in the Tashan coal mine in Datong, China, and has achieved a production of 10 Mtpa at a LLTCC mining operation in the ultra-thick coal seam. In the early twentieth century, the top-coal caving mining method was applied at steep seams in France, Spain and former Yugoslavia. Due to the low mechanical levels in mining, the method was actually an alternative of the high caving mining method, which was only used as a special mining method under complex geological conditions. At the end of forties and early fifties of the twentieth century, the top-coal caving mining method was used to extract the thick coal seams in the former Soviet Union, France and former Yugoslavia. With the progress of hydraulic support technology, the fully mechanized top-coal caving technology was improved and successfully applied in some countries.

In the late eighties of the last century, the top-coal caving technology was not widely applied and its potential was not fully achieved due to the competition from other energy industries, the changes of social and political systems, and no solutions for the difficulties of its application in difficult geological conditions. Up to 1992, fully mechanized top-coal caving faces had been stopped in all countries, with the last site in Russia. By that time, China was the only country using the LTCC mining method to extract coal from thick coal seams (Wang 2009). Currently, China is a world leader in developing and conducting the LTCC mining technology, which results in several large, safe, high production rate and high efficiency mining areas including Luan, Yanzhou, Yangquan and Suozhou (Fan et al. 2003; Wang 2011). In recent years, with the development of the LTCC mining technology in China, the technology and equipment is starting to be introduced in some other countries, such as Australia, and is successfully used in underground coal mines.

Although China was late to develop and apply top-coal caving mining technology, its development and applications are progressing very fast, showing significant economic potential and attracting attentions from other countries. In China, the top-coal caving mining method means the fully mechanized longwall top-coal caving mining method. A longwall panel is laid out at the bottom of the thick coal seam and extracted using a fully mechanized longwall mining method. At the same time, the remaining coal above the longwall face are fractured by ground stress and strain (manually fractured in some special cases), and caved through the sliding window at the support canopies into an additional scraper conveyor, and then transported out of the working face. There are approximately four stages for the development of LTCC technology in China.

## 1.1 Stage 1: Exploration stage (1982–1990)

Since 1982, the LTCC technology has been introduced and investigated in China. In 1984, the first industrial trial of the technology at a gentle inclined seam was conducted at Northern Area 3 in Puhe mine, Shenyang Province, China (Yan and Fu 2003). Due to the problems with support design and equipment, and lack of experience in production management, the trial was not successful. However, the subsequent trials at steep inclined coal seams in the No. 2 mine of Yaojie, Meihekou mine of Liaoyuan, and Liudaowan mine in Urumqi, China, were all successful. Up until 1990, although the trials on the technology at gentle inclined coal seams continued in Northeastern China and Pingdingshan, there were no breakthroughs. In the second half of 1990, the LTCC face 8603 at the No. 1 coal mine in Yangquan produced 140,000 t/m, doubling the production from a sub-level coal face and exceeded 80 % of coal recovery from the face. The dip of the LTCC face was 3°–7°, the thickness was 6 m and the face width was 120 m. The trial at Yangquan found a way to achieve high production, high efficiency at a LTCC face, demonstrated the potential with LTCC technology, and laid a solid foundation for the development of LTCC technology. The feasibility of high production capacity and high efficiency of the technology has been proven at this stage.

## 1.2 Stage 2: Gradual maturation (1990–1995)

The key achievement at this stage was that the LTCC face at Xinglongzhuang mine in Yanzhou, China, reached the high production of 3 Mtpa. In addition, there was a breakthrough for LTCC technology at “three soft” coal seams, "large dip" coal seams (approximately 30°), and "high gassy" coal seams, which will enable a wide application of the technology in China. At this stage, the LTCC technology developed quickly and made some coal mining companies in China realize that the LTCC technology was a technological step-change for the coal mining industry. In addition, the research and studies were very active in the areas of ground control, support-strata relationship, cavability of top coal, and methods of top-coal caving, which provided various theories and practices.

## 1.3 Stage 3: Technical maturation and promotion (1995–2005)

Due to the huge technical advantages demonstrated, LTCC technology has attracted great attention from mining companies in China. Also with the removal of some technical difficulties in using LTCC technology, LTCC technology was widely and quickly applied in the coal mining industry in China. In 1995, LTCC technology was selected as one of five key technologies for further research and promotion during the period of the ninth five-year national economic plan by the Ministry of China Coal Industry. Several major technical issues associated with the LTCC mining method were named as key topics for research. Furthermore, in 1997, China National Nature Science Foundation launched a research project of "Basic study of whole seam coal extraction in thick coal seams". Various achievements were obtained at this stage. In some coal mines that meet appropriate geological conditions i.e., simple geological conditions, large coal reserves, fewer natural hazards, 6–9 m coal seams, and medium hard coals, the annual coal production and profit at LTCC faces increased substantially. For instance, in 1997, the coal production rate at the LTCC face in Dongtan mine in Yanzhou, China, achieved 4.1 Mtpa, and 208 t/manpower. In 1998, at the same face, the coal production rate reached 5.4 Mtpa, and the manpower efficiency was at 235 t/manpower, which was regarded as a world level in that time. In addition, at this stage, the LTCC technology was developed to extract some difficult coal seams, such as "three soft", "two hard", "large dip", "high gassy", "spontaneous combustion-prone", and "ultra-thin seams", etc. The various technologies were obtained from the above development.

During the period of the tenth five-year national economic plan, a project called "the research and experiment on LTCC technology and equipment with a production capacity of 6 Mtpa" was completed in Yanzhou, China. The study enabled a higher than 6 Mtpa production rate of the LTCC face for six consequent years, which showed that LTCC technology in China had reached a new high level.

## 1.4 Stage 4: Improvement (2005 to present)

In 2005, during the study of safe and high efficiency mining technologies for high gassy ultra-thick coal seams, the causes of problems that stagnated the production of high gassy LTCC faces were analyzed. In addition, the feasibility of further increasing the coal cutting height was investigated for coal extraction using LTCC technology at ultra-thick coal faces. In 2006, Li et al. (2006) presented some characteristics and potential of designing top-coal caving hydraulic support with large mining heights. In terms of equipment capacities, Lu et al. (2006) conducted a study on a complete set of mining equipment with a cutting height of 3.5 m. Currently, in order to overcome the difficulties in mining high gassy and ultra-thick coal seams, some mining companies in China, such as Tunliu mine and Wangzhuang mine of Luan Group, and Tashan mine of Datong Group, conducted various LTCC mining experiments with large mining heights and studies on the ground control at LTCC faces. Because LTCC mining technology with large mining height is a new coal mining method, however, there is still a lack of related theories and studies; for instance, the applicable conditions for a large mining height LTCC mining operation, the movement of the top coal and the roof strata, stress distribution around the face, and a complete set of equipment for a large mining height LTCC face.

In terms of LTCC mining operations, the characteristics of ground pressure, the movement of the top coal and roof strata, and the relationship between the support and surrounding rock are the main topics. They are also the main criteria for the selection of face equipment, mining parameters and support parameters.

The studies on ground pressure and the movement of the top coal and roof strata are limited in countries other than China. Limited literatures exist that describe top coal movement and top coal cavability (Hu 1995), while there is less description on roof structure, face pressure, and roof control, etc. Since the application of LTCC technology, there have been many studies on the movement characteristics of overlying strata, which has resulted in a large amount of achievements.

Kang Lijun (Kang 1990; 1995; 1996; 1998; 1999; Kang and Qi 1998; Kang et al. 1998; 1999) divided the roof movement into two stages, the non-complete extraction stage and the complete extraction stage. At the non-complete extraction stage, the periodic pressure from the main roof is mainly caused by the combination impact or individual impact from the broken cantilever beam roof in the irregular caving zone, and the broken or overturned overlying beam roof fixed at the two ends. But at the complete extraction stage, the periodical pressure from the main roof is mainly caused by the periodical broken, overturn and unstable arch beam roof in the regular caving zone. The strength of periodic pressure at the non-complete extraction stage is higher than that at the complete extraction stage. A case study on the roof movement of a LTCC face at the No. 4 mine in Yangquan, China, further described the roof movement at the two stages (Kang et al. 1997). Based on the movement characteristics of overlying strata at the LTCC face, Yan (1996) introduced a mechanical theory of limited deformation and proposed a balance structure of macro continuous "compressed arch beam" of overlying strata at the upper location.

Deng Guangzhe et al. from the Xi'an Mining Institute (Deng 1994) investigated the characteristics of "arch structure" of overlying strata movement and ground control law based on the observation and measurement at LTCC face and the analysis of 3D analogue modelling. Using mechanical analysis of the shell structure, the arch structure of the overlying strata at LTCC face was preliminarily analyzed. The analysis concluded that the formation of the arch structure at overlying strata relies on some external conditions. When there are no stable skewbacks, the arch structure becomes unstable. The caving of the arch structure of strata shows an abruptness. Zhang (1999) believe that after the immediate roof caved, an unstable "arch similarly" structure may be formed within 1.0–1.2 times of mining height above the coal face, and its stability is random. On the other hand, after the caving of the immediate roof above the unstable range, a stable "arch similarly" structure may be formed due to limited space. This type of "arch similarly" structure may be formed and caved with the advance of the coal face, resulting in periodical ground pressure.

Jiang Fuxing et al. proposed a concept of spatial structure of the overlying strata. Based on the different mining boundaries at different mining areas, the main roof and overlying strata may form four types of 3D structures after caving, including type "θ", "O", "S" and "C". The spatial structure type of overlying strata in mining regions or mines is initially determined by design, and then varies with the mining operation. It is determined by roof property, buried depth, coal pillars between the working face and the mining area, and fault protection pillars. In addition, it varies at different mining stages (Ma 2005; Jiang 1995; 2006; Wang 2006b; Hou et al. 2009; Liu2010).

In terms of the movement characteristics of overlying thick hard strata, Shi Hong (Shi 2005; Shi and Jiang 2004; 2005; Shi et al. 2005) regard the hard strata as a simple "beam fixed at two ends" structural model and analyzed the broken characteristics of thick hard strata before the initial fracture of the main roof. Using the stress distribution in the strata, Shi Hong, et al., proposed a mechanical criterion for three broken modes of thick hard rock, and predicted the initial fracture and the ground pressure interval of the main roof.

Based on the "elastic plate and articulated plate" mechanical model, Jia Xirong of Taiyuan University of Technology et al. (Jia et al. 1998) extended the ground pressure calculation method in medium thick coal seams into the calculation of ground pressure at LTCC face roof. According to the structural properties of roof strata and mining conditions, the strata with no self-support capability after fracture (no self-support strata) are defined as immediate roof. The strata with support structure, but without sufficient self-support capability after fracture (transition strata) are defined as main roof. The strata with self-support capability after fracture (complete support strata) are defined as roof overlying strata. In addition, they presented the basic assessment criteria for complete support strata, transition strata and no self-support strata.

Xie Guangxiang (Xie 2005; 2006; Xie and Luo 2005; Xie et al. 2006a, b; 2007a, b; 2009) believe that there is a “stress shell” composed of high stress beams in the surrounding rock space of mines. The maximum principal stress in the “stress shell” is greater than the principal stress in the strata inside and outside the “stress shell”. The stress shell bears and transfers the load and pressure from the overlying rock, and is a major support body while the main roof bears only partial load. Based on the findings on the “stress shell” and its mechanical properties, the 3D mechanical properties of the surrounding rock at LTCC faces were found, including the effect of mining height, the mechanism of pillar width and the response of advance rate. Furthermore, the mechanical properties of ground pressure abate and the mechanisms of dynamic hazard mitigation were obtained.

Some researchers have completed various studies on the theory of ground control and the law of roof movement at LTCC face (Buddery and Oldroyd 1992; Zhang 1995; Wu 1998; Wang et al.2001; Yasitli and Unver 2005; Ren 2005; Liu et al. 2006; Nan et al. 2008; Liu and Huang 2009; Xie and Zhao 2009a, b; Altounyan and Taljaard 2001; Alehossein and Poulsen 2010; Chen et al.2010; Miao and Lai 2011; Yu et al. 2011; Zhang et al. 2011), including seismic monitoring (Liu2008a, b; Kong et al. 2009; 2010a, b, c), analogous material (Kang et al. 2007a, b), numerical modelling (Wang et al. 2007; Zhu and Yan 2011), theoretical analysis (Meng 2007; Yang 2007; Fu 2008; Wu 2008; Zhang and Liu 2008; Zhou and Su 2008; Li and Xu 2009; Shi et al. 2009; Xing et al. 2009; Liu 2010; Meng et al. 2010; Wang 2010b) and site observations (Cheng 2008; Duan et al. 2008; Liu 2008a, b; Su 2008; Song et al. 2010).

The research results above are all based on the characteristics of ground pressure, and the models of “beam”, “arch”and “shell”. In addition, theoretical analysis and analogous (numerical) modelling were used to establish the model of overlying strata structure. Subsequently the models were validated on site. As a stable structure is formed in the strata at higher locations, its deformation and fracture will not affect or have little effect on the ground pressure at working face. Although there are some differences in studying methods and aspects, the ultimate purposes of the models derived are to explain the ground pressure during the LTCC operation and maintain a high efficient safe production. In recent years, however, the strong ground pressure at a large mining height LTCC face in ultra-thick coal seam cannot be explained by previous experiences and knowledge accumulated at a normal LTCC face. Therefore, based on the LTCC operation in ultra-thick coal seam of more than 14 m, this paper proposes a "cantilever beam-articulated rock beam" structural model. Based on the model proposed, the resistance force of support was calculated and the top coal and roof movement were monitored and analyzed.

In the study on the relationship between support and surrounding rock, to overcome the difference between the actual measurement and the traditional theory, Qian Minggao (Liu 1996; Qian et al. 1996a, b; Liu et al. 2002) regarded the key blocks of the Voussoir beam as the top boundary condition of the immediate roof, and believed that the support resistance force is mainly from "the pressure of loose blocks" and "the deformation pressure of overturned blocks" caused by the "S–R" movement of the "Voussoir beam". The deformation of immediate roof results in the overturned deformation load of the immediate roof inserted by the Voussoir beam absorbed by the fractured immediate roof (including top coal) and the non-existence of double curve relationship in the "$P–\Delta L$" relationship. Based on the mechanical properties and effect of various components in the support and surrounding rock system, the mechanical model of support and surrounding rock was established and provided a basis for further investigation on the relationship between the support and surrounding rock.

With the development of LTCC technology, the comprehensive mechanical model for LTCC mining face has been greatly improved. Liu Changyou, et al. used site observation, finite element numerical calculation, and the analogous material modelling method to investigate the comprehensive mechanical properties of the immediate roof and their effect on the relationship between support and surrounding rock. By considering the immediate roof as a variable body, the characteristics of deformation and fracture of the immediate roof and the structural mechanical and stiffness properties of the immediate roof were studied. They proposed that the load of the immediate roof is regionalized, and provided a calculation method for the stiffness of the immediate roof. In addition, based on the stiffness characteristics of the immediate roof with a rectangle shape face, the immediate roof is divided into three categories as stiffness similar, zero stiffness and medium stiffness. When the immediate roof stiffness is zero, the support is in the status of a "given load" or a "limited load". When the immediate roof is in a stiffness similar status, the support is in a "given deformation" status. When the immediate roof is in a medium stiffness status, the "$P–\Delta L$" curve shows a typical double curve relationship. When the immediate roof is in a zero stiffness status, the rational resistance force of support is mainly determined by its effect on the stability of the face ends.

The thickness variation of the immediate roof (including top coal) also affects the load bearing capacity of the immediate roof. Cao Changsheng et al. (Liu et al. 1997; 2002; Cao and Liu 1997; Cao et al. 1998; 1999; Cao et al. 1999) presented a concept on the critical thickness of the immediate roof and believed that the "$P$–$\Delta L$" double curve flattens when the immediate roof thickness exceeds a critical thickness. In other words, the variations of support resistance and main roof overturn angles have little effect on the roof subsidence.

Shi Yuanwei et al. (Kang et al. 1991; Shi and Chen 1993; Shi et al. 1993) presented and analyzed the critical thickness of the immediate roof and its effecting factors. They state that when critical thickness is greater than actual thickness, or when the immediate roof in front of the face enters a plastic zone, the immediate roof would lose its load bearing capacity after it enters the roof control zone. Therefore, the mechanical relationship of support and surrounding rock will show a variation. In contrast, the immediate roof will maintain a certain deformation capacity.

Fang (2002) simulated the effect on the roof stability at face ends by support type using discrete element software and believes that under soft coals, the critical issue is to control the distance from the support tip to the coal wall, which must be controlled within the distance limit. Under the conditions of medium hard coals, the constraint distance from the support tip to coal wall is relatively large and thus there will be a rational arrangement for the tip to wall distance and support resistance force. For hard coals, the study focus should be on improving the top coal caving ability. In the study on the mechanical relationship of support and surrounding rock in a soft coal extraction, Huang (2002) found that the increase of support resistance can reduce the tensile stress range in the top coal between support tip and coal wall, increase the self-support capacity from the top coal between support tip and coal wall, and suppress the movement and fracture of top coals. Nevertheless, the increase of support resistance has a limited effect on the improvement of subsidence of unsupported zone between the support tip and coal wall.

Jin et al. (2002) state that under the condition of hard roof and hard coal, the LTCC face shows the characteristics of hard roof, and demonstrates the characteristics of top coal cushion effect at LTCC face. The rational support resistance force should be based on the cantilever beam model with a modification by the coefficient of cushion effect.

Wu Jian et al. (Wu and Yan 1995; Wu and Fu 1998; Wu and Zhang 2001) suggest that the traditional ground control theory could not explain the interaction relationship between the support and surrounding rock. The key support parameters in the support and surrounding rock relationship includes the vertical support force, the horizontal support force, the distance between the supporting point of resultant force and the coal wall, and the distance between the support tip and coal wall. There are obvious effects from these parameters, sometimes obvious only when they interact.

Yang et al. (2009) state that the key to the interaction system of the support and surrounding rock is the interaction between the support and top coal. Under hard coal conditions, the overturn of the immediate roof is affected by the support and top coal system, and the turning angle of the lower strata is less than the turning angle of the main roof. Under the medium hard coals and soft coals, the immediate roof can equally transfer the overturn deformation of the main roof to top coals and the support system. With the consideration of the immediate roof as the top boundary of support-top coal systems, the mechanical model for two-leg shield support and surrounding rock can be established.

The studies on the relationship between roof support and surrounding rock provide theories for the design and selection of LTCC roof support, the improvement of support-surrounding rock status and effective roof control (including top coals). In this paper, based on the relationship between roof support and surrounding rock, the authors propose a 3D dynamic optimal design method with hydraulic support and surrounding rock coupling, and subsequently the determination of the working resistance of hydraulic support at the No. 8105 coal face in Tashan mine in Datong, China, and test on site.

In terms of the study on mining equipment for LTCC operation, the improvement of the production rate at a fully mechanized coal face mainly depends on the increase of longwall width and shear cutting depth, fast advance and the extension of applicable range. In particular, the application of electromechanical heavy equipment enables the increase of the production rate, including high powered electric traction shearer, large capacity conveyor, electric-hydraulic controlled hydraulic support, non-stop self-moving stage loader and conveyor end, and high voltage power supply for face equipment. Currently the mining equipment manufactured in China for the fully mechanized longwall face and the LTCC face can meet the requirements and demands for high production and high efficiency in the Chinese coal industry.

In the early years, China imported a large amount of shearers including chain haulage type and hydraulic haulage type. Since the 1970s, China has started to manufacture shearers. In the eighties, the hydraulic haulage shearers met the requirements for extracting coal seams with heights from 1.5 to 4.5 m. In addition, the difficulties in integrating all mining equipment had been overcome. There were about 50 types of shearers. Up to the 1990s, large power hydraulic haulage shearer developed in China has gone into mass production. Furthermore, the high performance electric haulage shearer had been developed, and is currently at an advanced level in the world, with a cutting height of 5.5 m. In China, the application of large power electric haulage shearers enables the increase of coal production at a fully mechanized face from 1 Mtpa to 4 Mtpa or even 10 Mtpa. Currently, several series of electric haulage shearers are manufactured in China. In addition, the electric shearers are equipped with intelligent monitoring, control and protection systems, and applied with information processing and sensor technologies to achieve electro-mechanization.

Top-coal caving hydraulic support is a key equipment for LTCC operations. During the last 20 years, top-coal caving hydraulic support was gradually developed from high position top-coal caving support, middle position top-coal caving support, to low position top-coal caving support. Currently, the low position top-coal caving support is widely used, which is a chock-shield hydraulic support with positive four-link bar, reverse four-link bar and single swing link bar.

In terms of the scraper conveyor, there has been significant improvement every 10 years in China. In the 1980s, there were various types of scraper conveyors with two series of chute width of 730 mm and 764 mm. In 1994, the SGZ880/800 cross-side unloading scraper conveyor with an entirely cast-welded chute was developed by the Taiyuan Branch of China Coal Research Institute and Northwestern Mining Equipment Manufactory, which had a capacity of 7000 t/d. During the same period, Zhangjiakou Mining Equipment Manufactory introduced some casting and processing equipment and manufactured scraper conveyors with entirely cast-welding chutes.

During the period of the ninth five-year national economic plan, with the cooperation of Zhangjiakou and Northwestern Coal Mining Equipment Manufactory, using CAD technology, the Taiyuan Branch of China Coal Research Institute developed the first scraper conveyors for LTCC face with retractable end chain adjusting device. They were the SGZ960/750 front scraper conveyor and the SGZ900/750 rear scraper conveyor, and also stage loader and crusher. The equipment developed met the requirements from Yankuang Group for a coal production of 10,000–13,000 t/d. During the period of the tenth five-year national economic plan, Yankuang Group, the Taiyuan Branch of China Coal Research Institute and Northwestern Benniu Group jointly developed the SGZ1000/1200 and the SGZ1200/1400 long distance high reliability front scraper conveyor and rear scraper conveyor. Currently, the SFZ1200/1400 long distance high reliable rear scraper conveyor is an ultra-heavy scraper conveyor for LTCC faces, which is characterized by its highest power level, widest chute and longest length. Furthermore, it integrated various advanced technologies, including automatic extension of the conveyor end, hydraulic motor chain tensioner, speed adjustment hydraulic coupler and compact chain. In the 1990s, its main specifications reached an advanced level accepted worldwide. The SGZ1000/1200 front scraper conveyor is currently the largest front scraper conveyor, and can be integrated with various powerful shearers and hydraulic supports. Its installed power is 2 × 600 kW. The development of the SGZ1000/1200 and the SGZ1200/1400 scraper conveyors enables not only the technical advance in scraper conveyor technology, but also in LTCC technology.

In order to promote the development of large mining height LTCC technology and equipment for ultra-thick coal seams, and to achieve safe, high efficiency and high recovery mining of ultra-thick coal seams, in 2008, the Ministry of Science and Technology of China launched a significant R&D project called "the study of large mining height LTCC technology and equipment" The project was supported by the national science and technology plan. With 14–20 m thick coal seams, the project has developed a large mining height LTCC mining method (LLTCC mining method), a complete set of mining equipment, roadway drivage and support technology and equipment, and mine safety warrant technology and equipment (Wang 2013a,b). In 2011, the technologies and equipment developed were tested at the No. 8105 coal face of Tashan mine in Datong, China, with a production of 1.0849 Mtpa. The success of the project marked a new level for large mining height LTCC technology and equipment for ultra-thick coal seams in China. In this paper, the major research achievements, case studies and technical economical results from this project are presented.

## 2 GEOLOGICAL AND MINING CONDITIONS AT THE TASHAN COAL MINE

### 2.1 Brief description of the mine

The Tashan coal mine is a large modern coal mine in Datong extracting the coals from Permo-Carboniferous system in the Datong coal field. The mine is located at the middle edge of Eastern Datong coal field in Shanxi Province, China, Fig. 1. The strike length of the mine is 24.3 km, the dip width is 11.7 km and the total area is 170.9 km$^2$. The mine extracts five coal seams including seam 2, 3, 4, 5 and 8. The mine has 5070 Mt of geological coal reserve, 4760 Mt of industrial coal reserve and 3070 Mt of mineable coal reserve. In 2007, the mine had a nominal production capacity of 1.5 Mtpa, and a life of 140 years.

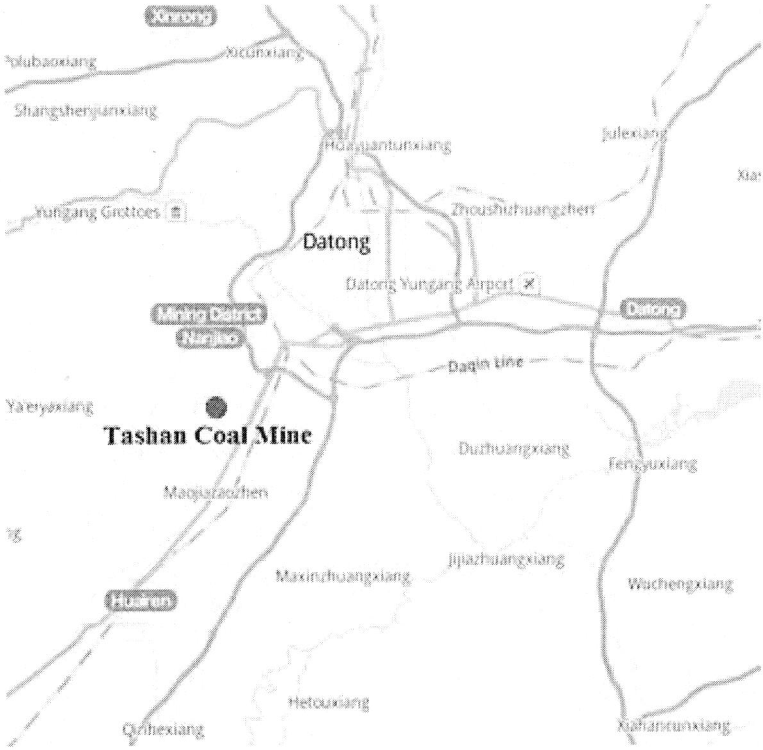


**Figure 1.**Locality of Tashan coal mine

## 2.2 Geological conditions of the mine

The main coal seams extracted at Tashan coal mine are coal seam 3–5; their buried depth ranges from 347 to 447 m; average seam thickness is 16.8 m and maximum is 20 m; and average seam dip is 4°. The protodyakonov coefficient F of the coal seams ranges from 2.7 to 13.7. There are 4–14 plies partings, and their lithologies consist of grey brown kaolinite, kaolinitic mudstone, grey and black carbonaceous mudstone, sandy mudstone, and locally dark grey siltstone.

The top of coal seam 3–5 is a 0.33 m thick false roof of grey black carbonaceous mudstone. The top part of the immediate roof consists of brown grey kaolinitic mudstone, magmatic rock and the seam 2. The middle part of the immediate roof is composed of shed coal and silicified coal. The bottom part consists of grey black carbonaceous mudstone, kaolinite and magmatic rock. The thickness of the immediate roof ranges from 2.4 to 6.3 m. From top to bottom, the upper roof consists of seam 4, magmatic rock, silicified coal, siltstone, fine sandstone, kaolinitic mudstone and sandy mudstone. The thickness of the upper roof varies from 11.31 to 27.36 m. The immediate floor consists of grey brown kaolinitic mudstone and sandy mudstone. It is brittle, fragile and contains coal bits. The lower floor is dark grey siltstone with local fine sandstone. The length of the No. 8105 LLTCC face is 207 m. The face is affected by igneous rock. Thus, there are some metamorphism and silicification in the seam 3-5. The seam structure is complex. The coal with metamorphism and silicification is hard, broken and with well-developed cleats. Mixed coal is lose and fragile. A lower coal seam is stable and hard, and forms a structure like a sandwich, shown in Fig. 2.

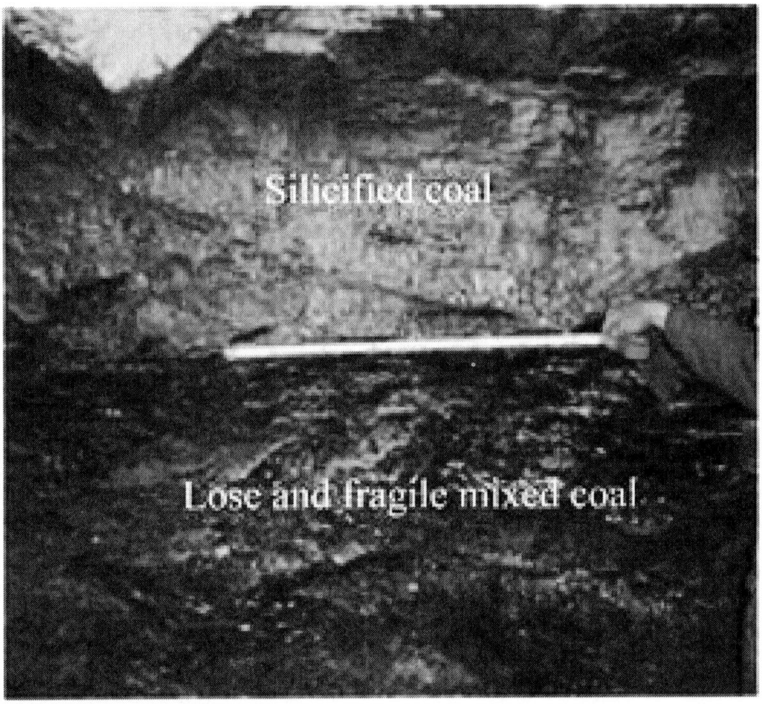


**Figure 2.** The upper seam structure at No. 8105 working face

The relative gas emission at coal seam 3–5 in Tashan coal mine is 1.95 $m^3$/t, which is classified as a low gas mine. However, the coal dust has the possibility of a dust explosion, with an explosion index of 37 %. The period of spontaneous combustion is 68 days. There is no high temperature heat hazard area. The geothermal gradient is 2.41 °C/100 m.

## 2.3 Geotechnical measurement and analysis of coal and rock masses

In order to fully understand the geotechnical properties of the surrounding rock, the measurement of geotechnical properties was systematically and comprehensively conducted, including the underground measurement of ground stress, rock strength test and rock structure observations. The measurement contents are listed in Table 1.

**Table 1.** Geotechnical measurement of surrounding rock at Tashan coal mine

| Order number | Measurement contents | Measurement instrument | Number of measurement points |
|---|---|---|---|
| 1 | Ground stress | SYY-56 ground stress monitor with hydraulic fracture | 3 holes |
| 2 | Rock strength | WQCZ-56 measurement instrument of rock strength | 8 holes |
| 3 | Rock structure | KDVJ-400 borehole camera | 13 holes |

### 2.3.1 Measurement results of in situ stresses

Using the hydraulic fracturing method, the in situ stress of rock in the roof of the seam 3–5 at Tashan coal mine was measured. The measurement results are shown in Table 2. These results show that the maximum horizontal principal stress is greater than the vertical principal stress. The type of stress field is the $\sigma_H > \sigma_V > \sigma_h$ type. Therefore, the stress field tested is mainly a structural stress field, and maximum horizontal principal stress is the principal stress.

**Table 2.** Test results of ground stress

| Order number | Roadway name | Buried depth (m) | Vertical stress (MPa) | Maximum horizontal principal stress (MPa) | Minimum horizontal principal stress (MPa) | Direction of maximum horizontal principal stress |
|---|---|---|---|---|---|---|
| 1 | 1070 auxiliary transport roadway | 467 | 11.44 | 12.00 | 6.40 | N26.7°E |
| 2 | 5102 gate road | 467 | 11.44 | 12.40 | 8.22 | N24.8°E |
| 3 | 2102 gate road | 467 | 11.44 | 12.90 | 7.24 | N19.0°E |

### 2.3.2 Test results of surrounding rock strength

The surrounding rock strength was directly measured in the borehole underground using the WQCZ-56 instrument. There were eight boreholes at four test stations, including four roof holes and four wall holes. Figures 3 and 4 show the test results in the No. 2102 roadway that was the closest station to the No. 8105 working face.

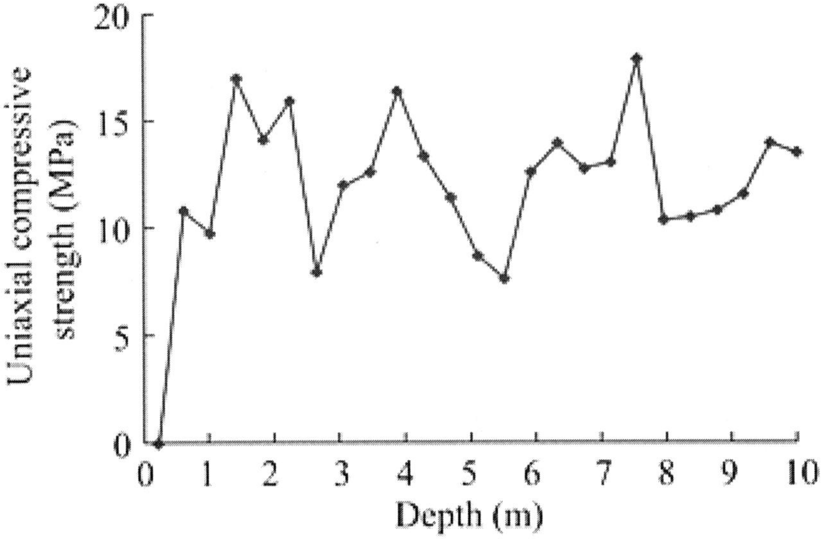


**Figure 3.** Test results of surrounding rock strength at roof of No. 2102 roadway

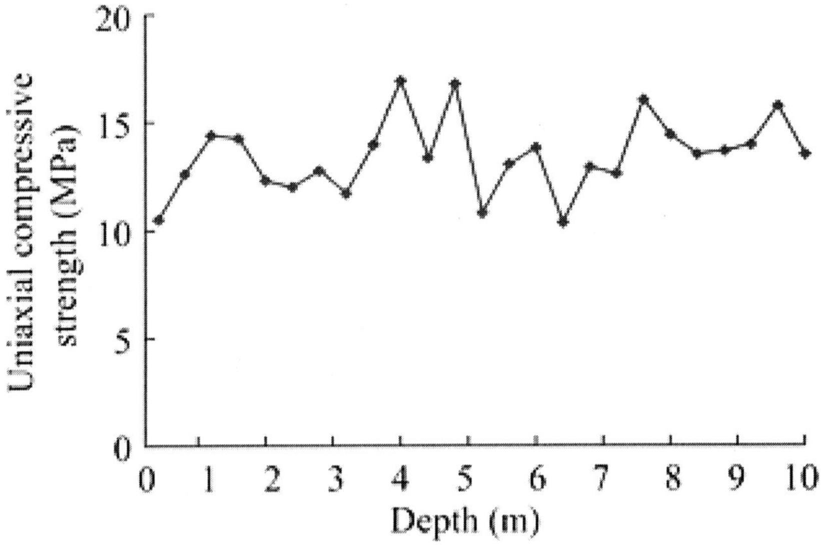


**Figure 4.** Test results of surrounding rock strength at wall of No. 2102 roadway

The test station was located in the No. 2102 roadway and 500 m away from the intersection of the No. 2102 roadway and the No. 1070 return airway. At this location, the roof holes and wall holes were all in coal seams and the coal strength was measured in detail. A 0.4 m fractured zone at roof holes was ignored and thus the maximum strength of the coal was 17.85 MPa, the minimum was 7.65 MPa, and the average was 12.43 MPa. The average coal strength in wall holes was 13.43 MPa.

### 2.3.3 Observations of the surrounding rock structure

The development of cleavage and fracture of the surrounding rock was directly observed in the boreholes underground using a KDVJ-400 borehole camera. The observations of 13 boreholes demonstrated that the cleavage and fracture in the top coal and immediate roof at the Tashan coal mine were well developed. In addition, there were various degree of layer separation at shallow roof strata and there was a trend to extend the layer separation into the upper strata. Figure 5 shows the photos of cleavage and fracture in boreholes.

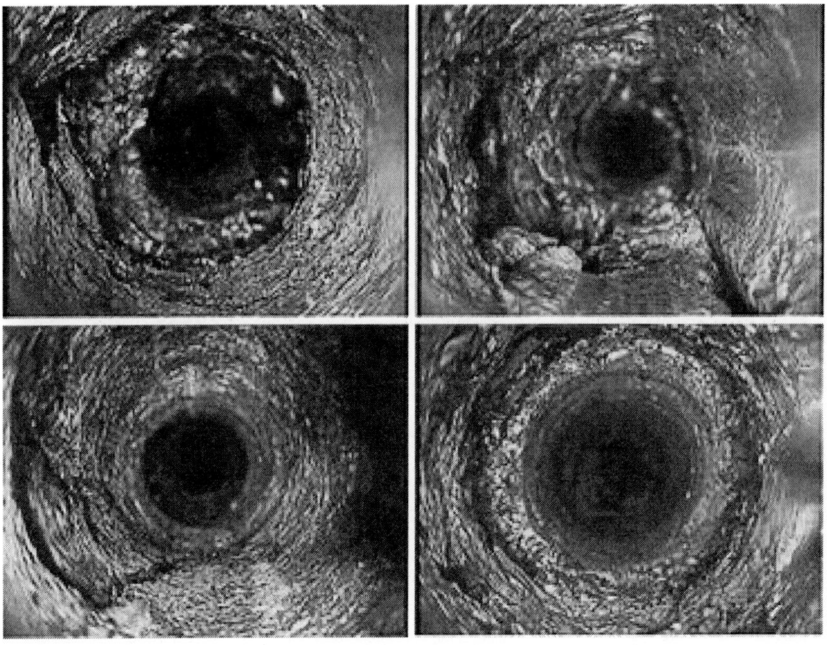

**Figure 5.** Typical photos inside boreholes at roof of roadway in Tashan coal mine

# 3 MINING METHOD AND GROUND CONTROL TECHNOLOGY FOR LLTCC OPERATION IN ULTRA-THICK COAL SEAMS

## 3.1 LLTCC in ultra-thick coal seams

In a conventional fully mechanized top-coal caving longwall face, the coal cutting height is normally 3.0–3.5 m. Based on the rule of cutting to caving ratio 1:3, the conventional top-coal caving height is 9–10.5 m. In other words, the maximum thickness of coal extraction is 12–14 m. In terms of ultra-thick coal seams with thicknesses greater than 14 m, if the cutting height remains as 3.0–3.5 m, there will be many problems. For instance, the cutting to caving ratio will be too low (1:4.7 if cutting height is 3.5 m in a 20 m thick coal seam); it would be difficult to cave top coals, and the coal recovery will be low. At the same time, the increase of coal production will result in the increase of gas emission and the difficulties in removing gas due to limited cross-section area at the coal face.

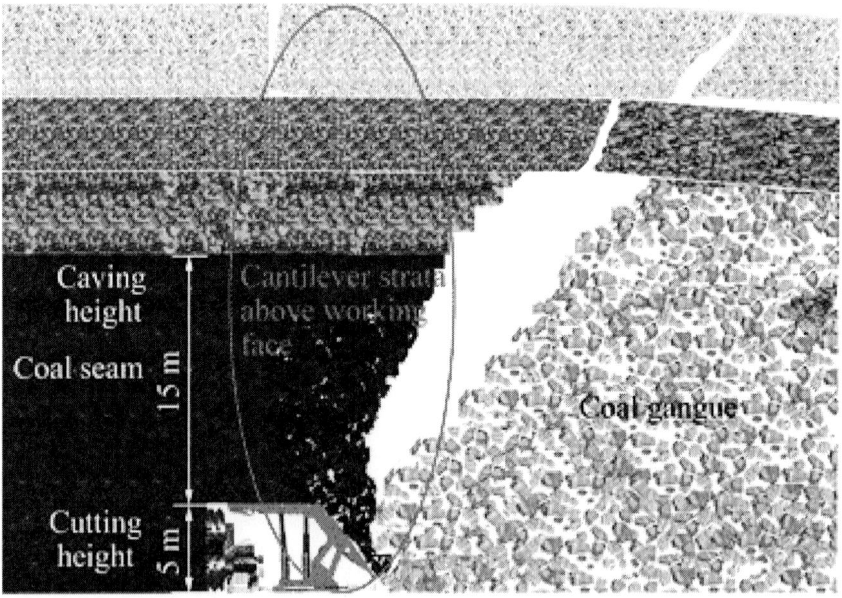


**Figure 6.** LLTCC mining method in ultra-thick coal seam

In order to overcome the problems mentioned above, the authors propose a LLTCC mining method, that is to increase the coal cutting height to 5 m, the top coal caving height to 15 m, and the total coal extraction height to 20 m, shown in Fig. 6. The LLTCC mining method involves a large coal cutting height, a large coal caving height and a large extraction space, that will result in some additional problems including coal wall spalling, difficulties in top-coal caving, and strong ground pressure. Those problems require comprehensive, in-depth and systematic research and testing.

### 3.2 3D spatial structural model of the roof in LLTCC mining

Because of the large thickness of the coal seam extracted through LLTCC mining in ultra-thick coal seams, the range of ground control should also be extended. After the completion of top coal caving operation, it is not possible for the roof rock to cave and fill in the goaf in a short time. Therefore, the immediate roof will form a "cantilever beam", and the upper roof will form a stable "articulated beam". In other words, a "cantilever beam–articulated beam" will be formed in a LLTCC coal face. In a general case, the overlying strata does not simply follow the movement from lower layer to upper layer, and instead forms various combinations of structures and moves with some laws. Figures 7 and 8 show the structural model of the roof.

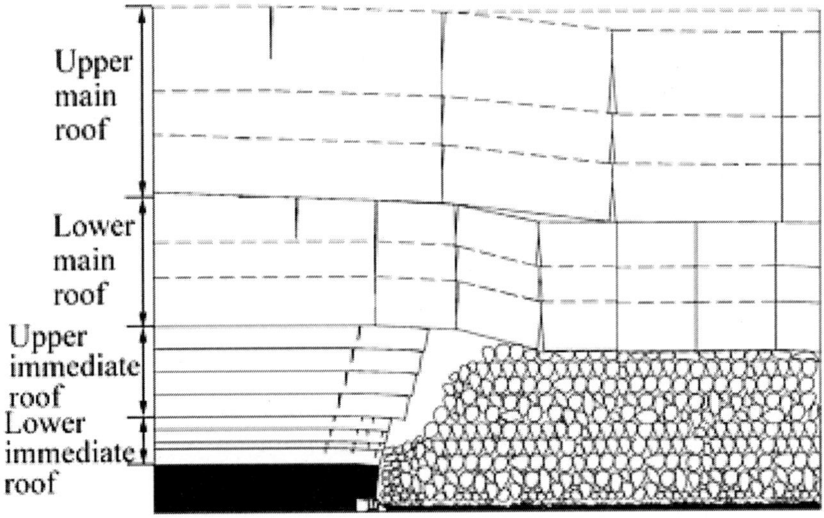


**Figure 7.** Strike cross-section of a LLTCC face

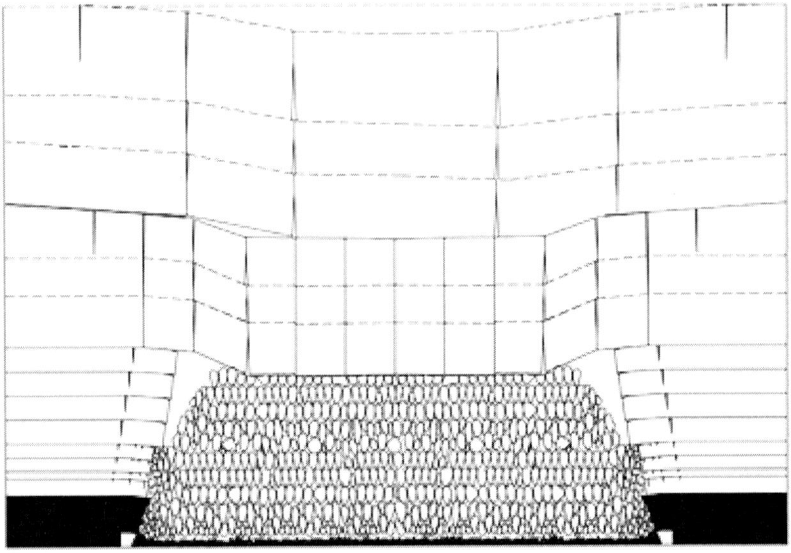

**Figure 8.** Dip cross-section of a LLTCC face

Based on the study discussed above, a "cantilever beam–articulated beam" structural model for overlying strata at a LLTCC face has been developed, shown in Fig. 9. The strata that need to be controlled are the strata that cannot be supported by caved rocks before they cave. They are in the form of a "cantilever beam" and defined as immediate roof. Above the immediate roof, the strata that are supported by caved rocks are called the upper roof with an "articulated beam" structure. The roof strata satisfying the $\Delta_j - \Delta_m \leq 0$ condition are defined as immediate roof while the roof strata satisfying the $\Delta_j - \Delta_m > 0$ condition are defined as upper roof. $\Delta_j$ is the ultimate subsidence.

$$\Delta_j = h - \frac{ql^2}{2kh\sigma_c} \tag{1}$$

where $h$ is the strata thickness analyzed, $k$ is a dimensionless coefficient ($k = 0.1\,h$), $q$ is the line load, $l$ is fracture length of the strata analyzed, $\sigma_c = (0.30 - 0.35)R_c$ ($R_c$ is compression strength), $\Delta_m$ is the possible subsidence (Yan 2009),

$$\Delta_m = (h_c + h_f)(1 - p_1) + (1 - k_p)h_m \tag{2}$$

where $p_1$ is the coal loss rate; $h_c$ is the coal-cutting height; $h_f$ is the coal caving height; $k_p$ is the expansion coefficient; $h_m$ is thickness of the immediate roof.

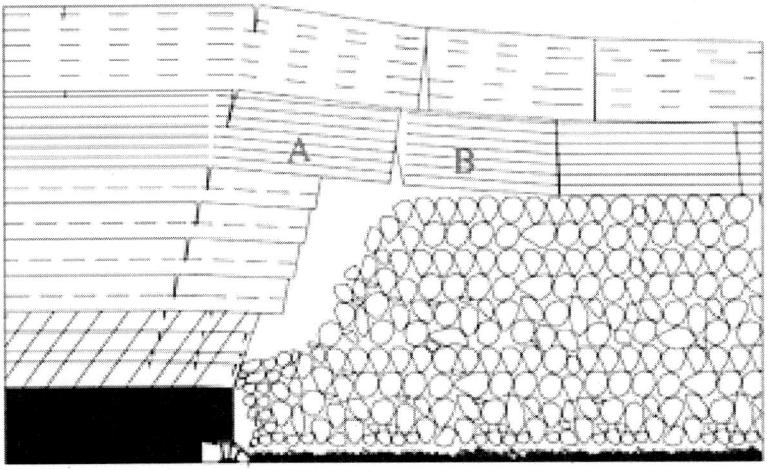


**Figure 9.** Structural model of “cantilever beam–articulated beam”

## 3.3 Determination of working resistance of the LLTCC hydraulic support

The top coal body of the LLTCC face in ultra-thick coal seams can be regarded as a “semi-rigid top coal body” that can transfer the roof deformation. The deformation effect of the part of the immediate roof enables the top coal body becoming “semi-rigid top coal body”. In terms of pressure on the support, this part of the strata can be called “no deformation pressure strata”. Through the “semi-rigid top coal body”, the pressure generated by the deformation of immediate roof and upper roof is transferred to hydraulic support. This part of the strata can be called “deformation pressure strata” (Yan 2009). The loads on the support are the combination of the weight of the top coal and the pressure generated by roof deformation. The force analysis of the immediate roof with deformation pressure is shown in Fig. 10. The force analysis of the upper roof is shown in Fig. 11.

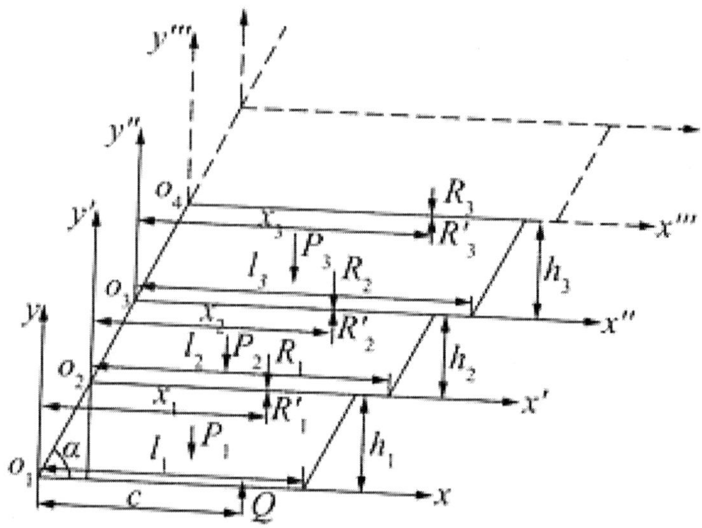


**Figure 10.** Force analysis and calculation of the immediate roof

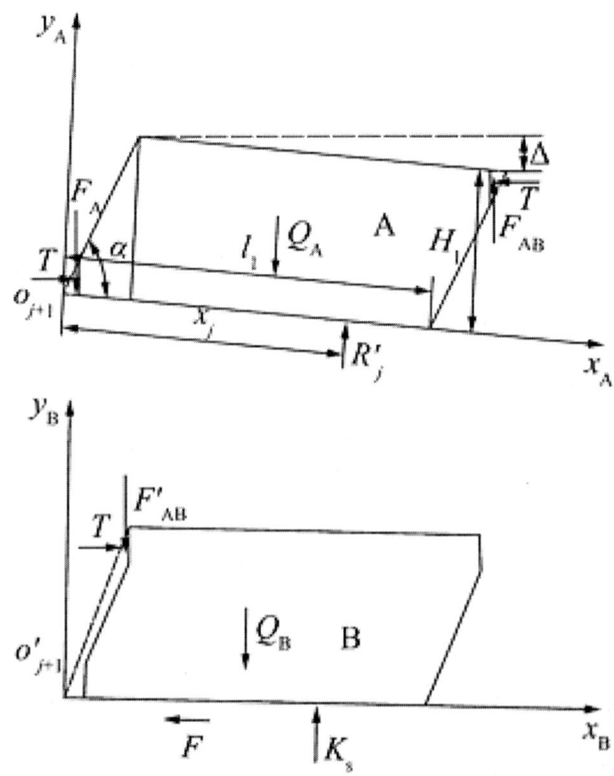


**Figure 11.** Force analysis of rock in main roof

Force analysis of the immediate roof with deformation pressure.

According to $\sum M_{oi} = 0$ ($i = 1, 2, 3, \ldots, j$), get:

$$P_1\left(\frac{l_1}{2}+\frac{1}{2}h_1\text{ctan }\alpha\right)+R_1x_1-Qc=0$$

$$P_2\left(\frac{l_2}{2}+\frac{1}{2}h_2\text{ctan }\alpha\right)+R_2x_2-R_1'(x_1-h_1\text{ctan }\alpha)=0$$

$$P_3\left(\frac{l_3}{2}+\frac{1}{2}h_3\text{ctan }\alpha\right)+R_3x_3-R_2'(x_2-h_2\text{ctan }\alpha)=0$$

$$\cdots\cdots\cdots\cdots$$

$$P_j\left(\frac{l_j}{2}+\frac{1}{2}h_j\text{ctan }\alpha\right)+R_jx_j-R_{j-1}'\left(x_{j-1}-h_{j-1}\text{ctan }\alpha\right)=0 \tag{1}$$

The *j* formulas above are combined, and which will get:

$$Qc=\frac{1}{2}\sum_{i=1}^{j}P_i(l_i+h_i\text{ctan }\alpha)+\sum_{i=1}^{j-1}R_ih_i\text{ctan }\alpha+R_jx_j \tag{3}$$

where $Q$ is the deformation pressure on support, kN; c is the distance from resultant force of support to coal wall, m; $P_i$ is the rock weight of immediate roof of ith layer with deformation pressure, kN; $h_i$, $l_i$ are the rock thickness and length of the immediate roof of *i*th layer with deformation pressure respectively, m; $\alpha$ is the rock fissure angle, (°); $R_j$is the additional force of upper strata, kN; $x_j$ is the distance from additional force of upper strata to caving point of *j*th layer immediate roof, m.

During the analysis of the large roof structure, the roof with deformation pressure is regarded as an entire body, and the interaction of internal layers can be ignored. Therefore, the Eq. (3) can be simplified as follows:

$$Qc=\frac{1}{2}\sum_{i=1}^{j}P_i(l_i+h_i\text{ctan }\alpha)+R_jx_j \tag{4}$$

(2)Analysis of rock A in main roof with deformation pressure.

During the analysis of rock A in main roof, assume that the broken distance of main roof A exceeding immediate roof $P_j$ is hjctan αhjctan α, thus, $\sum M_{j+1} = 0$ to get:

$$R_jx_j=Q_A\left(\frac{L}{2}+\frac{1}{2}H\text{ctan }\alpha\right)-T(H-\Delta) \\ -F_{AB}(L+H\text{ctan }\alpha) \tag{5}$$

where $Q_A$ is the weight of rock A in main roof with deformation pressure, kN; $T$ is the compression force between rocks, kN; $H$, $L$ is the strata thickness and broken distance of main roof with deformation pressure respectively, m; $\Delta$ is the subsidence of rock A in main roof with deformation pressure, m; $F_{AB}$ is the friction force between rock A and B, kN.

Substitute Eq. (2) into Eq. (3), to get:

$$Qc = \frac{1}{2}\sum_{i=1}^{j} P_i(l_i + h_i\text{ctan }\alpha) + Q_A\left(\frac{L}{2} + \frac{1}{2}H\text{ctan }\alpha\right) - T(H - \Delta) - F_{AB}(L + H\text{ctan }\alpha)$$

$$Qc = \frac{1}{2}\sum_{i=1}^{j+1} P_i(l_i + h_i\text{ctan }\alpha) - T(h_{j+1} - \Delta) - F_{AB}\left(l_{i+1} + h_{j+1}\text{ctan }\alpha\right) \tag{6}$$

(3)Analysis of rock B in main roof.

Force balance in vertical direction:

$$F'_{AB} = Ks - Q_B \tag{7}$$

In Eq. (5), F’AB=TfFAB’=Tf, F’AB=FABFAB’=FAB, therefore:

$$T = \frac{Ks - Q_B}{f} \tag{8}$$

where $K$ is the rigidity of gangue in goaf, N/m; $s$ is the compression of gangue in goaf, m, (s=(k1−k2)∑i=1jhi,k1s=(k1−k2)∑i=1jhi,k1 is the expansion coefficient, $k_2$ is the residual expansion coefficient); $f$ is the friction coefficient among rocks; $Q_B$ is the weight of key block B in main roof (assume $Q_B = Q_A$), kN.

Substitute Eq. (8) into Eq. (6), to get:

$$Q = \frac{f\sum_{i=1}^{j+1} P_i(l_i + h_i\text{ctan }\alpha) - 2(Ks - Q_B)(h_{j+1} + fl_{i+1} + fh_{i+1}\text{ctan }\alpha - \Delta)}{2cf} \tag{9}$$

In summary, the calculation formula of hydraulic support for LLTCC mining is as follows:

$$P_z = K_d B(G_d + Q) = K_d B\left[L_d h_d \gamma_m + \frac{f\sum_{i=1}^{j+1} P_i(l_i + h_i \text{ctan } \alpha) - 2(Ks - Q_B)(h_{j+1} + fl_{i+1} + fh_{i+1}\text{ctan } \alpha - \Delta)}{2cf}\right] \quad (10)$$

where $P_z$ is the working resistance force of LLTCC support, kN; $K_d$ is the dynamic load coefficient; $G_d$ is the weight of top coal, kN; $B$ is the distance between the centers of two supports, m; $L_d$ is the distance of roof control, m; $h_d$ is the thickness of top coal, m; γmγm is the bulk density of top coal, kN/m$^3$.

The equation for calculating the support external load obtained from the theoretical study discussed above was tested and validated at the No. 8105 coal face in Tashan coal mine in Datong, China. The borehole analyzed was WEI 1403 at the No. 8105 coal face in Tashan coal mine. Table 3 shows the structure of the strata in borehole, and Table 4 shows the physical and mechanical parameters.

**Table 3.** Structure of rock strata in WEI 1403 borehole

| Layer No. | Layer thickness (m) | Rock name | Layer No. | Layer thickness (m) | Rock name | Layer No. | Layer thickness (m) | Rock name |
|---|---|---|---|---|---|---|---|---|
| C1 | 4.49 | Mudstone | C22 | 2.40 | Siltstone | C43 | 7.25 | Coarse sandstone |
| C2 | 1.33 | Coal | C23 | 2.24 | Kaolinitic mudstone | C44 | 1.70 | Fine conglomerate |
| C3 | 2.97 | Sandy mudstone | C24 | 1.40 | Siltstone | C45 | 10.15 | Sandstone |
| C4 | 3.17 | Sandstone | C25 | 14.39 | Kaolinitic mudstone | C46 | 20.52 | Fine conglomerate |
| C5 | 15.67 | Sandy mudstone | C26 | 4.10 | Siltstone | C47 | 10.18 | Fine sandstone |
| C6 | 1.12 | Mudstone | C27 | 2.40 | Fine conglomerate | C48 | 4.95 | Siltstone |
| C7 | 1.78 | Coal | C28 | 3.70 | Coarse sandstone | C49 | 4.58 | Fine sandstone |
| C8 | 5.37 | Sandy mudstone | C29 | 3.00 | Siltstone | C50 | 2.16 | Fine conglomerate |
| C9 | 1.10 | Coarse sandstone | C30 | 14.13 | Sandy mudstone | C51 | 9.34 | Fine sandstone |
| C10 | 1.3 | Siltstone | C31 | 4.10 | Siltstone | C52 | 1.40 | Siltstone |
| C11 | 1.55 | Kaolinitic mudstone | C32 | 1.70 | Fine sandstone | C52 | 8.60 | Fine conglomerate |
| C12 | 5.03 | Siltstone | C33 | 7.96 | Sandy mudstone | C54 | 5.90 | Fine sandstone |
| C13 | 1.00 | Coarse sandstone | C34 | 2.66 | siltstone | C55 | 1.70 | siltstone |
| C14 | 1.10 | Siltstone | C35 | 1.65 | Fine sandstone | C56 | 1.00 | Fine sandstone |
| C15 | 5.37 | Kaolinitic mudstone | C36 | 3.50 | siltstone | C57 | 12.28 | Sandstone |
| C16 | 1.25 | Siltstone | C37 | 5.35 | Sandy mudstone | C58 | 10.20 | Siltstone |
| C17 | 2.93 | Coarse sandstone | C38 | 1.60 | Kaolinitic mudstone | C59 | 5.34 | Sandy mudstone |
| C18 | 0.90 | Siltstone | C39 | 0.65 | Coarse sandstone | C60 | 10.68 | Fine sandstone |
| C19 | 1.10 | Coarse sandstone | C40 | 13.64 | Siltstone | C63 | 122.56 | |
| C20 | 4.43 | Kaolinitic mudstone | C41 | 7.72 | Fine sandstone | to | | |
| C21 | 2.70 | Fine sandstone | C42 | 2.00 | Sandy mudstone | surface | | |

**Table 4.** Lithological parameters of rock strata

| Rock strata | Volume force ($kN/m^3$) | Tensile strength (MPa) |
|---|---|---|
| Coal | 14.50 | 2.50 |
| Mudstone | 25.10 | 2.90 |
| Sandy mudstone | 26.20 | 3.10 |
| Kaolinitic mudstone | 25.13 | 3.30 |
| Siltstone | 25.80 | 5.10 |
| Fine sandstone | 26.50 | 4.30 |
| Sandstone | 24.10 | 3.70 |
| Fine conglomerate | 26.50 | 4.23 |
| Coarse sandstone | 25.80 | 4.10 |

The determination on the working resistance force of hydraulic support for LLTCC mining in ultra-thick coal seams:

(1)Based on criteria of immediate roof.

$\Delta_{mi}$ is the possible subsidence of $i$th layer, $i = 1, 2,\ldots,12$.

$$\Delta_{m1} = 10.73\ \text{m}$$

$$\Delta_{j1} = h - \frac{ql^2}{kh\sigma_c} = 3.87\ \text{m} < \Delta_{m1}$$

Thus rock strata C1 is in the immediate roof.

……

$$\Delta_{m11} = 1.89\ \text{m}$$

$$\Delta_{j11} = h - \frac{ql^2}{kh\sigma_c} = 0.56\ \text{m} < \Delta_{m11}$$

Thus, rock strata C11 is in the immediate roof.

$$\Delta_{m12} = 0.63\ \text{m}$$

$$\Delta_{j12} = h - \frac{ql^2}{kh\sigma_c} = 4.32\ \text{m} > \Delta_{m12}$$

(2)Determination of rock strata without deformation pressure.

$\sum_{i=1}^{n}(\Delta_j)_i = \Delta_d, \Delta_d$ is a total deformation of coal body in roof control zone, Δd=ηhd(1+λ)Δd=ηhd(1+λ) (Yan 2009); *η* is the porosity of top coal, η=(1−γd/γ)×100%η=(1−γd/γdγγ)×100%, γdγdis the dried bulk density of coal seam, *γ* is the bulk density of coal seam, *λ* is the coefficient of horizontal pressure (measured value at Tashan coal mine is 1.13).

$$\Delta_d = \eta h_d(1+\lambda) = 0.3 \times 10.61 \times (1+1.13)$$
$$= 6.78\,\text{m} \sum_{i=1}^{4}(\Delta_j)_i = 5.50\,\text{m} < \Delta_d;$$

$$\sum_{i=1}^{5}(\Delta_j)_i = 12.48\ \text{m} > \Delta_d;$$

Rock strata C5 is divided into two parts, $C5^{-1} = 10.17$ m, $C5^{-2} = 5.50$ m.

$$\sum_{i=1}^{5^{-1}}(\Delta_j)_i = \Delta_d$$

Thus rock strata C1–$C5^{-1}$ is rock strata without deformation pressure.

(3)Determination of working resistance force.

To maximize Eq. (10):

$$P_z = K_d B\left[L_d h_d \gamma + \frac{f\sum_{i=1}^{j+1}P_i(l_i + h_i \cot\alpha)}{2cf}\right] \tag{11}$$

Analyze Table 3, refer to the mechanical property of each rock stratum, and take C12–C16 as a whole. Substitute the basic data of C5-2, C6, C7,…,C16 into Eq. (11), get:

$$P_z = K_d B \left[ L_d h_d \gamma + \frac{f \sum_{i=1}^{j+1} P_i (l_i + h_i \cot \alpha)}{2cf} \right]$$
$$= 1.6 \times 1.75 \times (923.07 + 4378.11)$$
$$= 14843.3\,\text{kN}$$

Therefore, based on the geotechnical conditions of rock strata at the Tashan coal mine, the working resistance force of hydraulic support for the No. 8105 LLTCC face at ultra-thick coal seam in Tashan coal mine was determined as 15,000 kN. The ZF15000/28/52 hydraulic support for LLTCC face was selected.

## 3.4 Analysis on the applicability of hydraulic support type

The dynamic change characteristics of the ZF15000/28/52 fully mechanized high strength LLTCC hydraulic support in a shift is shown in Fig. 12. The figure shows that the variation of working resistance was not large, implying that the support had a very high reliability.

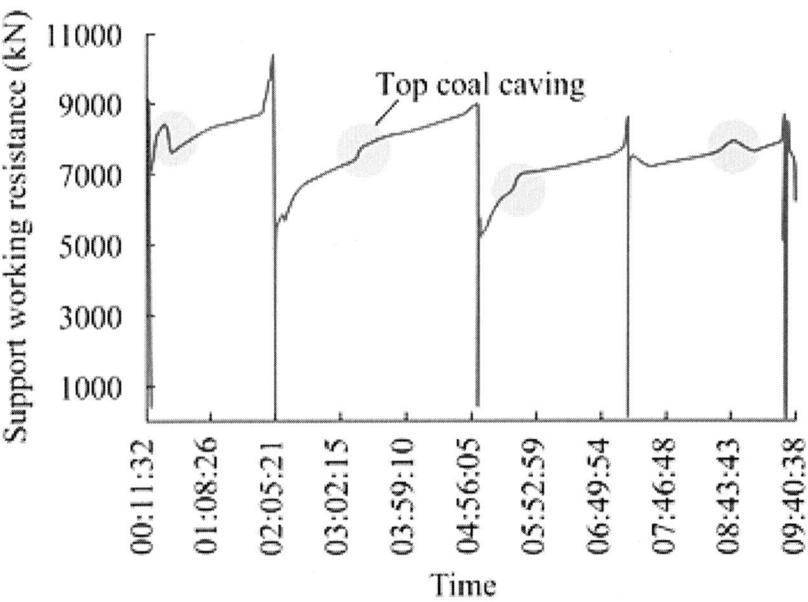


**Figure 12.** Periodical change of support working resistance at the middle of the face

Figure 13 shows the 3D support resistance variation at the end of the circle in the No. 8105 face. The impact range of the initial caving and periodical caving of the upper roof was extensive and covered the whole working face. In a normal working period, the average working resistance is 9073.06 kN. Table 5 shows that there was almost no effect on supports, although the dynamic load coefficient is large during loading period, indicating that the impact resistance of support is high. When load is high, and the working resistance force exceeds nominal resistance force, the relief valve can be activated in a timely manner, showing the stability of the support is good.

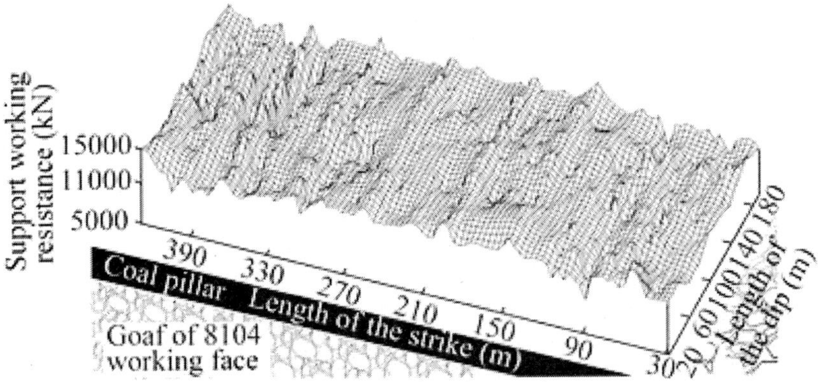


**Figure 13.** Distribution of ground pressure at the working face

The percentage of support resistance at different intervals was described as a histogram (Fig. 14). Figure 14 shows that the distribution of working resistance of hydraulic support was rational, and appeared as a distribution of sine wave. The support resistance was mostly within 8000–13,000 kN. In summary, the selection of support was reasonable and their utilization was high. The support selected was suitable for the roof conditions in the working face.

## 3.5 Analysis of the characteristics of top coal and roof movement in a LLTCC coal face

In order to study the movement law of top coal and roof at a LLTCC coal face, some boreholes were drilled into the top coal and roof of the tailgate at the No. 8105 LLTCC coal face in Tashan coal mine. Basic anchors were installed at different layers inside the boreholes. GUW300 tracking instruments were installed at the opening of the boreholes. The first monitoring station was setup at the location 300 m away from the box cut of the No. 8105 face. The

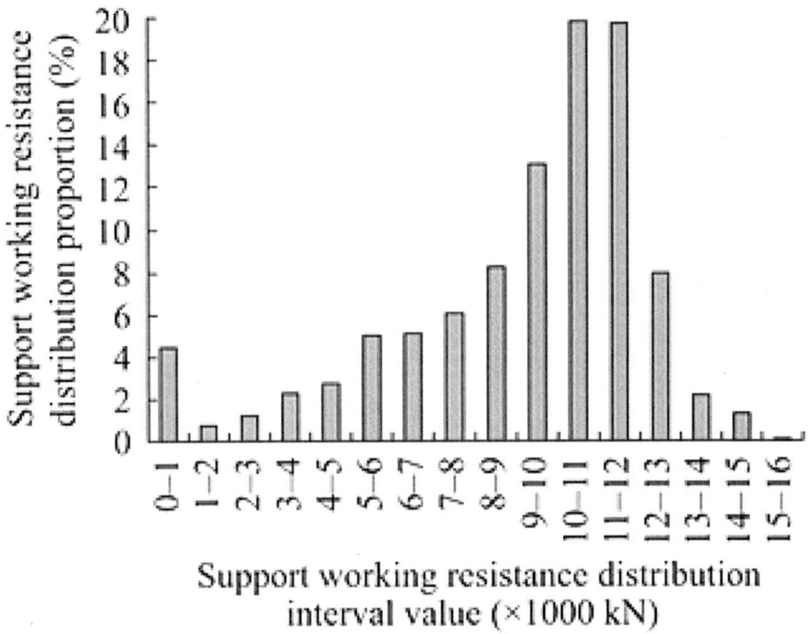


**Figure 14.** Histogram of support working resistance

second monitoring station was 15 m away from the first station. At each station, four boreholes were drilled into the top coal and roof, two deep base points were installed inside each hole, eight deep base points in total were installed, and four GUW300 deep base point movement tracking instruments were installed. The intersection angle of borehole and tailgate was 45°. The angles of from No. 1 to No. 4 boreholes with horizontal level were 40°, 30°, 20° and 10° respectively. The heights of borehole positions from No. 1 to No. 4 with floor were 2.4, 2.1, 1.8 and 1.5 m respectively. Figure 15 shows the layout of the boreholes. Figure 16 shows the layout of eight deep base points in each monitoring station with four points in the top coal and four points in the roof (Table 5).

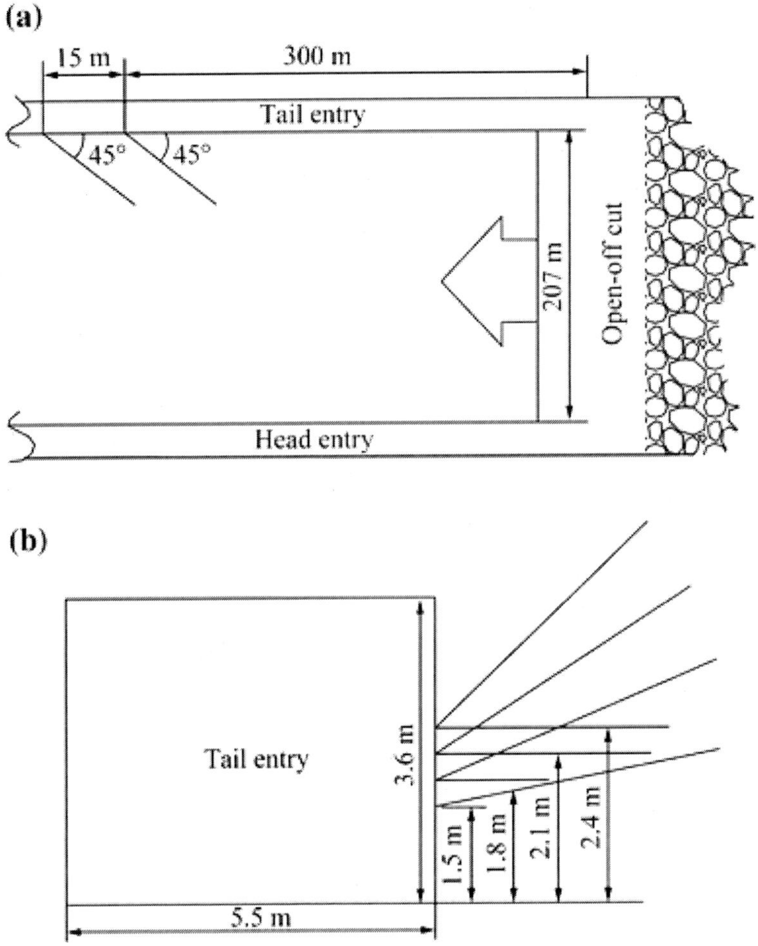


**Figure 15.** Boreholes layout. **a** Top view of boreholes layout, **b** vertical cross-section diagram

**Table 5.** Statistics of dynamic loading coefficient of upper roof

| Support No. | 20 | 21 | 63 | 64 | 95 | 96 |
|---|---|---|---|---|---|---|
| Dynamic loading coefficient at initial loading | 1.51 | 1.57 | 1.56 | 1.58 | 1.62 | 1.49 |
| Average dynamic loading coefficient at initial loading | 1.56 | | | | | |
| Dynamic loading coefficient at Ith periodical loading | 1.43 | 1.58 | 1.58 | 1.58 | 1.49 | 1.50 |
| Dynamic loading coefficient at IIth periodical loading | 1.54 | 1.58 | 1.57 | 1.56 | 1.55 | 1.46 |
| Dynamic loading coefficient at IIIth periodical loading | 1.30 | 1.51 | 1.66 | 1.41 | 1.41 | 1.40 |
| Dynamic loading coefficient at IVth periodical loading | 1.38 | 1.51 | 1.64 | 1.52 | 1.59 | 1.37 |
| Dynamic loading coefficient at Vth periodical loading | 1.44 | 1.52 | 1.63 | 1.56 | 1.57 | 1.46 |
| Average dynamic loading coefficient at periodical loading | 1.43 | 1.55 | 1.61 | 1.54 | 1.54 | 1.45 |
| Total average dynamic loading coefficient at periodical loading | 1.52 | | | | | |

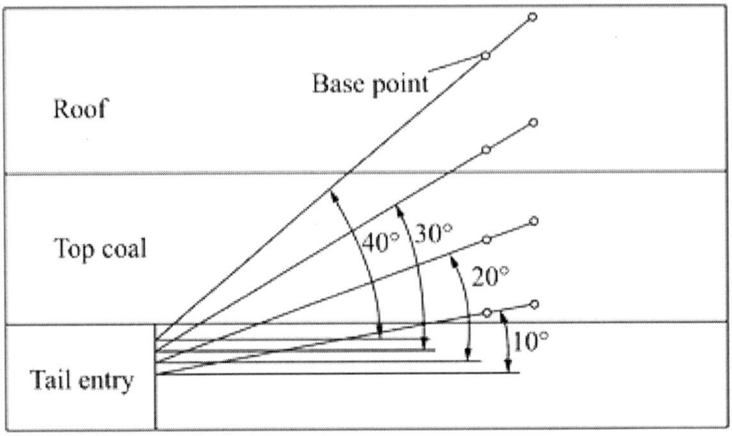


**Figure 16.** Layout of deep base points

Figure 17 shows the basic parameter geometry of the boreholes layout. Tables 6 and 7 show the parameters of deep base points. Basic geometry is described as Eq. (12).

$$X = \sqrt{(L\cos\alpha)^2 - (L\sin\beta)^2} \tag{12}$$

where $L$ is the depth of base point, m; $\alpha$ is the angle of elevation, (°); $\beta$ is the angle between borehole and tailgate, (°); $X$ is the horizontal length from borehole opening to deep base point and parallel to tailgate, m; $Y$ is the horizontal length from borehole opening to deep base point and perpendicular to tailgate, m; $Z$ is the vertical height from floor to deep base point, m; $H$ is the vertical height from floor to borehole opening, m.

From Figs. 18, 19, 20 and 21 show the movement of top coal and roof from two monitoring stations at the No. 8105 working face.

As shown from Figs. 18, 19, 20 and 21, among the initial displacement positions of eight top coal deep base points at two monitoring stations, the distance ahead of the coal wall at the working face ranged from 34 to 48 m with an average of 38 m; among the initial displacement positions of roof deep base points, the maximum distance ahead of the coal wall at the working face ranged from 22 to 34 m, with an average of 28.6 m.

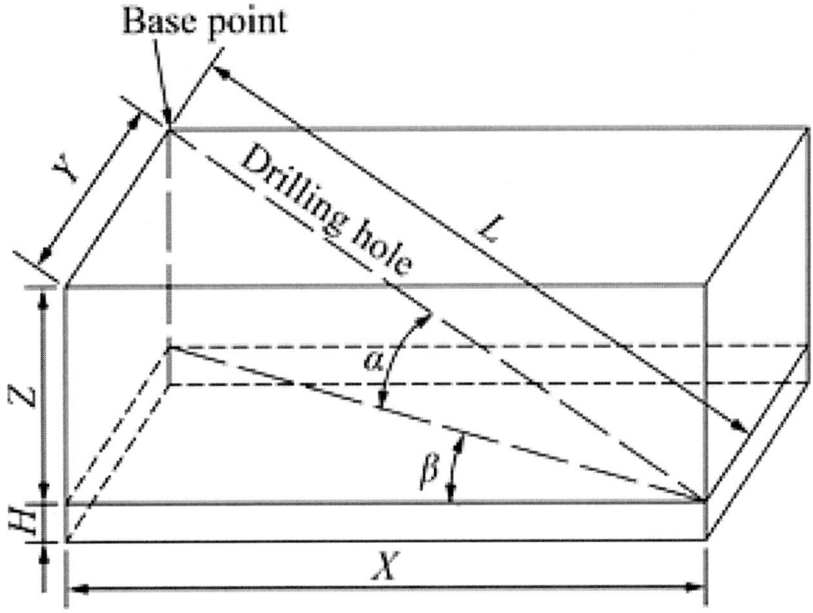


**Figure 17.** Geometry of deep base point parameters

**Table 6.** Parameters from first monitoring station

| Hole No. | Height from floor to hole opening (m) | Base point No. | Angle of elevation (°) | Height to floor (m) | Height to hole opening (m) | Depth to base point (m) | Horizontal projection of base point (m) | Distance of tailgate projection (m) |
|---|---|---|---|---|---|---|---|---|
| 1 | 2.4 | 11 | 40 | 32.1 | 29.7 | 46.2 | 35.4 | 25.0 |
| | | 12 | | 26.1 | 23.7 | 37.0 | 28.3 | 20.0 |
| 2 | 2.1 | 21 | 30 | 22.5 | 20.4 | 40.9 | 35.4 | 25.0 |
| | | 22 | | 18.4 | 16.3 | 32.7 | 28.3 | 20.0 |
| 3 | 1.8 | 31 | 20 | 14.7 | 12.9 | 37.7 | 35.4 | 25.0 |
| | | 32 | | 12.1 | 10.3 | 30.1 | 28.3 | 20.0 |
| 4 | 1.5 | 41 | 10 | 7.7 | 6.2 | 35.9 | 35.4 | 25.0 |
| | | 42 | | 6.5 | 5.0 | 28.7 | 28.3 | 20.0 |

**Table 7.** Parameters from second monitoring station

| Hole No. | Height from floor to hole opening (m) | Base point No. | Angle of elevation (°) | Height to floor (m) | Height to hole opening (m) | Depth to base point (m) | Horizontal projection of base point (m) | Distance of tailgate projection (m) |
|---|---|---|---|---|---|---|---|---|
| 1 | 2.4 | 11 | 40 | 32.1 | 29.7 | 46.2 | 35.4 | 25.0 |
| | | 12 | | 26.1 | 23.7 | 37.0 | 28.3 | 20.0 |
| 2 | 2.1 | 21 | 30 | 22.5 | 20.4 | 40.9 | 35.4 | 25.0 |
| | | 22 | | 18.4 | 16.3 | 32.7 | 28.3 | 20.0 |
| 3 | 1.8 | 31 | 20 | 14.7 | 12.9 | 37.7 | 35.4 | 25.0 |
| | | 32 | | 12.1 | 10.3 | 30.1 | 28.3 | 20.0 |
| 4 | 1.5 | 41 | 10 | 7.7 | 6.2 | 35.9 | 35.4 | 25.0 |
| | | 42 | | 6.5 | 5.0 | 28.7 | 28.3 | 20.0 |

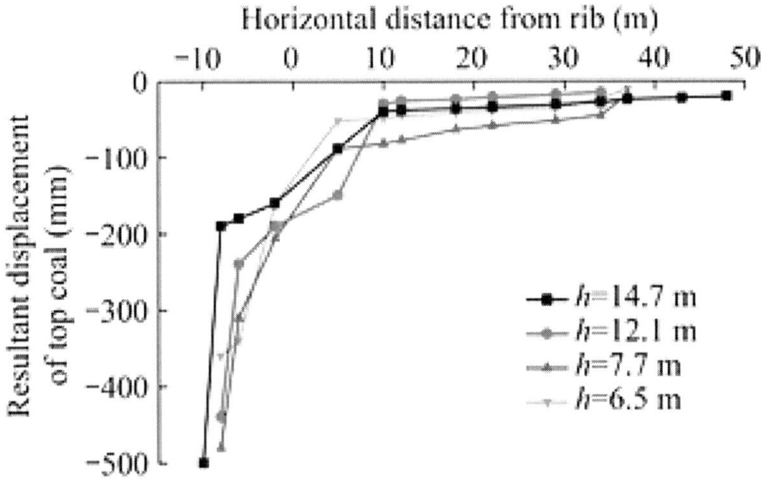


**Figure 18.** Top coal displacement at first monitoring station

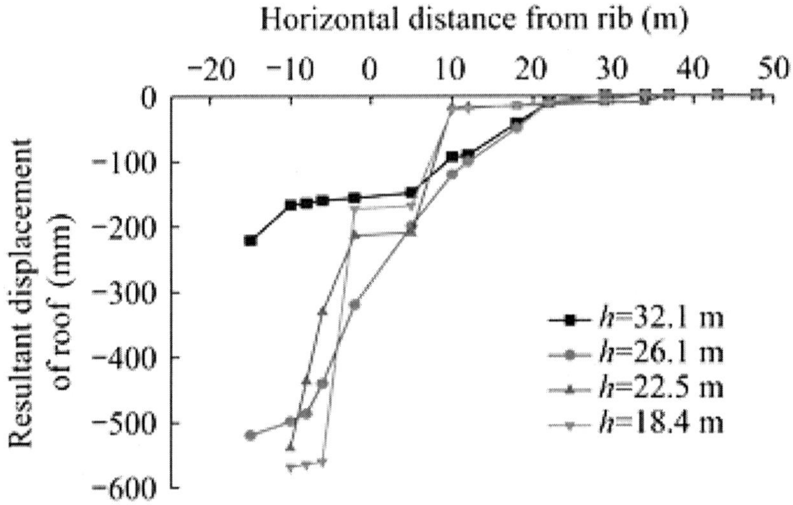


**Figure 19.** Roof displacement at first monitoring station

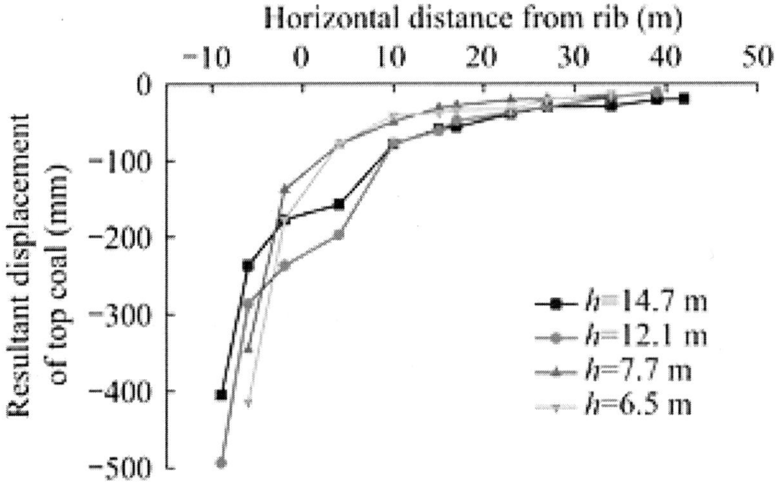


**Figure 20.** Top coal displacement at second monitoring station

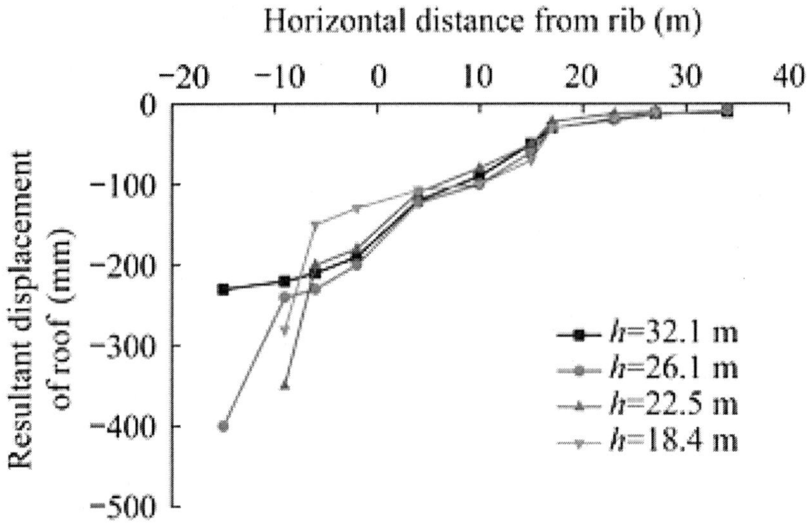


**Figure 21.** Roof displacement at second monitoring station

The average measured displacement at the top coal base points in front of the coal wall was 114.88 mm, accounting for 26.6 % of total displacement. The average measured displacement at the top coal base points behind coal wall was 317.63 mm, accounting for 73.4 % of total displacement. The total displacement was 432.5 mm. Average measured displacement at the roof base points in front of the coal wall was 149 mm, accounting for 38.3 % of the total displacement. Average measured displacement at roof base points behind coal wall was 240.25 mm, accounting for 61.7 % of total displacement. The total displacement was 389.25 mm. Although from initial displacement position, the top coal base points were affected by abutment pressure in front of the face, that lasted a long period and affected a long distance, the accumulated displacement of the top coal and roof was relatively small due to the constraint from limited space before entering the roof control zone. After entering the roof control zone, the movement of the top coal and roof followed the movement law of vertical subsidence after caving.

In front of the coal wall at the working face, the movement of the top coal and roof mainly showed a horizontal deformation under the abutment pressure due to the vertical constraints of the top coal and roof. At the rear of the coal wall which was under the repeated loading and unloading actions, the vertical constraints on the lower part of the top coal exhibited subsidential weakening with the advance of coal cutting resulting in a large space. Therefore, the movement of roof appeared as fracture subsidence and the movement of the top coal appeared as vertical displacement caused by the roof fracture subsidence. There was a large difference in accumulated top coal and roof displacement in the front and in the rear of the coal wall. In addition, the difference of displacement per unit advance was relatively large. The displacement rate of the top coal in front of the coal wall was 2.63 and 42.29 mm/m at rear of the coal wall. The displacement rate of the roof in front of the coal wall was 5.4 mm/m, and 21.35 mm/m at rear of coal wall. It demonstrated that the horizontal deformation rate of the top coal and roof caused by abutment pressure in front of the coal wall was much less than the vertical subsidence rate of the top coal and roof at rear of coal wall.

At eight base points in the top coal in two monitoring stations, from the coal wall to the gulf, the distance between the caving position to the coal wall ranged between 6 and 10 m, with an average of 7.8 m. Assume the average distance of the roof control was 6.5 m, the average caving position of the top coal was greater than the average distance of the roof control. In particular, the average caving position was 9 m in the middle or upper part of the top coal ($h$ = 12.1 m, or$h$ = 14.7 m), that indicated that there was a delay of the middle or upper part of top coal caving, the average distance of delay was 2.5 m, and the top coal was caved in a form of inverted step. From the point view of eight base points at two monitoring stations, the roof base points at$h$ = 18.4 m, $h$ = 22.5 m and $h$ = 26.1 m caved in time with the top coal caving. The displacement of the roof started to increase at the roof base point of $h$ = 32.1 m and 15 m at the rear of the coal wall. Therefore, the immediate roof was not completely caved or caved on time, and formed an immediate roof in the form of a cantilever beam above the coal seam. Based on the position of the top coal caving, the caving angle of the top coal can be approximately calculated, i.e., 64.3° for the first monitoring station, 70.1° for the second monitoring station, and 67.2° for an average caving angle.

## 3.6 Spalling of coal wall at a LLTCC coal face

### 3.6.1 Factors of coal wall spalling at a LLTCC coal face

At different stages of non-periodical ground pressure and periodical pressure, as the differences in mining height, advance speed and distance from the support tip to the coal wall, the spalling depth and spalling ratio were different at a LLTCC coal mining face (Yan 2008; Yin et al. 2008; Zhang et al. 2010). In order to better understand the spalling mechanism at a LLTCC coal mining face, the coal wall spalling were examined under different conditions including mining heights, advance rates, distances from the support tip to the coal wall, and ground pressure stages.

Using the numerical simulation method, the horizontal displacements of the coal wall with mining heights of 3.5, 4.5, 5.0 and 5.5 m were simulated and the results are shown in Fig. 22.

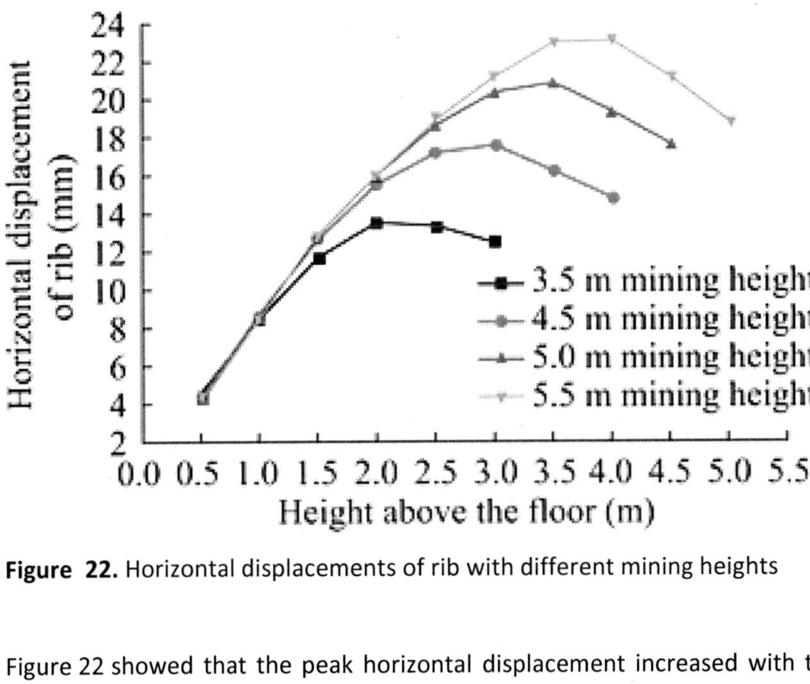


**Figure 22.** Horizontal displacements of rib with different mining heights

Figure 22 showed that the peak horizontal displacement increased with the increase of mining height. Considering the normal mining height was 4.0–4.5 m, the point of peak horizontal displacement to floor was approximately 2.5–3.0 m. Therefore, the rational height of the wall guard plate of support was 1.5 m. Based on simulated results, the second level wall guard plate was installed on a high reliable extendable beam and articulated front beam to prevent the spalling of the coal wall. Its structure is shown in Fig. 23.

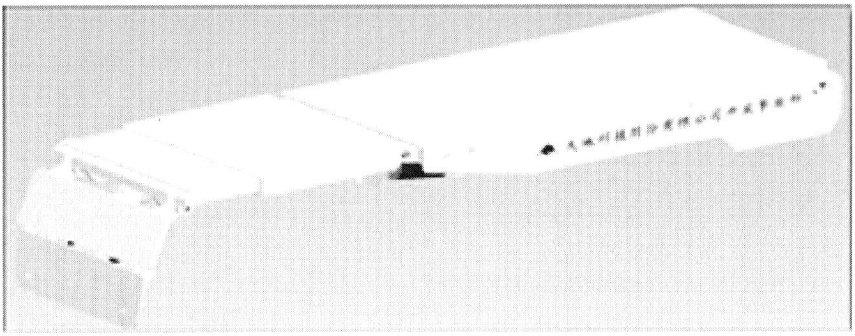

**Figure 23.** Structure of the second level wall guard plate installed on the extendable beam

The face advance speed also significantly affected wall spalling. The observations at the No. 8105 coal face demonstrated that with the increase of face advance speed, there was a reduction of damage area around the coal wall, and a reduction of wall horizontal displacement. In other words, the spalling of coal wall was suppressed. It is therefore suggested that the face advance speed should be rationally increased to reduce the exposure time and spalling of coal wall. Nevertheless, the effectiveness of controlling coal wall spalling was limited through the increase of face advance speed. With a large amount of observations on site, the effect of increasing face advance speed on coal wall spalling was found. If the advance speed is too high, the coal spalling might increase.

With the increase of the distance from support tip to coal wall, the peak abutment pressure in front of the face decreased. Subsequently, the displacement at support tip increased significantly, and the damage zone in front of the face also increased, redulting in significant spalling. Undoubtedly, the distance from the support tip to the coal wall should be reduced appropriately.

Coal cutting height, face advance speed and distance from support tip to coal wall were three factors that had substantial effects on coal wall spalling. Their weighted effects might be ordered as coal cutting height > face advance speed > distance from support tip to coal wall.

The effect on coal wall spalling from the caving and displacement of the top coal and the roof had an obvious regular pattern. The coal wall spalling clearly appeared before ground pressure commenced, increasing to maximum with ground pressure, and decreased to a minimum after ground pressure disappeared. During periodical ground pressure, the average spalling ratio of the coal wall increased to 24.58 %. With a low face advance speed, the effect on coal wall spalling would be obvious from periodical ground pressure. Therefore, the maintenance of the coal wall should be enhanced during the period of periodical pressure occurring.

The seriousness of coal wall spalling is different at different positions. Coal wall spalling was found to be most serious at the middle part of the face, less serious at the lower part of the face and better at the upper part of the face.

According to the observation at the No. 8105 LLTCC face, the position of peak abutment pressure in front of the coal face was between 10 and 25 m, the relative stress concentration coefficient $k$ was 1.3–6.5 during the peak period, and the average was 2.13. From the 10–25 m zone in front of the coal face to the coal wall was the stress release zone, and the effected zone by abutment pressure was 80 m.

With the analysis on the characteristics of coal wall spalling at the LLTCC face under different conditions, including mining height, face advance speed, distance from support tip to coal wall, ground pressure, and different positions at the coal face, the authors have developed a comprehensive spalling control technology of controlling the face advance speed, increasing initial support power, and improving the support capacity for wall protection. The technology developed has been tested and applied at the No. 8105 coal face.

### 3.6.2 Observation plan of coal wall spalling at the No. 8105 face

The observation of coal wall spalling consisted of two aspects:

(1)During the non-periodical pressure period, under different face advance speeds, the coal wall spalling ratio and depth are at different positions of the face.

(2)During the periodical pressure period, under different face advance speeds, the coal wall spalling ratio and depth are at different positions of the face.

The observation plan of coal wall spalling was as follows: the length of the No. 8105 face was 207 m, and the number of supports was 121. The face was divided into three observation zones including upper part, middle part and lower part (upper part: No. 1–No. 30 supports, middle part: No. 31–No. 89

supports and lower part: No. 90–No. 121 supports). Figure 24 shows the observation zones.

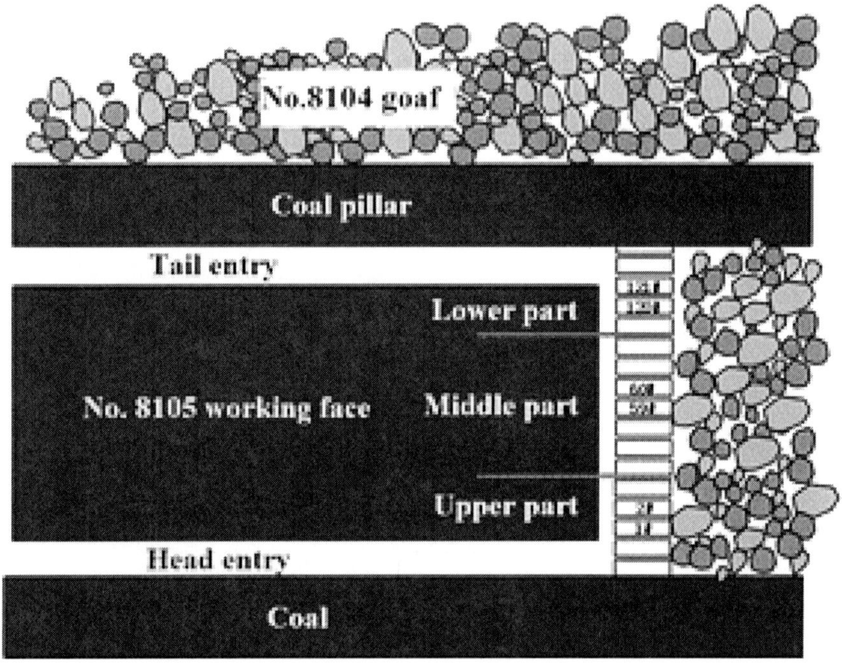


**Figure 24.** Observation plan

### 3.6.3 Analysis of coal wall spalling during non-periodical pressure period

(1)Coal wall spalling at the upper part of the face.

Observation results of coal wall spalling at the upper part of the face (non-periodical pressure period) are shown in Table 8 and Fig. 25.

In the non-periodical ground pressure period, the depth of coal wall spalling increased with the face advance speed at the upper part of the face, and eventually maintained at a certain depth range. When the face advance speed reached 3.05 m/d, the coal wall spalling length and depth reached their maximum values of 35 m and 0.6 m respectively, and the maximum spalling ratio was 66.67 %. The relationship between spalling length, depth, ratio and the face advance speed displayed a significant range. But generally, the values tended to increase with the face advance speed.

**Table 8.** Characteristics of coal wall spalling at the upper part of the face (non-periodical ground pressure period)

| Face advance speed (m/d) | Average spalling depth (m) | Spalling length (m) | Spalling ratio (m) | Maximum spalling depth (m) |
|---|---|---|---|---|
| 2.05 | 0 | 0 | 0 | 0 |
| 2.25 | 0 | 0 | 0 | 0 |
| 2.25 | 0.40 | 31.50 | 60.00 | 0.50 |
| 2.40 | 0.35 | 31.50 | 60.00 | 0.50 |
| 3.00 | 0.20 | 14.00 | 26.67 | 0.30 |
| 3.05 | 0.40 | 35.00 | 66.67 | 0.60 |
| 3.10 | 0.35 | 22.75 | 43.33 | 0.60 |
| 3.15 | 0 | 0 | 0 | 0 |
| 3.40 | 0.35 | 7.00 | 13.33 | 0.40 |
| 3.60 | 0 | 0 | 0 | 0 |
| 3.85 | 0.30 | 1.75 | 3.33 | 0.30 |
| 3.90 | 0.30 | 17.50 | 33.33 | 0.40 |
| 4.00 | 0.40 | 17.50 | 33.33 | 0.40 |
| 4.50 | 0.25 | 17.50 | 33.33 | 0.40 |
| 4.60 | 0 | 0 | 0 | 0 |
| 4.75 | 0.25 | 1.75 | 3.33 | 0.30 |
| 5.00 | 0.30 | 28.00 | 53.33 | 0.30 |
| 5.40 | 0.30 | 26.25 | 50.00 | 0.50 |
| 5.50 | 0.25 | 14.00 | 26.67 | 0.30 |
| 5.65 | 0 | 0 | 0 | 0 |
| 5.75 | 0.20 | 12.25 | 23.33 | 0.30 |
| 6.00 | 0.25 | 14.00 | 26.67 | 0.30 |
| 6.15 | 0 | 0 | 0 | 0 |
| 6.25 | 0 | 0 | 0 | 0 |
| 6.50 | 0 | 0 | 0 | 0 |
| 7.00 | 0 | 0 | 0 | 0 |
| 8.50 | 0.30 | 15.75 | 30.00 | 0.50 |

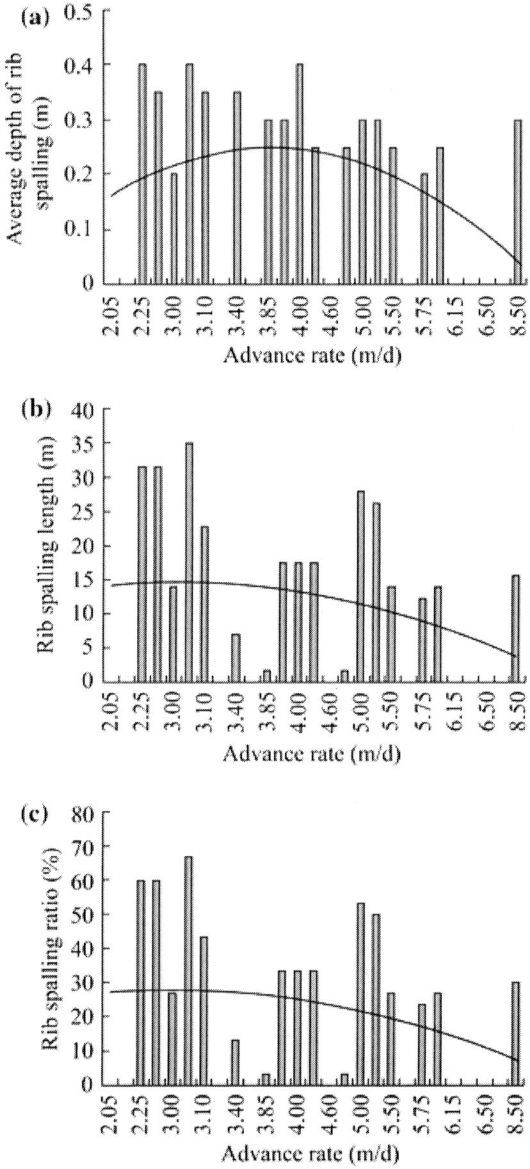


**Figure 25.** elationship *curves* between coal wall spalling and face advance speed at the upper part of the face (non-periodical ground pressure). **a** Relationship between average rib spalling depth and face advance rate, **b** relationship between rib spalling length and face advance rate, **c** relationship between rib spalling ratio and face advance rate

(2)Coal wall spalling in the middle part of the face.

Observation results of coal wall spalling at the middle part of the face (non-periodical pressure period) are shown in Table 9 and Fig. 26.

**Table 9.** Characteristics of coal wall spalling in the middle part of the face (non-periodical ground pressure period)

| Face advance speed (m/d) | Average spalling depth (m) | Spalling length (m) | Spalling ratio (%) | Maximum spalling depth (m) |
|---|---|---|---|---|
| 2.05 | 0.30 | 29.75 | 28.81 | 0.40 |
| 2.25 | 0.30 | 24.50 | 23.73 | 0.30 |
| 2.40 | 0.35 | 22.75 | 22.03 | 0.50 |
| 3.00 | 0.35 | 28.00 | 27.12 | 0.60 |
| 3.05 | 0.40 | 42.00 | 40.68 | 0.60 |
| 3.10 | 0.40 | 15.75 | 15.25 | 0.70 |
| 3.15 | 0.45 | 21.00 | 20.34 | 0.70 |
| 3.40 | 0.35 | 31.50 | 30.51 | 0.50 |
| 3.60 | 0.35 | 50.75 | 49.15 | 0.50 |
| 3.85 | 0.30 | 33.25 | 32.20 | 0.30 |
| 3.90 | 0.35 | 26.25 | 25.42 | 0.50 |
| 4.00 | 0.30 | 17.50 | 16.95 | 0.30 |
| 4.50 | 0.30 | 50.75 | 49.15 | 0.40 |
| 4.60 | 0.25 | 14.00 | 13.56 | 0.30 |
| 4.75 | 0.30 | 12.25 | 11.86 | 0.40 |
| 5.00 | 0.40 | 8.75 | 8.47 | 0.40 |
| 5.40 | 0.30 | 22.75 | 22.00 | 0.40 |
| 5.50 | 0.20 | 15.75 | 15.25 | 0.20 |
| 5.65 | 0.30 | 14.00 | 13.56 | 0.30 |
| 5.75 | 0.35 | 29.75 | 28.81 | 0.50 |
| 6.00 | 0.35 | 19.25 | 18.64 | 0.30 |
| 6.15 | 0.30 | 26.25 | 25.42 | 0.40 |
| 6.25 | 0.20 | 7.00 | 6.78 | 0.30 |
| 6.50 | 0.30 | 33.25 | 32.20 | 0.30 |
| 7.00 | 0.20 | 8.75 | 8.47 | 0.30 |
| 8.50 | 0.25 | 7.00 | 7.00 | 0.40 |

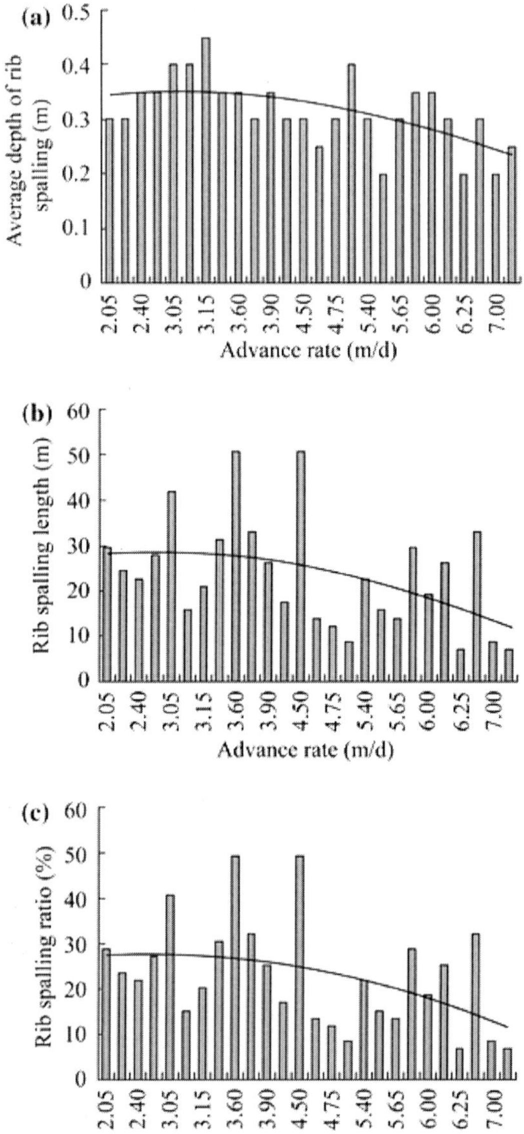


**Figure 26.** Relationship *curves* between coal wall spalling and face advance speed in the middle part of the face (non-periodical ground pressure). **a** Relationship between average rib spalling depth and face advance rate, **b** relationship between rib spalling length and face advance rate, **c** relationship between rib spalling ratio and face advance rate

During the non-periodical pressure period, being similar to the coal wall spalling at the upper part of the face, the depth of coal wall spalling decreased with the increase of face advance speed in the middle part of the face, the spalling ratio showed a trend of non-linear decrease with the increase of face advance speed.

(3)Coal wall spalling at the lower part of the face.

Observation results of coal wall spalling at the lower part of the face (non-periodical pressure period) are shown in Table 10 and Fig. 27.

**Table 10.** Characteristics of coal wall spalling at the lower part of the face (non-periodical ground pressure period)

| Face advance speed (m/d) | Average spalling depth (m) | Spalling length (m) | Spalling ratio (%) | Maximum spalling depth (m) |
|---|---|---|---|---|
| 2.05 | 0.30 | 26.25 | 46.88 | 0.40 |
| 2.25 | 0.25 | 24.50 | 43.75 | 0.30 |
| 2.40 | 0 | 0 | 0 | 0 |
| 3.00 | 0.45 | 8.75 | 15.63 | 0.70 |
| 3.05 | 0 | 0 | 0 | 0 |
| 3.10 | 0.20 | 15.75 | 12.50 | 0.30 |
| 3.15 | 0.45 | 21.00 | 20.34 | 0.70 |
| 3.40 | 0.35 | 8.75 | 15.63 | 0.50 |
| 3.60 | 0.40 | 14.00 | 25.00 | 0.50 |
| 3.85 | 0.30 | 7.00 | 12.50 | 0.30 |
| 3.90 | 0.35 | 8.75 | 15.63 | 0.50 |
| 4.00 | 0.30 | 12.25 | 21.88 | 0.30 |
| 4.50 | 0.30 | 21.00 | 37.50 | 0.40 |
| 4.60 | 0.25 | 10.50 | 18.75 | 0.30 |
| 4.75 | 0.30 | 3.50 | 6.25 | 0.40 |
| 5.00 | 0 | 0 | 0 | 0 |
| 5.40 | 0.30 | 19.25 | 34.00 | 0.40 |
| 5.50 | 0 | 0 | 0 | 0 |
| 5.65 | 0.40 | 8.75 | 15.63 | 0.50 |
| 5.75 | 0 | 0 | 0 | 0 |
| 6.00 | 0.50 | 14.00 | 25.00 | 0.70 |
| 6.15 | 0.30 | 17.50 | 31.25 | 0.40 |
| 6.25 | 0.25 | 15.75 | 28.13 | 0.40 |
| 6.50 | 0.30 | 14.00 | 25.00 | 0.30 |
| 7.00 | 0.30 | 15.75 | 28.13 | 0.40 |
| 8.50 | 0.30 | 8.75 | 16.00 | 0.40 |

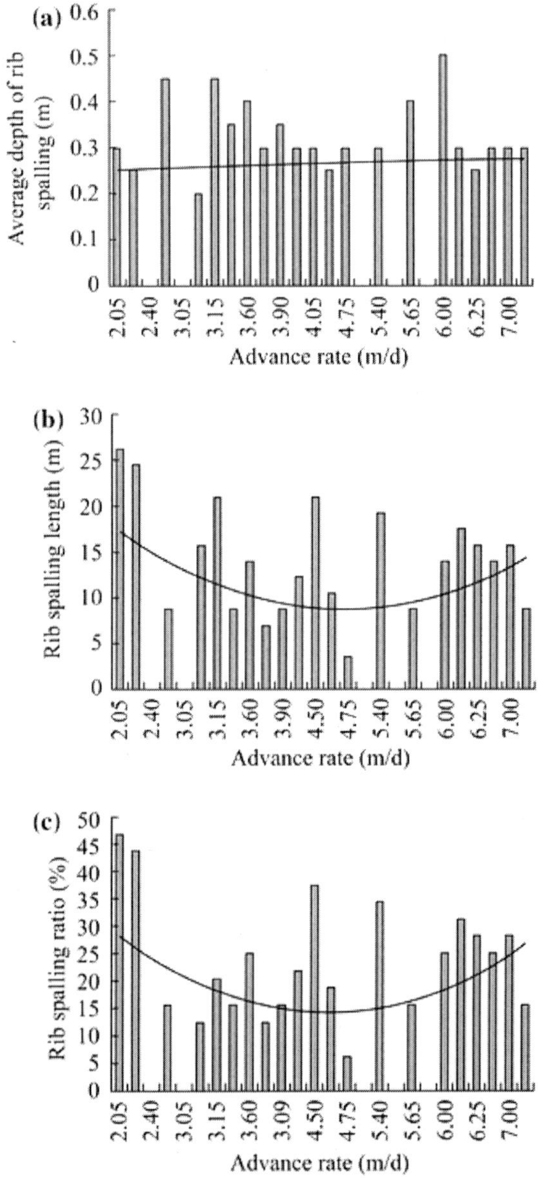


**Figure 27.** Relationship *curves* between coal wall spalling and face advance speed at the lower part of the face (non-periodical ground pressure). **a** Relationship between average rib spalling depth and face advance rate, **b** relationship between rib spalling length and face advance rate, **c** relationship between rib spalling ratio and face advance rate

During the non-periodical pressure period, at the lower part of the face, the relationship between coal wall spalling and face advance speed showed a certain degree of randomness. When the face advance speed reached 2.4, 3.05, 5, 5.5 and 5.75 m/d, there was no spalling occurring. In general, the depth of coal wall spalling showed less variation with face advance speed at the lower part of the face, the average spalling depth concentrated within 0.3–0.4 m. With the increase of face advance speed, the spalling length and ratio showed a trend of decrease early, to increase at a later time.

(4)Comparison of coal wall spalling at different face positions during non-periodical ground pressure period.

Figure 28 shows the comparison of the depth of coal wall spalling at different face positions during non-periodical ground pressure period. Table 11 lists the statistical analysis results of coal wall spalling at different face positions during the non-periodical ground pressure period. Based on the analysis and comparison, the spalling depth was 0.2 m at the upper part of the face, 0.32 m in the middle part of the face and 0.26 m at the lower part of the face, suggesting that the spalling depth was deepest in the middle part of the face, less deep at the lower part and least deep at the upper part.

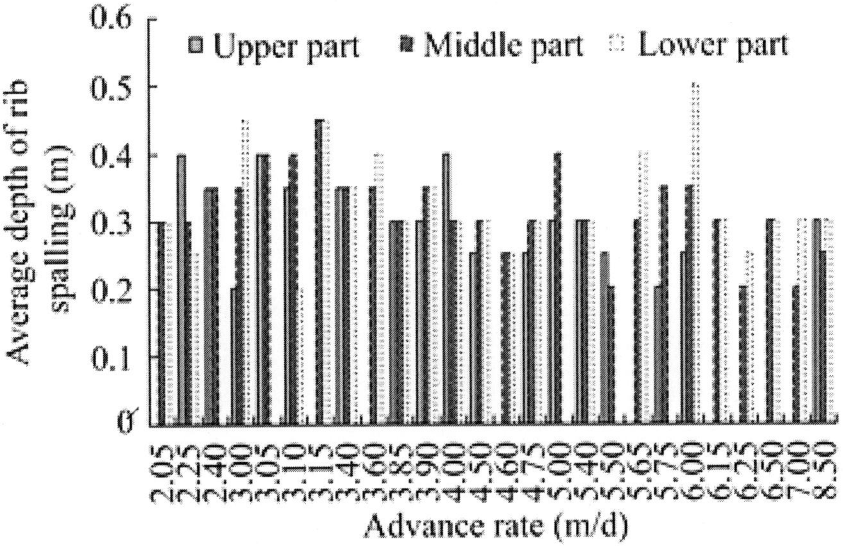


**Figure 28.** Comparison of average spalling depth at different face positions (non-periodical ground pressure period)

**Table 11.** Statistical analysis results of spalling depth at the upper, middle and lower parts of the face (non-periodical ground pressure period)

| Face advance speed (m/d) | Average spalling depth (upper) (m) | Average spalling depth (middle) (m) | Average spalling depth (lower) (m) | Average spalling depth (m) |
|---|---|---|---|---|
| 2.05 | 0 | 0.30 | 0.30 | 0.20 |
| 2.25 | 0.40 | 0.30 | 0.25 | 0.32 |
| 2.40 | 0.35 | 0.35 | 0 | 0.23 |
| 3.00 | 0.20 | 0.35 | 0.45 | 0.33 |
| 3.05 | 0.40 | 0.40 | 0 | 0.27 |
| 3.10 | 0.35 | 0.40 | 0.20 | 0.32 |
| 3.15 | 0 | 0.45 | 0.45 | 0.30 |
| 3.40 | 0.35 | 0.35 | 0.35 | 0.35 |
| 3.60 | 0 | 0.35 | 0.40 | 0.25 |
| 3.85 | 0.30 | 0.30 | 0.30 | 0.30 |
| 3.90 | 0.30 | 0.35 | 0.35 | 0.33 |
| 4.00 | 0.40 | 0.30 | 0.30 | 0.33 |
| 4.50 | 0.25 | 0.30 | 0.30 | 0.28 |
| 4.60 | 0 | 0.25 | 0.25 | 0.17 |
| 4.75 | 0.25 | 0.30 | 0.30 | 0.28 |
| 5.00 | 0.30 | 0.40 | 0 | 0.23 |
| 5.40 | 0.30 | 0.30 | 0.30 | 0.30 |
| 5.50 | 0.25 | 0.20 | 0 | 0.15 |
| 5.65 | 0 | 0.30 | 0.40 | 0.23 |
| 5.75 | 0.20 | 0.35 | 0 | 0.18 |
| 6.00 | 0.25 | 0.35 | 0.50 | 0.37 |
| 6.15 | 0 | 0.30 | 0.30 | 0.20 |
| 6.25 | 0 | 0.20 | 0.25 | 0.15 |
| 6.50 | 0 | 0.30 | 0.30 | 0.20 |
| 7.00 | 0 | 0.20 | 0.30 | 0.17 |
| 8.50 | 0.30 | 0.25 | 0.30 | 0.28 |
| Average | 0.20 | 0.32 | 0.26 | 0.26 |

Figure 29 shows the comparison of the spalling ratios at different face positions during the non-periodical ground pressure period. The spalling ratio showed a trendency of reduction with the increase of face advance speed during the non-periodical ground pressure period. As shown in Table 12, the coal wall spalling ratio was 22.56 % at the upper part of the face, 22.81 % in the middle part of the face, and 19.05 % at the lower part of the face, that indicated that the spalling ratio was largest in the middle of the face, less at the upper part of the face, and the least at the lower part of the face.

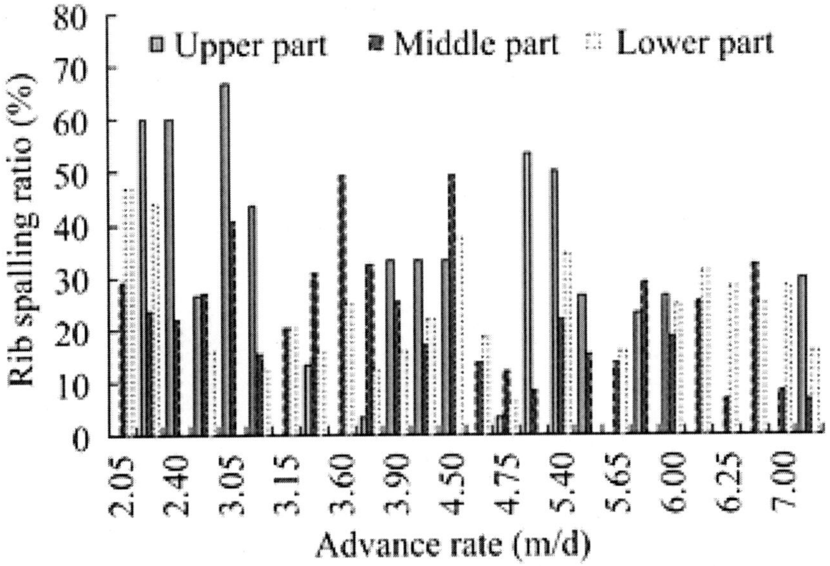


**Figure 29.** Comparison of average spalling ratio at different face positions (non-periodical ground pressure period)

### 3.6.4 Analysis of coal wall spalling during the periodical ground pressure period

(1)Coal wall spalling at the upper part of the face.

Observation results of coal wall spalling at the upper part of the face (during the periodical ground pressure period) are shown in Table 13 and Fig. 30.

**Table 12.** tatistical analysis results of spalling ratio at the upper, middle and lower parts of the face 8108 (non-periodical ground pressure period)

| Face advance speed (m/d) | Average spalling ratio (upper) (%) | Average spalling ratio (middle) (%) | Average spalling ratio (lower) (%) | Spalling ratio (%) |
|---|---|---|---|---|
| 2.05 | 0 | 28.81 | 46.88 | 27.05 |
| 2.25 | 60.00 | 23.73 | 43.75 | 38.89 |
| 2.40 | 60.00 | 22.03 | 0 | 26.21 |
| 3.00 | 26.67 | 27.12 | 15.63 | 24.52 |
| 3.05 | 66.67 | 40.68 | 0 | 37.20 |
| 3.10 | 43.33 | 15.25 | 12.50 | 26.21 |
| 3.15 | 0 | 20.34 | 20.34 | 20.29 |
| 3.40 | 13.33 | 30.51 | 15.63 | 22.83 |
| 3.60 | 0 | 49.15 | 25.00 | 31.28 |
| 3.85 | 3.33 | 32.20 | 12.50 | 20.29 |
| 3.90 | 33.33 | 25.42 | 15.63 | 25.36 |
| 4.00 | 33.33 | 16.95 | 21.88 | 22.83 |
| 4.50 | 33.33 | 49.15 | 37.50 | 43.12 |
| 4.60 | 0 | 13.56 | 18.75 | 11.84 |
| 4.75 | 3.33 | 11.86 | 6.25 | 8.45 |
| 5.00 | 53.33 | 8.47 | 0 | 17.75 |
| 5.40 | 50.00 | 22.00 | 34.00 | 32.97 |
| 5.50 | 26.67 | 15.25 | 0 | 14.37 |
| 5.65 | 0 | 13.56 | 15.63 | 10.99 |
| 5.75 | 23.33 | 28.81 | 0 | 20.29 |
| 6.00 | 26.67 | 18.64 | 25.00 | 22.83 |
| 6.15 | 0 | 25.42 | 31.25 | 21.14 |
| 6.25 | 0 | 6.78 | 28.13 | 10.99 |
| 6.50 | 0 | 32.20 | 25.00 | 22.83 |
| 7.00 | 0 | 8.47 | 28.13 | 11.84 |
| 8.50 | 30.00 | 7.00 | 16.00 | 15.22 |
| Average | 22.56 | 22.81 | 19.05 | 22.60 |

**Table 13.** Characteristics of coal wall spalling at the upper part of No. 8105 face during periodical ground pressure period

| Face advance speed (m/d) | Average spalling depth (m) | Spalling length (m) | Spalling ratio (%) | Maximum spalling depth (m) |
|---|---|---|---|---|
| 3.00 | 0.20 | 15.75 | 30.00 | 0.30 |
| 4.50 | 0.25 | 15.75 | 30.00 | 0.50 |
| 5.00 | 0.40 | 21.00 | 40.00 | 0.50 |
| 5.50 | 0.25 | 29.75 | 63.33 | 0.30 |
| 6.50 | 0.35 | 15.75 | 30.00 | 0.50 |

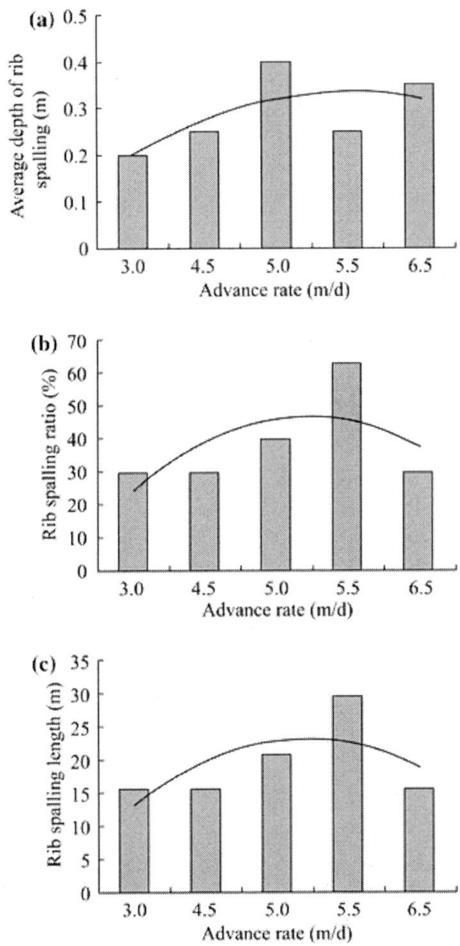


**Figure. 30,** Relationship curves between coal wall spalling and face advance speed at the upper part of the face (periodical ground pressure period). **a** Relationship between average rib spalling depth and face advance rate, **b** relationship between rib spalling ratio and face advance rate, **c** relationship between rib spalling length and face advance rate

During the period of ground pressure, the spalling depth, spalling length and spalling ratio at the upper part of the face had a similar variation trendency with the increase of face advance speed, i.e., increase early and decrease later. When the face advance speed reached 5.50 m/d, the spalling ratio was the largest at the upper part of the face at 63.33 %.

(2)Coal face spalling in the middle part of the face.

Observation results of coal wall spalling at the middle part of the face (during the periodical ground pressure period) are shown in Table 14 and Fig. 31.

**Table 14.** Characteristics of coal wall spalling in the middle part of No. 8105 face during periodical ground pressure period

| Face advance speed (m/d) | Average spalling depth (m) | Spalling length (m) | Spalling ratio (%) | Maximum spalling depth (m) |
|---|---|---|---|---|
| 3.00 | 0.40 | 29.75 | 28.81 | 0.60 |
| 4.50 | 0.25 | 50.75 | 49.15 | 0.30 |
| 5.00 | 0.30 | 19.25 | 18.64 | 0.30 |
| 5.50 | 0.20 | 19.25 | 18.64 | 0.20 |
| 6.50 | 0.30 | 29.75 | 28.81 | 0.40 |

During the period of periodical ground pressure, the spalling depth presented a trend of decrease early on, and increasing later with the increase of face advance speed. The spalling length and ratio presented a trend of gradual reduction with the face advance speed. In the middle part of the face, the spalling depth was 0.6 m, maximum spalling ratio was 49.15 % and maximum spalling length was 50.75 %.

(3)Coal wall spalling at the lower part of the face.

Observation results of coal wall spalling at the lower part of the face (during the periodical ground pressure period) are shown in Table 15 and Fig. 32.

**Table 15.** Characteristics of coal wall spalling at the lower part of No. 8105 face during periodical ground pressure period

| Face advance speed (m/d) | Average spalling depth (m) | Spalling length (m) | Spalling ratio (%) | Maximum spalling depth (m) |
|---|---|---|---|---|
| 3.00 | 0.45 | 7.00 | 12.50 | 0.70 |
| 4.50 | 0.30 | 21.00 | 37.50 | 0.40 |
| 5.00 | 0.40 | 21.00 | 37.50 | 0.50 |
| 5.50 | 0.25 | 7.00 | 12.50 | 0.30 |
| 6.50 | 0 | 0 | 0 | 0 |

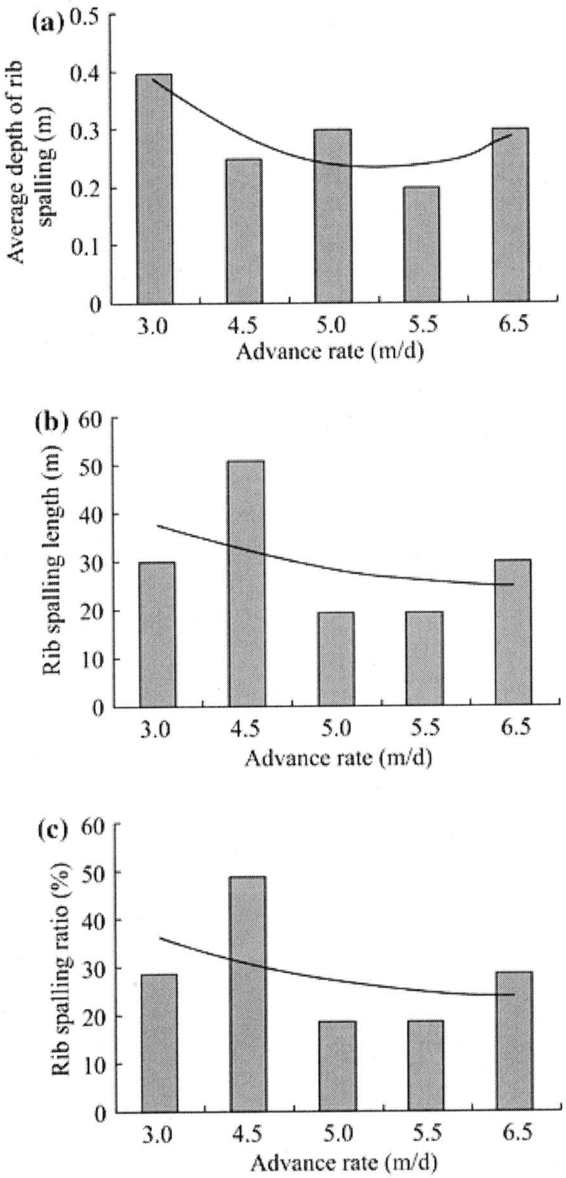


**Fig. 31** Relationship curves between coal wall spalling and face advance speed in the middle part of the face (periodical ground pressure period). **a** Relationship between average rib spalling depth and face advance rate, **b** relationship between rib spalling length and face advance rate, **c** relationship between rib spalling ratio and face advance rate

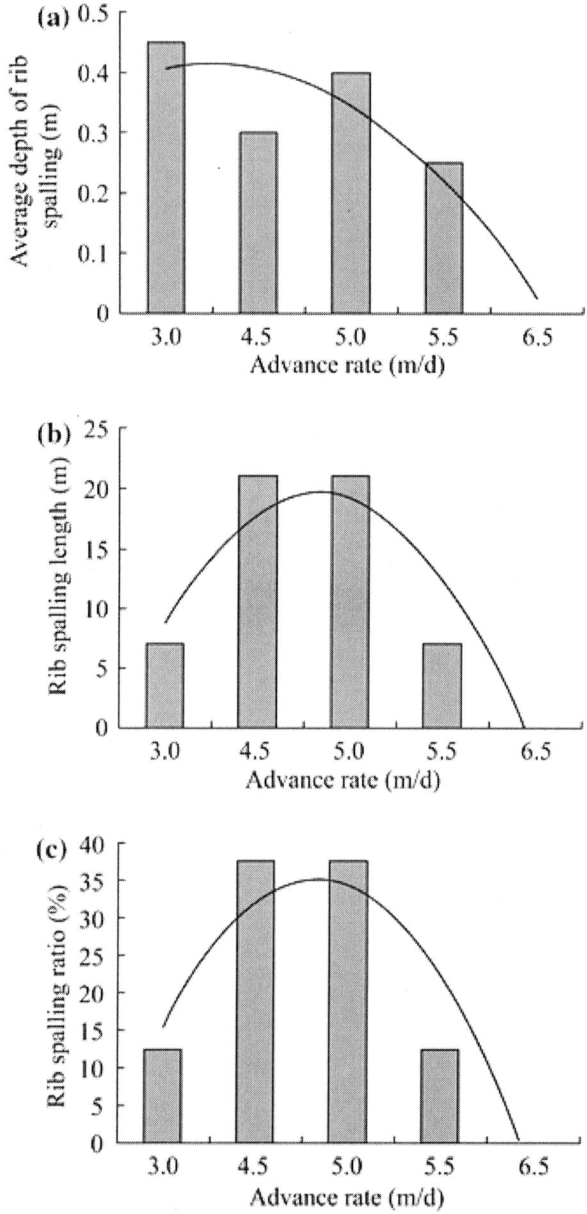


**Figure 32.** Relationship *curves* between coal wall spalling and face advance speed at the lower part of the face (periodical ground pressure period). **a** Relationship between average rib spalling depth and face advance rate, **b** relationship between rib spalling length and face advance rate, **c** relationship between rib spalling ratio and face advance rate

During the period of periodical ground pressure, the average coal wall spalling depth at the lower part of the face decreased with the increase of the face advance speed. Before the face advance speed reached 4.5 m/d, there was no distinct decrease of spalling depth, and the slope of the trend line was almost zero. When the face advance speed exceeded 4.5 m/d, there was a distinct decrease of spalling depth, thus the slope of the trend line increased.

As shown in Fig. 32b, c, during the periodical ground pressure period, the coal wall spalling ratio at the lower part of the face demonstrated a trend of increase early on, and decreasing later with the increase of face advance speed.

(4)Comparison of coal wall spalling at different face positions during the periodical ground pressure

As shown in Table 16, during the period of periodical ground pressure, the spalling depths at different face positions were almost identical, the average spalling depth was maintained at 0.29 m. The maximum spalling depth reached 0.7 m and the spalling depth exceeded 0.5 m, accounting for 30 %. During the period of periodical ground pressure, the spalling depth showed randomness, however, in general, presented a trend to decrease with the increase of face advance speed.

**Table 16.** Statistical analysis results of spalling depth at the upper, middle and lower parts of No. 8105 face (during periodical ground pressure period)

| Face advance speed (m/d) | Average spalling depth (upper) (m) | Average spalling depth (middle) (m) | Average spalling depth (lower) (m) | Average (m) |
|---|---|---|---|---|
| 3.00 | 0.20 | 0.40 | 0.45 | 0.35 |
| 4.50 | 0.25 | 0.25 | 0.30 | 0.27 |
| 5.00 | 0.40 | 0.30 | 0.40 | 0.37 |
| 5.50 | 0.25 | 0.20 | 0.25 | 0.23 |
| 6.50 | 0.35 | 0.30 | 0 | 0.22 |
| Average | 0.29 | 0.29 | 0.28 | 0.29 |

As shown in Table 17, during the occurrence of periodical ground pressure, the spalling ratio at the upper part of the face was the largest, reaching 38.67 %, less in the middle part at 28.81 %, and least at the lower part, 20.1 %. The average spalling ratio was 29.16 %.

**Table 17.** Statistical analysis results of spalling ratio at the upper, middle and lower parts of No. 8105 face (during periodical ground pressure period)

| Face advance speed (m/d) | Spalling ratio (upper) (%) | Spalling ratio (middle) (%) | Spalling ratio (lower) (%) | Average (%) |
|---|---|---|---|---|
| 3.00 | 30.00 | 28.81 | 12.50 | 23.77 |
| 4.50 | 30.00 | 49.15 | 37.50 | 38.88 |
| 5.00 | 40.00 | 18.64 | 37.50 | 32.05 |
| 5.50 | 63.33 | 18.64 | 12.50 | 31.49 |
| 6.50 | 30.00 | 28.81 | 0 | 19.60 |
| Average | 38.67 | 28.81 | 20.00 | 29.16 |

### 3.6.5 Comparison of coal wall spalling at different ground pressure periods

Figures 33 and 34 show spalling depth and spalling ratio at different ground pressure periods respectively (average 4.9 m/d).

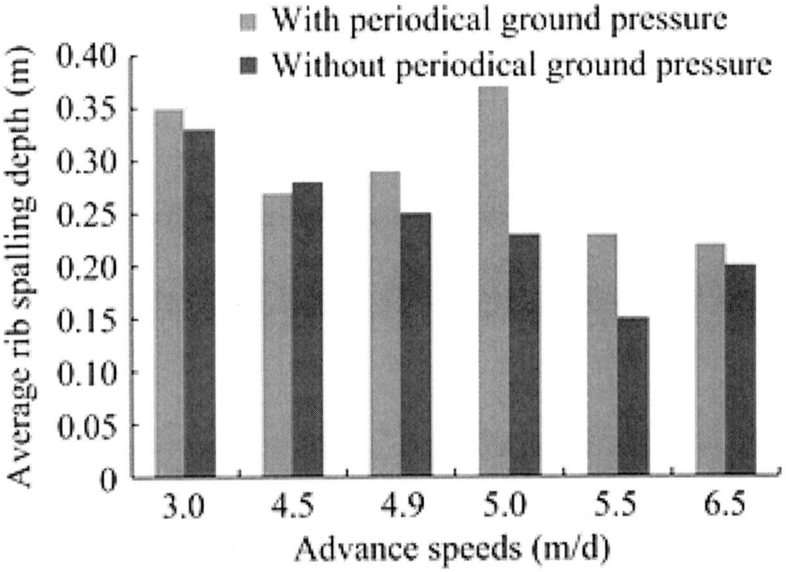


**Figure 33.** Comparison of average spalling depth at different ground pressure periods under different face advance speeds

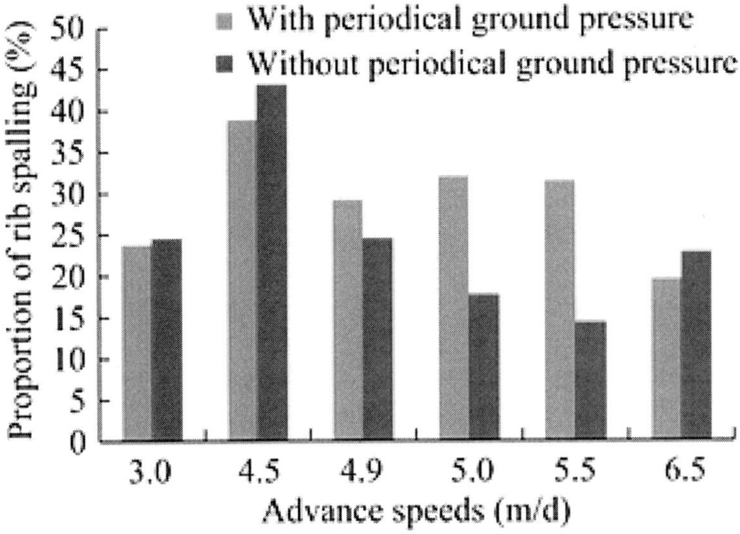


**Figure 34.**Comparison of spalling ratio at different ground pressure periods under different face advance speeds

As shown in Fig. 33, the average difference of spalling depth with periodical ground pressure was 0.05 m (under the same face advance speed, the difference of spalling depth with periodical ground pressure or without periodical ground pressure).

As shown in Fig. 34, the periodical ground pressure has limited influence upon the coal wall spalling ratio at the No. 8105 face. The difference of spalling ratio caused by the ground pressures was 4.64 % (at the same face advance speed, the difference between the spalling ratio during periodical ground pressure period and the spalling ratio during the non-periodical ground pressure period).

### 3.6.6 Conclusion of the observation on coal wall at No. 8105 LLTCC face

(1)During the non-periodical ground pressure period, the relationship between the coal wall spalling ratio and face advance speed presented randomness. However, in general, the spalling ratio reduced with the increase of face advance speed. There were some differences in the spalling ratio at different face positions. The statistical analysis of the spalling ratio showed: the spalling ratio in the middle part of the face > the spalling ratio at the upper part of the face > the spalling ratio at the lower part of the face.

(2)During the periodical ground pressure period, the spalling depth and ratio showed a decreasing trend with the increase of the face advance speed. The spalling depth showed a difference at different face positions, i.e., upper part > middle part > lower part.

(3)During the period of periodical ground pressure occurrence, the spalling ratio showed a trend of increase early and decreased later on with the increase of the face advance speed. The spalling ratios at different face positions were different.

Through the comparison of coal wall spalling with the neighbouring No. 8104 face, it was found that: during the period of non-periodical ground pressure occurring, the average coal wall spalling ratio was 33.08 % and the spalling depth varied from 0.2 to 0.3 m at the No. 8104 face; the average spalling ratio was 22.06 % and the spalling depth varied from 0.18 to 0.25 m at the No. 8105 face. During the period of periodical ground pressure, the spalling ratio was 36.18 % at the No. 8104 face, and 29.16 % at the No. 8105 face. Based on the statistical analysis, the spalling depth and length were the largest in the middle parts of the No. 8104 and No. 8105 faces. In comparison with the No. 8104 face, the spalling ratio at the No. 8105 face was 33.4 % less than that at the No. 8104 face, and the spalling depth was also 50 mm less than that at the No. 8104 face. Therefore, it can be concluded that the coal wall spalling was significantly reduced and the face achieved a fast advance speed due to the application of proposed comprehensive control technology at the No. 8105 face in Tashan coal mine in Datong, China, including controlling face advance speed, increasing support initial abutment force and increasing the wall protection capacity of support.

## 3.7 High efficient top-coal caving technology at a LLTCC operation

### 3.7.1 Study on rational top-coal drawing interval

It is important to select a rational top-coal drawing interval to improve coal recovery and reduce the percentage of gangue. If the drawing interval is too large, the top coals might be caved into the goaf, resulting in a coal loss. On the other hand, if the drawing interval is too small, the gangue might be mixed with coals and cave into the discharge window, which may not only affect the coal quality, but also be mistaken for top coal exhaustion and result in coal loss. The factors for determining the drawing interval consists of the thickness of the top coal, the discharge window length of support, the center height of the discharge window and the shearer's cutting depth. The principal for determining the drawing interval is to fracture and loosen the top coal in the range of the discharged coal, increase top coal recovery and reduce the percentage of gangue. In addition, the rational drawing interval should match the coal mining process and form an integer-times relationship with the shearer's cutting depth.

The drawing interval must be greater than the length of discharge window to avoid mixing the gangue with coal. The small drawing interval might result in the gangue in the goaf being mixed with caved top coals. The large drawing interval might result in top coal losses. A rational drawing interval will maintain the mixture of top coal with gangue and top coal losses in allowable limits. In a LLTCC face, the space for top coal fracturing becomes larger due to the increase in mining height, therefore, the effects of ground pressure on top coal fracture become greater. With the effects of ground pressure, the top coal will be fractured and broken thoroughly. The top coal fragment becomes smaller and has a better flowability.

The drawing interval has a significant influence on the coal and gangue flow and thus is a key parameter for the LLTCC process. Figure 35 shows the coal and gangue flow at different drawing intervals. The boundary of coal and gangue before and after top coal discharge is regarded as the starting line for starting coal discharge and the finishing line for finishing coal discharge. In the experimental test, three drawing intervals were tested including one cutting and one coal caving, two cuttings and one coal caving, and three cuttings and one coal caving. In the process of support shift and coal caving, the boundary of coal and gangue was moved forward and maintained in the same shape. With the increase of the drawing interval, the distance between the starting line and the finishing line also increased.

As shown in Fig. 35, with the increase in the top coal drawing interval, there were some variations in the boundary shape of coal and gangue before and after top coal caving. In other words, the initial caving point of top coal shifted forward, the distance between start line and finish line of top coal caving increased with the drawing interval. This indicated that the amount of coal discharged at each discharge circle increased with the increase of the drawing interval.

There were three kinds of coal and gangue mixtures near the discharge window of support after top coal caving using different drawing intervals:

(1)When the drawing interval is small, the gangue in the direction of the goaf reaches the discharge window earlier than the top coals do, and the discharged coals mix with gangue. Before coal discharge, the boundary between coal and gangue near the discharge window is beyond the lower boundary of the tail beam. Therefore, it results in the part of middle to top coals being unable to be discharged due to the enclosure of gangue and the tail beam. In this case, the gauge might enter the discharge window from the bottom of the window, and increase the percentage of gangue in the coals obtained.

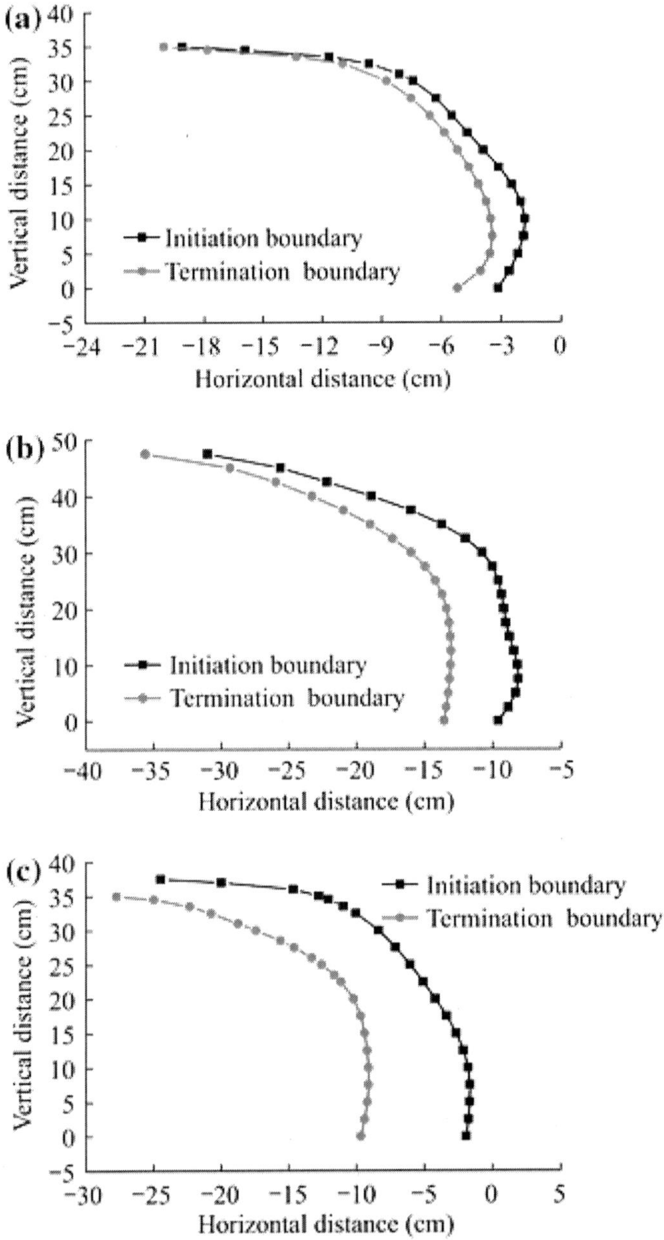


**Figure 35.** Boundaries between coal and gangue with different top coal drawing intervals. **a** One cutting and one drawing, **b** two cuttings and one drawing, **c** three cuttings and one drawing

(2)With a rational top-coal drawing interval, at initial coal discharge, the gangue in the goaf and top coal will reach the discharge window of the support at the same time. Before the coal discharge, the boundary between coal and gangue is behind the lower boundary of the tail beam, thus the horizontal movement of gangue in the goaf is small. In the process of top-coal caving and discharge, the coals can smoothly reach the discharge window. With the caving of the lower and middle part of the coals, the gangue above the coal seam caves as well, then there will be some mixture of coal and gangue during the discharge of the upper layer of top coal. The mixture gangue is mainly from the roof above the seam that enters the discharge window with the discharge of top coals.

(3)When the drawing interval is too large, at the beginning of coal discharge, top coals caved reach the discharge window earlier than gangue in the goaf. Before coal discharge, the boundary between coal and gangue is obviously behind the lower boundary of the tail beam, and the gangue in the goaf cannot reach the discharge window. With a LLTCC operation, the angle of the shield beam becomes larger, and the height of the discharge window becomes higher. During the process of coal discharge, the top coal above the discharge window can be discharged quickly and the gangue above the top coal also caves quickly. In this case, the coal and gangue in the goaf near the discharge window with natural angle of depose cannot flow toward the discharge window and be discharged, resulting in coal losses and low coal recovery.

Figure 36 shows the shape of residual top coals with different drawing intervals. As shown in the figures, the one cutting and one drawing method (drawing interval is 0.8 m) can lead to a high top coal recovery.

### 3.7.2 Study on rational coal discharge method

Top coal discharge method involves the combination of sequence of coal discharge, the times of coal discharge at each discharge window and the quantity of coal discharge, as well as the number of discharge window opened in the same time along the face. The sequence of coal discharge can be categorized as sequential coal discharge and alternated coal discharge. The times of coal discharge at each discharge window can be categorized as single, double and multiple coal discharges. The number of coal discharge window opened in the same time can be categorized as single window discharge and multiple window discharge. The number of simultaneously

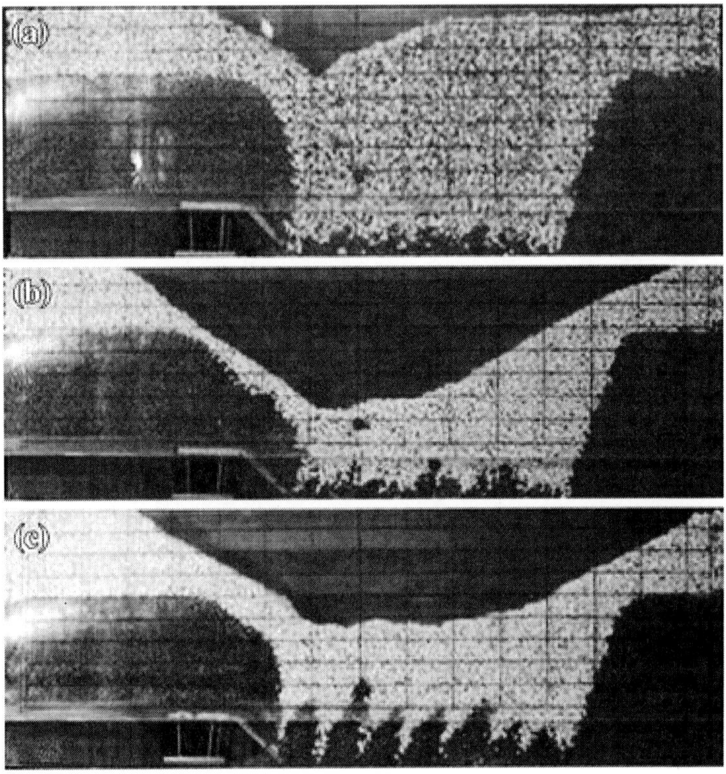

**Figure 36.** Shape of residual top coals with different drawing intervals. **a** One cutting and one drawing (drawing interval 0.8 m), **b** two cuttings and one drawing (drawing interval 1.6 m), **c** three cuttings and one drawing (drawing interval 2.4 m)

opened discharge window can be categorized as single coal discharge and multiple coal discharge. The quantity of coal discharge can be categorized as equal quantity and non-equal quantity. Because it is difficult to manage equal or non-equal quantity coal discharge in operation, and single or multiple coal discharge can be managed in labor planning, however the determination of the coal discharge method is mainly based on the sequence of coal discharge and the times of coal discharge at each discharge window. There are four main alternative methods including single sequential coal discharge, single alternated coal discharge, multi-round sequential coal discharge and multi-round alternated coal discharge. The geological conditions for different coal seams are different, and their capabilities are also different, thus, different coal discharge methods must be used, and the recovery of top coal is also varied.

A numerical analysis was conducted to simulate the top-coal caving and discharge by using the geological parameters of coal seams and the technical parameters of hydraulic supports at Tashan coal mine. In addition, the simulated loose thickness of the top coal was 10.50–11.17 m, and the simulated cutting heights were 4, 4.5 and 5 m. The top-coal caving and discharge operation was simulated including single sequential coal discharge, single alternated coal discharge and multiple alternated coal discharge method. The numerical results showed that the recovery of coal cutted and discharged was the lowest using single-time alternated multiple windows coal discharge, and highest using discharge in multi-round & multiple windows sequence alternately. In order to increase the recovery of top coal, the method of multiple-time alternated multiple window coal discharge was selected in the LLTCC operation at the No. 8105 face, Tashan coal mine in Datong, China.

# 4 KEY EQUIPMENT FOR THE LLTCC COAL MINING OPERATION

Key equipment for the LLTCC coal mining operation involves hydraulic support, shearer, front scraper conveyor, rear scraper conveyor, headgate belt conveyor and support hauler, etc. Prior to this project, there was no equipment for LLTCC coal mining operations in China or elsewhere in the world. Therefore, the various key equipment for LLTCC mining operation have been developed in this project.

## 4.1 Hydraulic support with large mining heights

Hydraulic support is one of key equipment for a LLTCC coal mining operation. The requirements for hydraulic support consist of rational structure, sufficient support resistance force, stable and shock resistance, sustainability of high efficient coal discharge and high coal recovery.

### 4.1.1 Support and rock coupling 3D dynamic optimization design method

In the design of hydraulic support, a support and rock coupling 3D dynamic optimization design method was used. The effects of surrounding rock on support structure, support intensity, and shift capability were fully considered. As the support and rock coupling based 3D dynamic parameter design commenced from roof movement, a simulation was conducted to simulate the transfer of fracture, subsidence, crash and the caving of roof into the pressure, torque, deformation and shift speed of the support. Using a series of conditions, support working resistance, support type and control parameters were dynamically determined to satisfy the requirements of roof movement and effective support on the roof. With the consideration of coal wall and floor characteristics, the forms and parameters of the auxiliary components for coal wall protection and bottom lift were determined. The advantages of the proposed method can be stated as: the dynamic characteristics of surrounding rock were fully considered through the dynamic interaction between supports and surrounding rock, the variation of roof subsidence and fracture was transferred to the support in the forms of pressure, torque and constraints. Hydraulic support responded in terms of forms and characteristic parameters, and the response results fed back to rock in the forms of support resistance force and torque. Therefore, the roof caving and the distribution of stress and strain could be controlled.

In terms of the technique for the support design, a 3D parametric dynamic design method from top to bottom was used. In the design process, the requirements of support from surrounding rock were gradually satisfied. The flowchart of support design is shown in Fig. 37. The method proposed achieves seamless integration between the optimization of structural parameters and the 3D modelling. Furthermore, the method improves the design efficiency, provides an integrated platform for structure optimization and parametric design, and improves the applicability of support.

### 4.1.2 Determination of support technical parameters

Based on the geological conditions at the No. 8105 coalface in Tashan coalmine, the composition of support working resistances during their calculation was analyzed. Using the numerical modelling method, the numerical model was built based on the occurrence conditions of coal seams. Subsequently, the model was used to simulate the support intensity of 0, 0.5, 0.9, 1.2, 1.3, 1.4, 1.5, and 1.6 MPa, respectively. The analysis on the vertical stress at the coalface showed that the increase of support intensity could not change the distribution of abutment stress in the front of the coalface. The front peak abutment stress was approximately 10 m from the coal wall. With the increase of support intensity, the area of peak abutment stress in the front of the coal face decreased and became closer to the coal wall.

In order to obtain the relationship curve between support intensity and roof subsidence ($P$–$\Delta L$curve) within the roof control range, the subsidence of the roof at a position 3 m away from the coal wall were measured, and simulated with the support intensity of 0.5, 0.9, 1.2, 1.3, 1.4, 1.5 and 1.6 MPa. The curve between support intensity and roof subsidence is shown in Fig. 38.

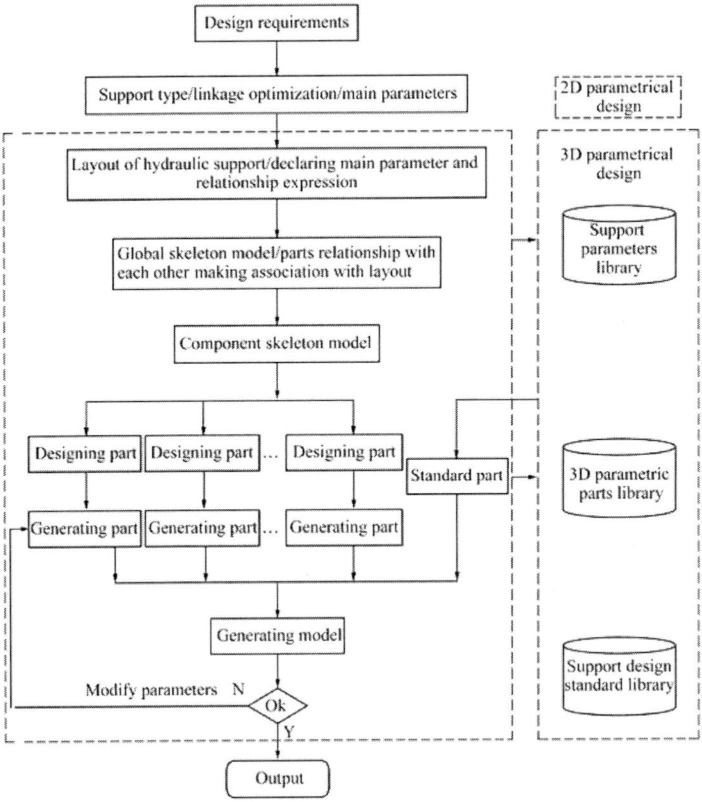


**Figure 37.** Flowchart of 3D parametric dynamic design of the hydraulic support from top to bottom

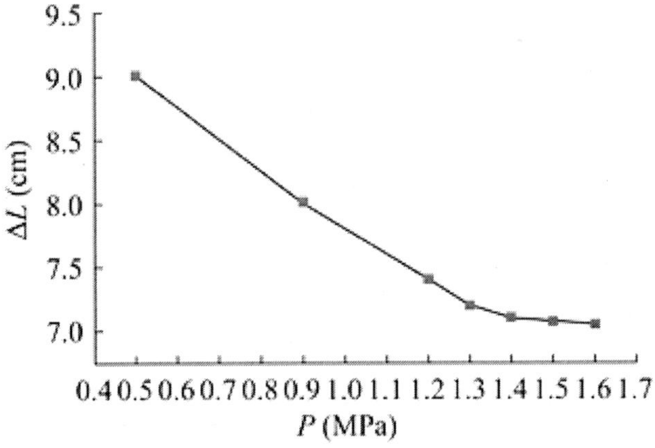


**Figure 38.** Relationship curve between support intensity and roof subsidence ($P$–$\Delta L$ curve)

As shown in the relationship curve between support intensity $P$ and roof subsidence $\Delta L$, the subsidence of the roof gradually decreases with the increase of support intensity. When the increase of support intensity reaches a certain level, the increase of support intensity have little effect on the roof subsidence. Nevertheless, if the support intensity is below a given level, the reduction of support intensity will have substantial impact on roof subsidence. The given level of support intensity can be selected as rational support intensity. When the support intensity reaches 1.4–1.5 MPa, the decrease of roof subsidence will not obvious with the increase of support intensity. As a result, the rational support intensity is determined as 1.4–1.5 MPa. With comprehensive analysis on the mining and face conditions, the support intensity of the hydraulic support was determined as 1.4 MPa in Tashan coal mine.

Determination of support resistance.

Nominal working resistance $F$ can be calculated as Eq. (13):

$$F \geq \frac{PB_cL}{\eta} \tag{13}$$

where $P$ is the nominal support intensity at the LLTCC face, 1.4 MPa; $L$ is the center distance, 1.75 m; $B_c$ is the roof control distance, 5.5 m; $\eta$ is the support efficiency, 0.98.

Substitute the parameters above into Eq. (13), get:

$$F \geq \frac{1.4 \times 5.5 \times 1.75}{0.98} = 13750 \text{ kN}$$

Considering the safety coefficient, the nominal support resistance was determined as 15000 kN, which is consistent with the calculation result from the "cantilever beam-articulated beam" structural mechanical model.

The support and rock coupling mechanical model (Wang 2009) was used to analyses the main technical parameters of hydraulic support at Tashan coal mine. The support parameters were optimized based on the support and rock coupling mechanical model. The structural parameters, i.e. the beam length of the support, the center distance of the support, and maximum and minimum heights, were used as optimizing variables, and the surrounding distribution of roof stress and the floor pressure of the support front were used as the optimizing objective. The optimizing expression was:

Objective functions:

$$\begin{cases} \Delta p = |p - p_j| \leq \lambda (j = 1, 2, \ldots n) \\ \min \delta \end{cases} \tag{14}$$

where $p_j = f(l, h_{max}, h_{min}, a, b)$, $\delta = k(l, h_{max}, h_{min}, a, b)$; $\Delta p$ is the absolute difference between support intensity $p_j$ calculated iteratively based on support parameters and the result calculated based on surrounding rock parameters. When $\Delta p$ is less than or equal to a given condition of convergence $\lambda$, the support intensity is regarded as rational. The optimizing objective of floor pressure at the support front is to minimize the floor pressure. Function $f$ and $k$ are the mechanical status expression of the surrounding rock affected by support parameters obtained from the analysis of the interaction of support and surrounding rock, respectively. In the objective function, $l$ is the length of top beam, $h_{max}$ and $h_{min}$ are maximum support height and minimum support height; $a$ is the support center distance, being selected as 1.5, 1.75 and 2.05 m, $b$ is the horizontal distance between the center of the top beam prop cup and the center of the base prop foot.

Before optimization, the support type should be selected. The parameters of support are used as the variables of optimization function, after which the multiple-objective optimization function is established. After the calculation results converge to a group of stable values, the rational optimization results are obtained. In the Tashan coal mine, during the process of the LLTCC mining operation in 14–20 m thick coal seams, the thickness of the top coal is large and the caving space is also large, therefore, the movement of roof increases, and the range of resultant force point of interaction between support and roof becomes large (Yu et al. 2012). According to the observation results of ground pressure at the No. 8104 LLTCC face in Tashan coal mine, the resistance alternately increased at the rear prop or front prop during the roof periodical ground pressure period. As a consequence, the positive four-link bar type of support was selected to better suit the ground pressure.

The average seam thickness at the No. 8105 face in Tashan coal mine is approximately 20 m. Based on the requirement of not exceeding the cutting to caving ratio 1:3, the cutting height reached 5 m. Based on the requirements of cutting height and the parameter optimization of support-rock coupling, the main technical parameters of support were determined as follows: the maximum support height is 5200 mm, the minimum support height is 2800 mm, the top beam length is 5615 mm, the support center distance is 1750 mm, the horizontal distance between top beam prop cup center and support prop base center is 402 mm, and the support working resistance is 15,000 kN. Figure 39 shows the LLTCC hydraulic support as developed.

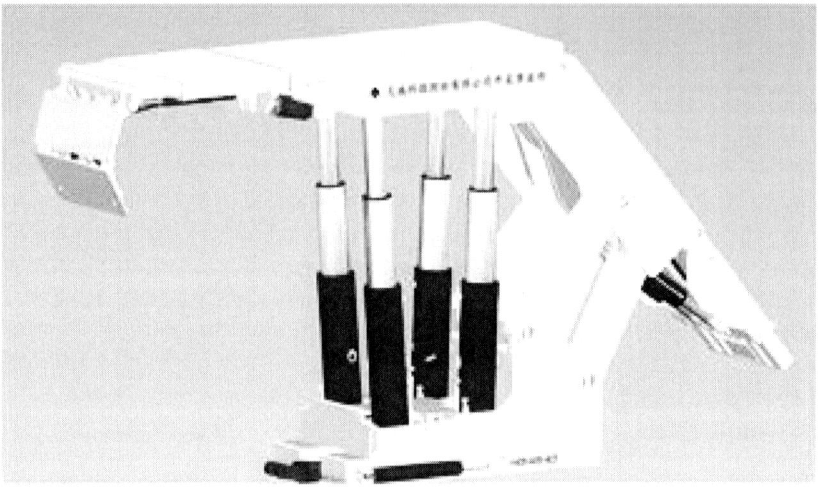

**Figure 39.** LLTCC hydraulic support with a height of 5.2 m

#### 4.1.3 Development of shock resistance components for LLTCC hydraulic support

In comparison to the fully mechanized longwall mining method and the fully mechanized LTCC mining method, the LLTCC mining method requires a higher standard for the shock resistance of hydraulic support. Thus, a large diameter double telescopic shock resistance prop was developed. Its main parameters are as follows: outer cylinder: cylinder diameter $\phi$360 mm, cylinder outer diameter $\phi$418 mm; middle cylinder: cylinder diameter $\phi$260 mm, cylinder outer diameter $\phi$340 mm; small cylinder: cylinder diameter $\phi$235 mm, cylinder outer diameter$\phi$145 mm; working resistance ($P_1/P_2$ = 43.2/82.3 MPa): 4400 kN.

A 1000 min$^{-1}$ large flow rate safety valve fast release device was developed to meet the requirement of a safety valve with a flow rate of 620 min$^{-1}$ when prop was under shock force. With the development of key components above, the shock resistance capacity of the hydraulic support increased approximately 10 %.

#### 4.1.4 High efficient coal discharge device for a LLTCC hydraulic support

At a LLTCC coal mining face in a coal seam with thickness greater than 10 m, the caving height is high after the top coals cave, and the size of coal block is relatively large. Therefore, the top coals might form an “arch” balance structure during top coal caving. To break the “arch” balance structure and enable the top coals to be easily discharged into the rear scraper conveyor is a key technology. Therefore, the technical issues discussed above must be solved for LLTCC hydraulic support, which provides the top coal control technology for a LLTCC hydraulic support.

As a result, the following method can be used for the LLTCC hydraulic support:

(1)The control of the size of the coal discharge window: The control of the discharge window is to control the coal discharge quantity at a single discharge window. Under the same flowability of caved top coals, the discharged quantity in a unit time is in proportion with the size of the discharge window. As a result, the centerline spacing of supports was modified from 1.5 m to 1.75 m to increase the size of discharge window along the inclined direction of the face (size in transverse direction). Simultaneously, the size of the discharge window in the longitudinal direction (along the strike direction of the face) was controlled.

The size of the coal discharge window is controlled by a coal discharge device (coal discharge sliding plate and tail beam). The size of the discharge window is the function of the extension length of the sliding plate and the swing angle of the tail beam. When the coal discharge window is completely opened, the maximum size of the discharge window in the longitudinal direction is equal to the coal-reception width of the rear scraper conveyor. In this case, the coal discharge rate of single support is determined by the chain speed of the rear scraper conveyor and the blockage coefficient of coal flow. The coal discharge rate of single support can be calculated using Eq. (15).

$$V_f = 60\, K_f F \gamma V_s \tag{15}$$

where $V_f$ is the coal discharge rate of single support, t/min; $K_f$ is the blockage coefficient of discharged coal flow, $K_f = 0.6$; $F$ is the carrying cross-section of the rear scraper conveyor, $m^2$; $\gamma$ is the loose coal density, $t/m^3$; $V_s$ is the chain speed of scraper conveyor, m/s.

(2)The time of multiple coal discharge and the control of coal discharge quantity: In respect of the LLTCC mining operation at Tashan coal mine, because the ply of the top coal is very thick and the top coal is very hard, after top coal caving, the upper top coals cannot fully break due to limited caving space. Some of top coals close to the roof cannot even cave. In this case, if the caved coals are discharged completely, there will be losses of large coal blocks and uncaved top coals. As a result, there should be multiple coal discharges, e.g., two or three times. The multiple coal discharges will provide time and space for the fracturing and caving of top coals, and enable the boundary of caved top coals and immediate roof gangue to be evenly subsided.

The purpose of multiple coal discharges is to provide time and space for the top coals and the immediate roof to fracture and cave. Therefore, the delay time of the second coal discharge cannot be too short. Generally, the second coal discharge should be more than 10 m away from the first coal discharge. It should be adjusted according to the movement of top coals and the roof.

The discharged coal quantity in a round is determined by the awaited discharge of top coals. The awaited discharge quantity of top coals can be calculated theoretically, as shown in Eq. (16).

$$Q_d = h_2 B S \gamma \eta_d \tag{16}$$

where $Q_d$ is the awaited discharged quantity of top coals in a support, t; $h_2$ is the thickness of top coals, m; $B$ is the width of support, m; $S$ is the discharge interval, m; $\eta_d$ is the recovery of top coals, %.

Because the discharged coal quantity in a unit of time at a discharge window cannot be calculated, the control of discharged coal quantity each time at a support is to control the time. After the start of a LLTCC operation, the coal discharge time at a discharge window should be calculated through several rounds of coal discharge operation. The time from the start of discharge until the gangue occurring in the discharge flow is the time of coal discharge in a round. When using two rounds of coal discharge, the time spent on one round of coal discharge should be half of the total coal discharge time, and 1/3 of the total coal discharge time for three rounds of coal discharge.

(3)During the process of coal discharge, the size of caved coal is suitable at the initial stage and the discharged coal flow is smooth. With the discharge of top coals, the large-size coals increase and form a balanced arch above the discharge window to block the coal flow. In this case, the base of the balanced arch should be broken using a coal discharge device. In addition, the large coal blocks should be crushed to enable the continuity of coal discharge. Therefore, the tail beam should be continuously swung up and down during the process of coal discharge to disturb the awaited top coals. The upswing of the tail beam can crush large coal blocks and the down swing can loosen the coal flow.

Caving and discharging the top coals and increasing coal recovery is the major objective of the present project. Based on the studies on the caveability of top coals and the laws of top coal caving, the support structure and the method of top coal caving and discharge were optimized. A new highly efficient coal caving and discharge device was developed to increase top coal recovery. Figure 40 shows the design of the coal discharge device.

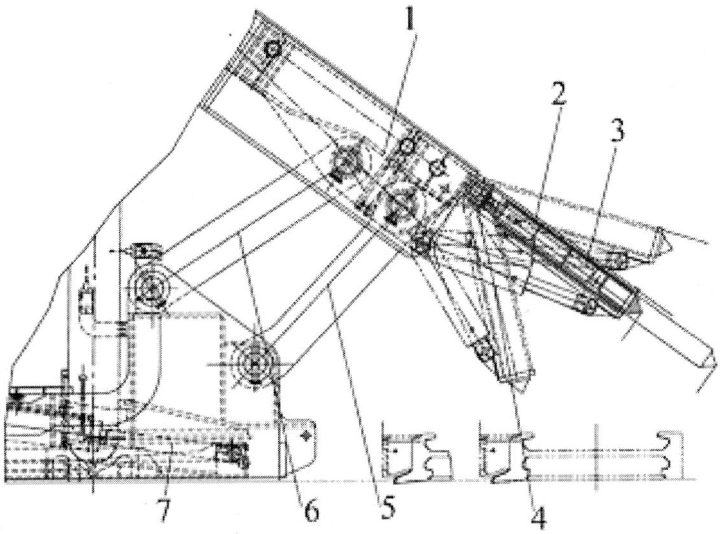


**Figure 40.** Coal discharge device. *1* shield beam, *2* tail beam-sliding plate, *3* pump of sliding plate, *4* pump of tail beam, *5* rear link bar, *6* front link bar, *7* base

Through the studies on previous coal discharge devices, the following problems were found:

(1)In previous type LTCC supports, the front link bar was the double link bar, and the rear link bar was the single link bar. The rear bar was fixed in the middle of the support base, which resulted in blocking the operator's sight and difficulty in observing the effects of top coal caving and discharge.

(2)There was no passage from the front to the rear of the support. Because the rear link bar was fixed in the middle of the support base, operators could not go through two supports from the front to the rear of the support. The only way was to go to the rear of the support via face ends, which resulted in difficulties in terms of safety and maintenance.

(3)The coal discharge device of the tail beam-sliding plate was easily jammed and hard to slide. Because the sliding plate was not slid back, the sliding plate occasionally cut the chain of the rear scraper conveyor when the tail beam swung.

In order to solve the above problems, a new type of coal discharge device was designed with a double rear link bar, middle passage and observation window for coal discharge through the optimization of support structure. In addition, the high efficient and high recovery coal discharge device had a strong disturbance capacity for releasing coals.

(1)A new type of coal discharge device with double front and rear link bars, middle passage and observation window.

Through the optimization of the four-link bar on support, on the basis of meeting the requirements on support movement and limited positions, the internal components, i.e., shield beam and base, were re-designed. A new type of coal discharge device was developed with new double front and rear link bar, middle passage, and observation window, as shown in Fig. 41.

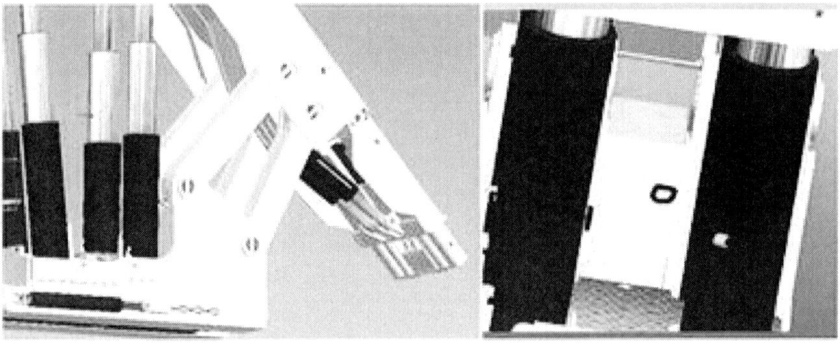

**Figure 41.** Middle passage in support

Under the ground pressure, the top coal is fractured and caved. The size of coal is different depending on the coal hardness. During the process of top coal discharge, the increase in large coals causes a balanced arch above the support discharge window and blocks the coal flow. In this case, the base of the balanced arch should be fractured using the coal discharge device. In addition, the large coal blocks should be crushed to enable the continuity of coal discharge. Therefore, a high efficient and high recovery coal discharge device was developed with a strong disturbance capacity. Two jacks with a cylinder diameter of $\phi$180 mm were installed on the tail beam for operation. The force of a single jack was 1000 kN ($P$ = 39 MPa) and 2000 kN with both. In order to increase the disturbance to top coals, the upswing of the tail beam can reach 19.5° to crush top coals, and the down swing can reach 41° to loosen coal flow. During the process of top coal discharge, the tail beam was swung continuously to disturb the awaited top coals and to achieve a high efficient and high recovery coal discharge.

## 4.2 High efficiency and high reliability electrical haulage shearer

### 4.2.1 Assessment of the overall reliability of electrical haulage shearer

The electrical haulage shearer is one of the key equipment in coal mining operations. High efficient continuous coal cutting is the shearer's main task, as the reliability and safety will affect coal production and operator safety. To meet the coal cutting requirements at the Tashan LLTCC coal mining operation, a new high efficiency, high reliability electrical haulage shearer had been developed. The shearer's specifications are as follows: cutting height 2.8–5.5 m, total installed power 1945 kW, coal cutting power 750 kW, maximum haulage speed 15–25 m/min, and maximum haulage power 2 × 570 kN, as shown in Fig. 42.

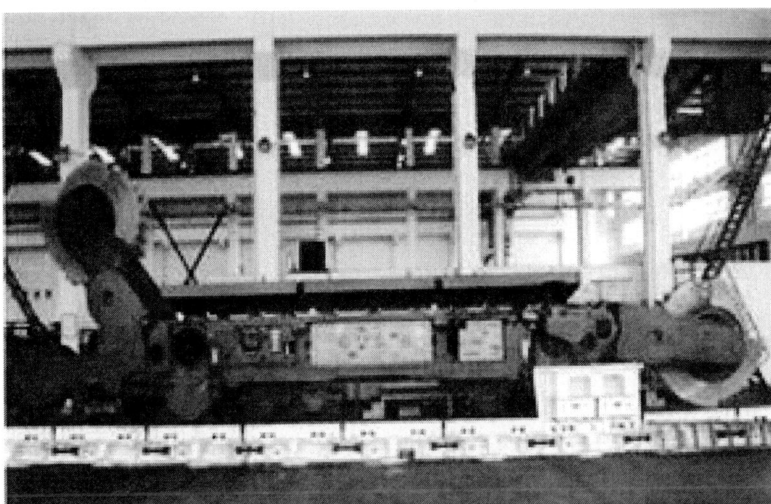

**Figure 42.** High efficiency and high reliability electrical haulage shearer

The reliability of the shearer is the key factor controlling normal mining operation. As a result, the assessment method for assessing shearer's reliability has been investigated. Table 18 lists 38 common faults of the electrical haulage shearer. A fault tree analysis method was used to analyses the reliability and design. Based on the theoretical analysis on component design, installation and the environment of usage, the main causes of component failure were investigated to find the weakest link in reliability, and improve the reliability and utilization of the shearer.

**Table 18.** Common faults of electrical haulage shearer

| No. | Fault | No. | Fault |
|---|---|---|---|
| 1 | Not reach correct position | 20 | Structure crash |
| 2 | Broken | 21 | Jam |
| 3 | Loosen | 22 | False open |
| 4 | Fall off | 23 | False close |
| 5 | Bending | 24 | Unusual wear |
| 6 | Twisting | 25 | Oil leakage |
| 7 | No input | 26 | Inappropriate gap |
| 8 | No output | 27 | Puncture |
| 9 | Circuit open | 28 | Plastic deformation |
| 10 | Short circuit | 29 | Poor contact |
| 11 | Unable to switch | 30 | Blockage |
| 12 | Unable to start | 31 | Poor sealing |
| 13 | False action | 32 | Peel off |
| 14 | Flow blockage | 33 | Burn out |
| 15 | False indicator | 34 | Worn |
| 16 | Unexpected operation | 35 | False connection |
| 17 | External leakage | 36 | Burn down |
| 18 | Internal leakage | 37 | Fractured |
| 19 | False action | 38 | Rusty |

The fault tree method for assessing the faults in electrical haulage shearer was divided into two stages:

1. (1)Establishment of fault tree for the electrical haulage shearer system.

①Collect and analyses the technical document of the electrical haulage shearer, including the drawings of the shearer, maintenance records, working environment and geological conditions, etc.

②Determine the contents and constraints of the electrical haulage shearer.

③Determine top events based on the electrical haulage shearer system.

④Analyze the causes and factors related with top events, the causes and factors related with each sub-system.

⑤Map the fault tree of the electrical haulage shearer system. Deductively analyses from top events, search for causes level by level until reaching the basic event, map the fault tree according to the their logical relationship

(2)Quantitative analysis of the electrical haulage shearer system.

①Simplify the fault tree, number the logical gates and basic events for further analysis.

②Calculate the failure rate of the basic event.

③Calculate the occurrence rate of the top event.

④Calculate the importance of parts of each basic event, including probability importance and criticality importance.

⑤Establish the main control measures on key components individually according to the importance of each sub-system and elements.

#### 4.2.2 Shearer load database and faults database

A remote data file submission scheme was developed to achieve a remote submission of shearer monitoring data by using the PHP language and B/S architecture. Through the automaton, the remote data was summarized and sent to database at headquarters to provide data for the simulation of shearer operation.

Using a new Browser/Server architecture, under Browser/Server three-layered architecture, the presentation, business logic and data service were divided into three individual units: presentation: Web browser; business logic: Web server with extension function of application program; data service: database server.

Monitoring objects are the monitored components in the shearer, which generate monitoring data. Monitoring data is the data converted from real-time signals generated by monitoring objects, which can be recognized by the computer. The graphic library in the monitoring system is composed of the instrument graphics of monitoring objects, which can be used by an application program. The relationship of three is shown in Fig. 43.

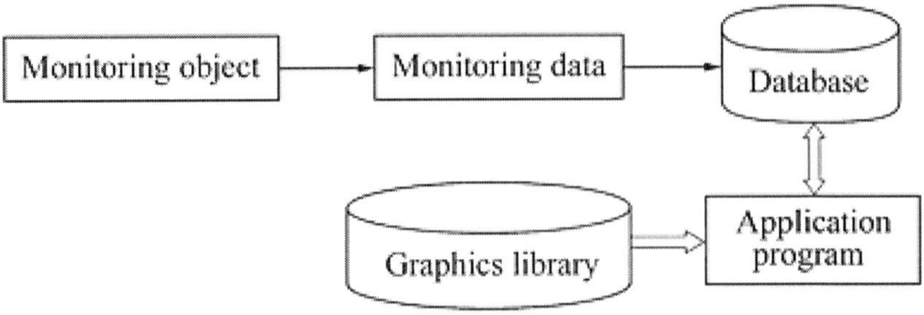


**Figure 43.** Relationship of monitoring objects, data and the graphic library

The parameters of the monitoring system of the electrical haulage shearer were mainly used to define the environmental parameters of system operations, including the parameters displayed at the client terminal and the parameters of network transmissions, and the geological parameters, mining parameters, gateroad parameters, the parameters of the scraper conveyor, the parameters of the hydraulic support, and the parameters of the shearer and its accessories.

Based on a whole configuration electric control system, the monitoring data of the shearer system is shown in Table 19.

**Table 19.** Data structure of the parameters of shearer operation condition

| Parameters | Variable type | Variable name | Note |
|---|---|---|---|
| Left cutting motor power | Float | LCMP | Left cutting motor power |
| Right cutting motor power | Float | RCMP | Right cutting motor power |
| Left haulage motor power | Float | LHMP | Left haulage motor power |
| Right haulage motor power | Float | RHMP | Right haulage motor power |
| Oil pump motor power | Float | OBMP | Oil pump motor power |
| Water pump motor power | Float | WBMP | Water pump motor power |
| Left cutting motor temperature | Float | LCMT | Left cutting motor temperature |
| Right cutting motor temperature | Float | RCMT | Right cutting motor temperature |
| Left haulage motor temperature | Float | LHMT | Left haulage motor temperature |
| Right haulage motor temperature | Float | RHMT | Right haulage motor temperature |
| Oil pump motor temperature | Float | OBMT | Oil pump motor temperature |
| Water pump motor temperature | Float | WBMT | Water pump motor temperature |
| Haulage direction | Bolean | HD | Haulage direction |
| Haulage speed | Float | HS | Haulage speed |
| Shearer position | Int | SP | Shearer position |

Four current transformers were used in the shearer's electric control system to monitor the single-phase current of each cutting motor. In this case, the loading status of the motor can be known. The DC0-10 V voltage signal output from the current transformer is sent to PLC for comparison to obtain the signals of the underload or overload. Pt100 thermal resistances are installed inside the motor windings of four cutting motors on the left and right, haulage motors on the left and right. The thermal resistances are directly connected with the RTD module of PLC. The data collected are stored in CF cards as .csv files for subsequent data analysis. The visualization system of monitoring data connects the .csv files to the application programs through the ADO, OLE, and ODBC methods. The application programs input the data into corresponding database tables to display the data in a graphic format.

Based on the analysis on the requirement for the functions of monitoring the data visualization system, the system case model was established for the system, as shown in Fig. 44.

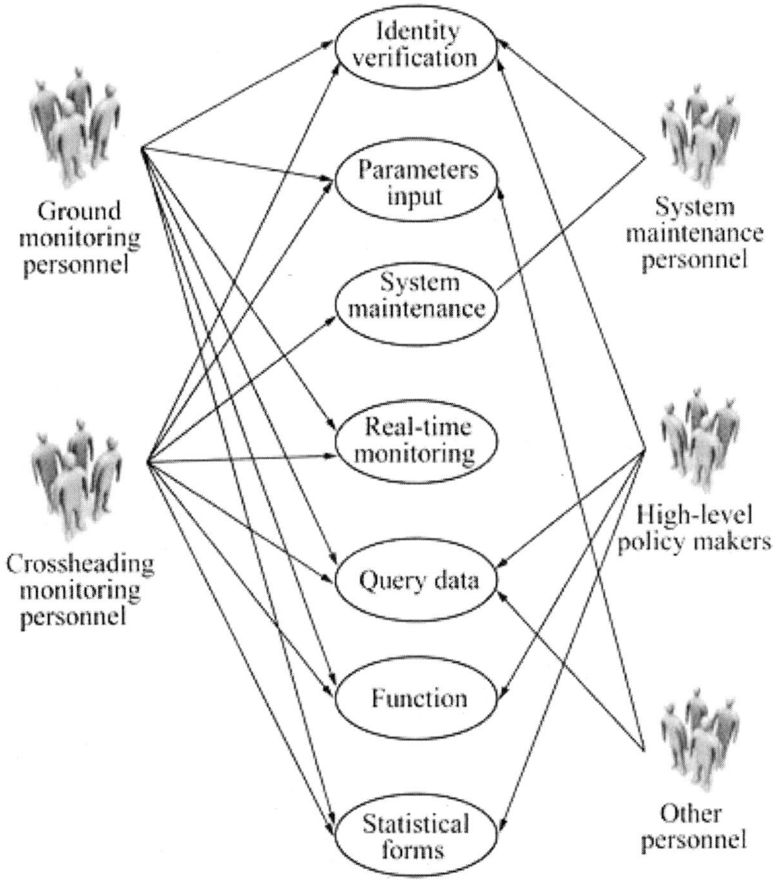


**Figure 44.** System case model for shearer monitoring data

The large amount of monitoring data generated during the shearer operation were compiled and transferred into the database. After being processed in the database, the relevant data was extracted to link with the graphic library. The visualization of data was achieved. The large amount of historical data was analyzed and mined to form a decision support system.

### 4.2.3 Development of 750 kW high reliable shearer ranging arm

Shearer's ranging arm shell (Fig. 45) is a power transmission part of drum rotary cutting and a supporting part of the curving movement of the drum. To enable the shearer's ranging arm maintaining its normal operation during the period of nominal coal cutting quantity (overhaul life maintenance), the arm shell should have excellent comprehensive mechanical properties, i.e., high tensile strength, high fatigue strength and hardness, and high impact toughness. As a result, a new material CrNiMo series of hardened and tempered steel was developed. The medium carbon CrNiMo series special cast steel material was selected because the alloy steel with Cr and Ni has a high strength, in addition to high plasticity and toughness. The addition of Mo can control the secondary temper brittleness, reduce overheating, increase temper stability and obtain high strength and toughness of steel after it is hardened and tempered. Because of the addition of Cr, Ni, Mo and other minor alloy elements in the alloy, the alloy steel has a high hardenability. In addition, due to the solid solution strengthening of Ni and Mo elements, and the carbide precipitation strengthening of Cr and Mo elements, Mo and Cr elements hinder the growth of austenite grain, which will improve the strength, hardness and worn resistance of the alloy steel.

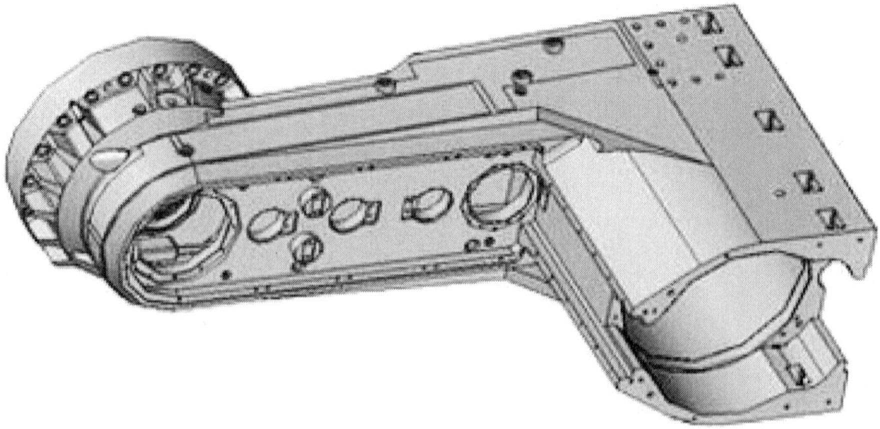

**Figure 45.** 3D model of shearer arm shell

The large power ranging arm shell is made of large heterotypic cast steel, thus, it is in an irregular shape with large internal space and a complex structure. Furthermore, the shell's thicknesses vary significantly. Therefore, if the cooling rate after high temperature austenite is too fast, the shell might have cracks. At the same time, the alloy steel of the arm shell has a high hardenability, and has a high hardness under air quenching (air cooling, normalizing) with modest cooling rate. Therefore, during the process of air quenching and high temperature tempering, the rate and method of increasing temperature and the temperature of air quenching need to be appropriately controlled to meet the mechanical property requirements from the arm shell body, and prevent the occurrence of cracks.

The heat treatment of the shearer's ranging arm shell is high temperature tempering after air quenching (normalizing), which is completed before the machining of the shell. The process is: check before heat treatment—air quenching—intermediate check—tempering—final check. Figure 46 shows the normalized curve.

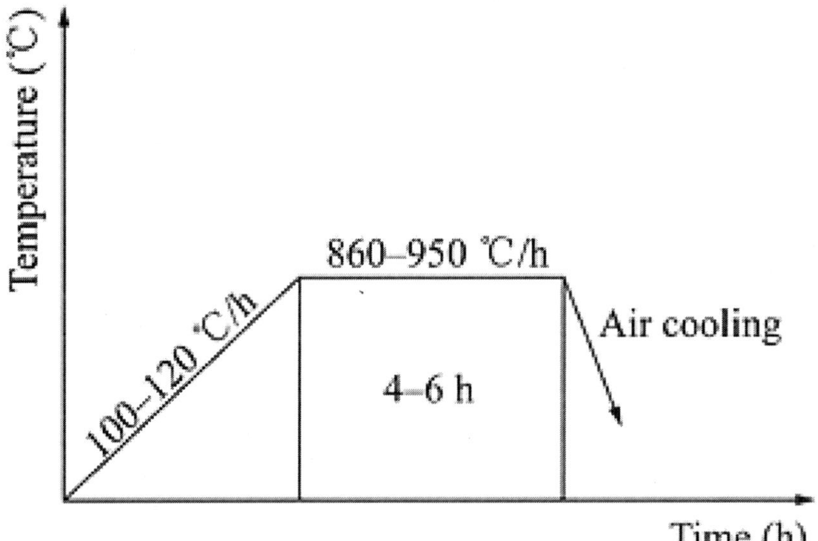


**Figure 46.** Normalizing curve

The shell cast outline of the split-type ranging arm is 2948 mm × 1434 mm × 961 mm, the minimum wall thickness is 45 mm, the maximum wall thickness is 119 mm, and the cast weight is 6380 kg. The position of water passage in the cast part needs to be tested in a hydrostatic test under eight standard atmospheric pressures, and the inner cavity is water leakage-proof. To make the castings with excellent mechanical properties, the density of the castings needs to be high and reaches GB 7233—87 II level in ultrasonic flaw detection. The geometry, allowance of machining, and dimensional deviation of the castings are consistent with the specifications of cast steel for engineering machinery JB/T 5939—1991. Therefore, based on ranging arm shell cast material composition based casting characteristics and structure, size, and casting weight level, the foundry program was determined, including the sand casting method and casting process (pouring position, parting surface, sand box structure and size). After the casting process was determined, the designs were conducted including the design of casting parameters, sand core design, gating system design, riser design, chill design, and vent design.

Ranging arm shell casting is a large heterotypic steel casting. A template sample manual molding was used. The molding sand is quartz sand with $SiO_2$ concentration greater than 96 %. The molding process used ester-hardened sodium silicate sand, core sand used 30–50 mesh of quartz sand, and binder used phenolic resin.

On the design of the outlet, sand core was used to make the exhaust channel, and the vent was reserved in sand mound. More vents were designed on the external mound upper box, in particular, on the sand mound upper box at the water jacket position of the ranging arm.

In terms of the design of feeding system, the gating and rising, and chill were appropriately laid out based on the modulus of each structural element by using the modulus method. The top insulation riser and side insulation riser were set up in the local area, and the external chill was placed. In addition, a riser subsidy was set up at necessary parts to feed castings.

With the computer numerical simulation of the process of shell mold filling and solidification, the casting process and parameters were optimized. Among them, the machining allowances were adjusted according to the JB/T5939—1991 the specifications of cast steel for construction machinery, and the shrinkage was set based on the inner cavity and external shape. In addition, using the lofting small casting test, the rationality and stability of the shell casting process was determined.

With the optimization of the casting process, the casting quality of the shell of the large power ranging arm was good in trial production. Through the process of heat treatment discussed above, the surface hardness test on the CrNiMo series casting steel of the ranging arm shell showed the hardness deviation in a reasonable arrange. The mechanical properties are as follows: Hardness HB200-240, tensile strength ≥700 MPa, yield strength ≥600 MPa, percentage elongation ≥18 %, area contraction ≥40 %, and impact toughness ≥70 J.

After using the technologies above, the performance of the shearer's ranging arm shells remained in good condition. The mechanical properties of the shell can meet the requirements of the high-power shearer.

In addition, the heat balance of the shearer ranging arm was investigated and a special forced lubrication and cooling device was developed. The heat of the shearer ranging arm comes mainly from the gears, bearings and stirring oil by gears. There are four main ways of heat dissipation for the shearer ranging arm: convective heat transfer between the ranging arm shell and air flow; heat removal by the cooling water of the ranging arms; heat absorption by the lube oil of the ranging arm; radial heat transfer between ranging arm and its connection devices.

With the significant increase of ranging arm power, and the working requirements of equipment continuous transshipment by high production and high efficiency working face, it is difficult to solve the problem of heat caused by the loss of transmission efficiency through traditional methods. Thus, a dedicated heat balance system was set for the ranging arm. The design of the water jacket for the ranging arm shell was optimized. A cooling pipe was installed in the gear chamber. The built-in cooler is shown in Fig. 47. A hydraulic gear pump system was installed for forced lubrication and cooling. In addition, the temperature sensor was installed, when temperature exceeded the limit, the alarm was triggered. The design forms a unique, advanced and reliable ranging arm heat balance system.

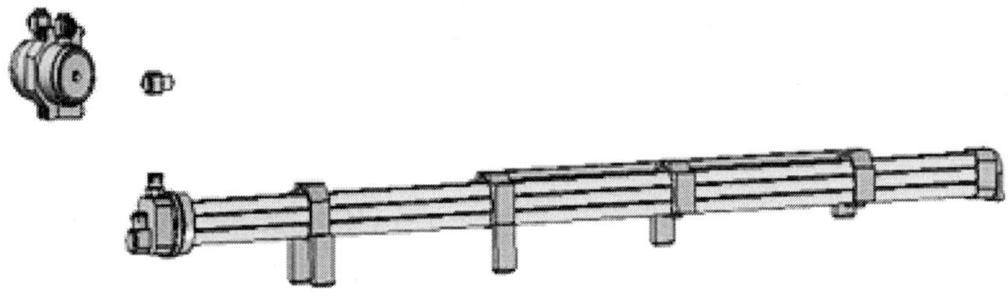

**Figure 47.** Built-in cooler

In order to increase the service life of gears and bearings inside the ranging arm, and increase the reliability of the shearer, the hydraulic system of the gear pump was installed for forced lubrication and cooling. The ranging arm gearbox was used as an oil tank for the automatic lubrication device. At the other side of shearer ranging arm I, screw pump 1 was mounted. In the gear oil tank, N320 middle load gear oil was injected. The gear on axial group I drives the gears on the gear pump, and the lubricating oil in the pump, under the action of centrifugal force, was pumped out through the oil tube to filter, which filters out impurities in the oil. After the cooling, the oil was transported by pipeline to the axial group III, axial group IV, axial group V, axial group VI and axial group VII. Each axial group and gear had special holes drilled, and the lubricating oil lubricated the mating surfaces through the hole as the gear turned.

In order to clearly describe the effect of heat radiation on the shearer ranging arm temperature field after optimizing the cooler, the heat radiation without the cooler was theoretically and numerically analyzed when the ranging arm angle is 0° and ambient temperature is 0°. The temperature rise curve of the ranging arm (Fig. 48) and the color cloud of stead temperature field (Fig. 49) were obtained.

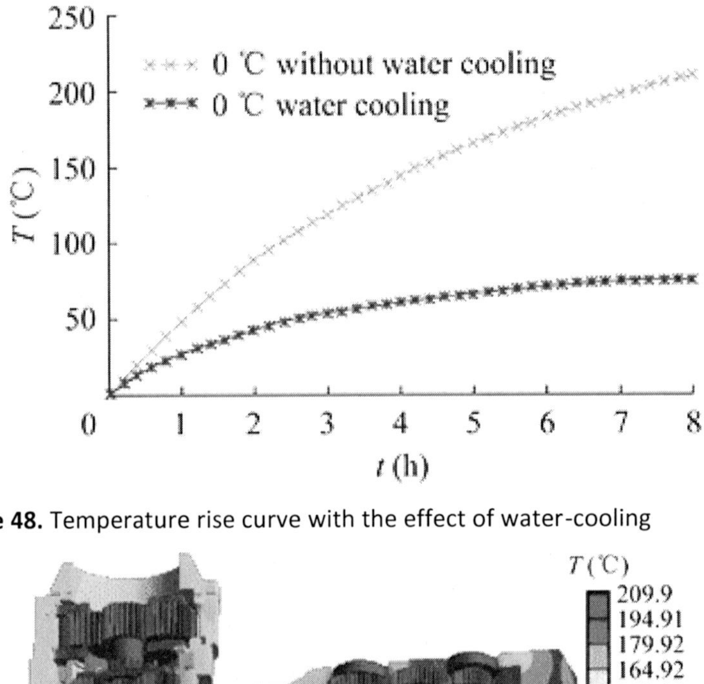


**Figure 48.** Temperature rise curve with the effect of water-cooling

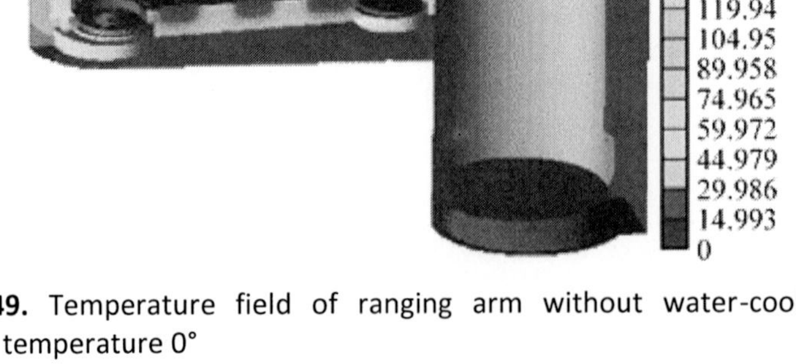


**Figure 49.** Temperature field of ranging arm without water-cooling at ambient temperature 0°

As shown in Fig. 48, the effect of the water cooler after optimization on the temperature rise of the ranging arm is significant. Without the water cooler, the acceleration speed of temperature increase is very large. Figure 49 shows the distribution of the ranging arm temperature field without the water cooler under working conditions. Without the water cooler, the temperature gradient generated between transmission shaft and box is very large. It indicates that the water cooler of ranging arm design has solved the overheating problem with the 750 kW ranging arm. In addition, it provides a reference for the study on the heat balance of large power ranging arms, and the optimization of cooler design.

In order to further improve the reliability of the shearer ranging arm, the seal performance of the shearer ranging arm was evaluated. In reality, the seal problems mainly appeared in moving seals. There are two moving seals in the ranging arm, one is the seal between drum connection sets and the gland at the output shaft of the ranging arm (low-speed shaft), the other is the seal between the ranging arm shaft I (high-speed shaft) and motor cavity body, as shown in Fig. 50.

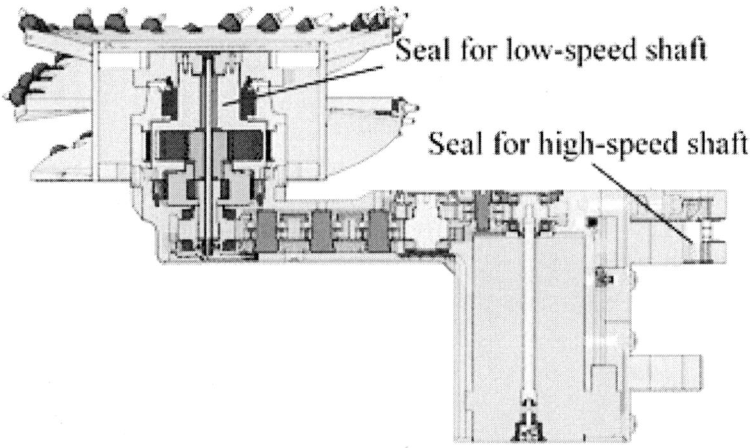


**Figure 50.** Locations of high speed and low speed seals on shearer ranging arm

Currently, a floating seal is used on the low-speed shaft seal of the ranging arm. The floating oil-seal is a sealing device combining dynamic and static sealing techniques. The floating oil-seal is composed of two identical metal rings (static floating seal ring and dynamic floating seal ring) and an "O" shape ring. In order to further understand the mechanism of the floating oil-sealing and optimize the assembly clearance, a test device of floating oil-seal was developed, as shown in Fig. 51. Figure 52 shows the photos of the test device.

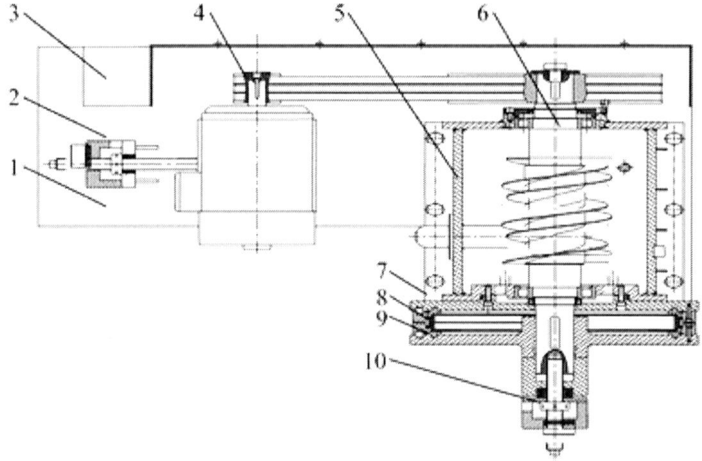


**Figure 51.** Major components of floating oil-seal test device. *1* Support, *2* 2 V belt tension device, *3*electric control console, *4* moter, *5* oil tank, *6* shaft, *7* static ring fixer, *8* float oil seal, *9*moving ring fixer, *10* axial loading device

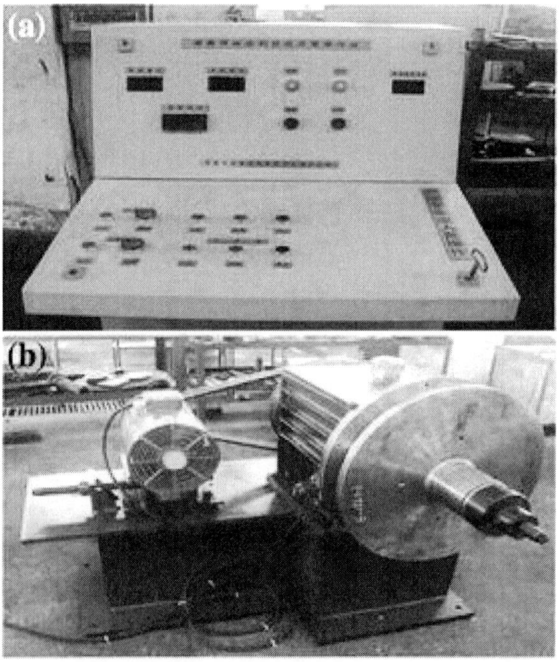


**Figure 52.** Floating oil-seal test device. **a** Electric control console, **b** mechanical parts of test device

The working principal of the floating oil-seal test device is as follows: a axial force is imposed on floating oil-seal through the axial loading device; the speed of floating oil-seal is adjusted through the electric control console, the oil temperature in floating oil-seal cavity and the test time of floating oil-seal are recorded; through the heater installed in the oil tank heat the oil in the tank, then the relationship between the axial force on floating oil-seal and assembly clearance can be measured; the floating oil-seal operation, and temperature increase and wear is monitored; and the oil leakage assembly clearance of floating oil-seal under static or dynamic status at a given temperature is detected. Main technical parameters of the test device are shown in Table 20.

**Table 20.** Main technical parameters of test device of floating oil-seal

| Output (V) | Motor power (kW) | Variable frequency speed adjustment range (r/m) | Maximum output torque (N m) | Floating oil-seal size |
|---|---|---|---|---|
| 380 | 3 | 0–200 | 265 | $\phi$293–$\phi$560 |

Based on the main factors that affect the performance of the floating oil-seal, and the working principal of the test device, the routine test items and methods were determined as follows: hardness test on "O" type ring; test on the relationship between pressure and shift; static oil leakage test; test on the elastic resilience of the static "O" type ring; test on dynamic temperature rise; test on the operation of the floating oil-seal; test on dynamic oil leakage; test on the wearing condition of the floating oil-seal; test on service life; and the comparison of performance of floating oil-seals from different manufacturers.

The main problem for using the framework oil-seal of ranging arm's high-speed shaft is its premature failure, i.e., the failure before the service life of the framework oil-seal. The main causes of the premature failure for the framework oil-seal at the ranging arm shaft I are as follows: poor quality framework oil-seal, e.g., poor quality port, and defects; poor quality of self-tightening spring; the magnitude interference between port inner diameter and shaft I outer diameter is too small, which results in low radial pressure; and the material of framework oil-seal is not good, which results in wearing out at port. Design and machining: there are some misalignments at some positions, such as ranging arm, shaft I and bearing cup; there is a low degree of finish at shaft I that amounted with framework oil-seal; and inappropriate heat treatment, etc. Assembly: damage on the port of framework oil-seal, inclination of bearing cup, loose spring, different type of grease or different quantify of grease on oil-seal port and shaft surface. To overcome the problems associated with the framework oil-seal of ranging arm shaft I, and to increase the sealing reliability of high-speed shaft of ranging arm, the following measures were taken: select high quality framework oil-seals; maintain the machining precision of key components; checking and maintenance on oil leakage of the framework oil-seal.

### 4.2.4 High speed ultra-powerful pin and rail haulage system

Based on the previous system, a high speed ultra-powerful chainless haulage system was developed. It has a rated traction of 2 × 570 kN and a traction speed of up to 20 m/min.

The clearance matching of chainless haulage system with a pitch of 147 mm was studied. First of all, the variable range of meshing central distance of the shearer walk wheel and scraper conveyor pin rail was determined. Its determination principles are: under the correct meshing situation, the minimum meshing central distance can warrant the no interference and no gear jam between walk wheel and pin rail (two section pin row connection), and it is usually approximately 10 mm less than the pitch radius of the walk wheel; the maximum meshing central distance must satisfy the rational meshing, the simulation shows that the increase of the meshing central distance has little effect, based on analysis and experience, the value is taken as 15 mm larger than the corresponding pitch radius of the walk wheel; a further increase of meshing central distance would cause: imprecise rolling, impact on gears from every contact and alteration, the wear of wheel gear and rack gear, etc.

The wear resistance of components in the chainless haulage system of maximum traction force 2 × 570 kN was investigated. In the study, four types of cladding materials A, B, C and D were studied; the cladding of substrate steel can dramatically improve the surface hardness and abrasion resistance of the substrate. Based on the analysis, the C type is the hardest cladding layer among the four types of cladding material, up to HRC66.9, the A cladding layer is a less hard layer, the B cladding layer is the least hard layer, with its hardness reaching HRC51. The friction and wear test showed that the four types of cladding layers have the same wearing manner, e.g., abrasive and adhesive wears. Among the four types of cladding materials, the wear resistance of A is the best, followed by B, C and D that have the same wear resistance. Cladding material is Fe-based alloy powder; its chemical composition is shown in Table 21.

**Table 21.** Chemical composition of cladding materials (wt %)

| Sample | C | Si | Ti | V | Cr | Mn | Ni | Fe |
|---|---|---|---|---|---|---|---|---|
| A | 1.12–2–1.25 | – | 0.2 | – | 3.6 | 0.7 | – | Remains |
| B | 1.0–1.2 | 0.15 | – | 0.33 | 5.8 | 0.6 | – | Remains |
| C | 1.45–1.7 | 0.35 | 0.4 | – | 12.3 | 0.88 | 0.21 | Remains |
| D | 1.12–2–1.25 | – | 0.24 | 0.27 | 3.7 | 1.03 | 1.16 | Remains |

The modified substrate steel after the cladding of Fe–Cr-Mn–Ti Fe-based alloy powder has an A cladding layer and a high hardness, excellent anti-wear properties, and a substrate with very good toughness, and is superior to any other alloy steel wear-resistant material. This modified substrate steel can be used as the shearer's guide sliding shoe material to meet the performance requirements of the shearer guide sliding shoe under complicated mining conditions.

### 4.2.5 Development of large-diameter, ultra-powerful and wear-resistance spiral drums with pick-shaped cutter and its components

The shearer's pick holder and welding process were investigated. In earlier years, the pick holder of a small power shearer was cast with medium carbon steel. The common damage of pick holders were: weld cracking; overall cracking along pin hole due to high substrate hardness, poor plastic toughness; surface wear due mainly to poor surface organization, low hardness, poor wear resistance; inner hole wear due to poor surface organization, low hardness, and poor wear resistance. Comparison of different materials for the pick holders is shown in Table 22.

**Table 22.** Comparison of material properties

| Property | ZG40Cr | 35CrMnSi | $15CrNi_3MoA$ |
|---|---|---|---|
| Material property | Not compact, many defects, low strength, low plasticity | High strength, good plasticity | High strength, excellent plasticity |
| Processing property | Poor hardnessability, high carbon-equivalent, poor welding property | Good hardnessability, high carbon-equivalent, poor welding property | Good hardnessability, low carbon-equivalent, good wielding property |
| Application property | Same surface hardness. In terms of the core, hardness is too high, poor plasticity, poor impact resistance; in terms of surface, hardness is too high, poor wear resistance | Same surface hardness. In terms of the core, hardness is too high, poor plasticity, poor impact resistance; in terms of surface, hardness is too high, poor wear resistance | After carburizing and quenching, the hardness at core is appropriate, good plasticity, high surface hardness, good wear resistance |

In order to better meet the working conditions of shearer's pick holders, a low carbon alloy steel 15CrNi3MoA was used to make the pick holder which was subsequently treated by carburizing and quenching. Because the carbon content of the material is low, its carbon equivalent is also low and its welding property is good. The total alloy element content is low, therefore it is low cost, but its hardenability is high. After carburizing and quenching, the carburized layer is martensite plus carbide, its hardness exceeds 58 HRC, so the surface wear resistance is good, and substrate is a thin lath martensite. A material with a hardness of approximately 300 HB, a strong toughness, and strong impact resistance, would be a more appropriate for making pick holders.

The wear process of the shearer drum helical vane was studied. In poor production conditions, the tail end of the shearer drum helical vane was often worn out. After a comparative study of several methods, the chrome SA1750CR wear-resistant composite plate was selected. The plate is made as follows: using the heap welding method, a layer of high chrome and carbide material are surfaced on a low alloy steel plate, and form a heap welding layer with high wear property, while the back of the plate has high toughness property; the large difference in the properties of front and back side of the composite plate results in the large improvement in the properties of bending, welding and mechanical processing of composite plate and original low carbon alloy steel plate.

### 4.2.6 Development of the prototype shearer and performance test

Based on earlier studies in June 2009, the Shanghai Branch of Tiandi Science & Technology Co., Ltd commenced the manufacture of the prototype shearer and completed in February 2010. The key process of its main components is described as follows:

As the MG750/1915-GWD shearer developed is a heavy-duty large power shearer, large casting shells, such as ranging arms and traction gearbox, are heavy in weight, and the cavity structure is complex and the thickness is uneven. Through software simulation, the parameters of the riser, such as number, size and position, were rationally designed to effectively avoid the casting defects, e.g. cracks and loose. To overcome the problem of blowholes in casting, in terms of process, a vent was made on the core and on the sand box. In addition, a well-shaped exhaust duct was made on the sand box. Large particles of synthetic quartz sand were used as the back sand. In these ways, the casting blowhole was effectively eliminated. In addition, the measures of a one-box multi-core combined tool and a core with multiple positioning were applied to ensure dimensional accuracy. In the machining process, the benchmark superposition method was used to achieve location accuracy. Before semi-finishing machining, a baseline was mapped properly, and the base surface was machined properly. Based on the correct baseline, the surface of each hole was machined in semi-finishing or finishing. To meet the requirements of geometric tolerances of some holes, a one clamping multichannel processing method was used to ensure the requirements of finishing size. A "casting-air quenching and high temperature tempering-rough-finishing-stress removal tempering-finishing" processing route was used to ensure the strength and dimensional stability of the castings. With the development of materials and the processing method, on the basis of solderability, the hardness of ranging arm shell reaches 200–240 HB, and the tensile strength reaches $\sigma_b \geq 700$ MPa, which greatly enhances the mechanical properties.

Before forging the gear, the oxidized layer and surface defects were removed using a hand sand wheel to effectively avoid the cracking phenomenon of forging residue. In the forging process, the procedures must be strictly followed; the forging temperature must be strictly controlled with the temperature difference not exceeding 300 °C. After forging, the forging part must be normalized under more than 950 °C and tempered less than 600 °C to eliminate forging stress and improve cutting performance. After a rough-machining of the gear blank, each part underwent an ultrasonic defect check. A grinding undercut large radius hob was used for gear grinding to increase gear root fillet, and improve the impact resistance and bearing capacity of gears. In the carburizing and quenching heat treatment process, the carbon potential concentrations were strictly controlled at 0.8 %–1.0 %. A "quenching + deep freezing + low temperature tempering" process was used to ensure that the gear surface hardness reached HRC58-62, surface carbide reached Grade 1–3, the depth of effective hardened layer reached 1.5–1.7 mm range (including grinding), core hardness reached HRC38 approximately, and retained austenite content was less than 9 %. All gears were ground in high precision grinding machine NILES, and some of the key components, such as planetary gear and sun gear, were under tip relief operation. At the same time, the accuracy of gear machining was one level higher than the specified level on the drawings to ensure a good meshing of the gears. The ground gears were treated by strengthened shot blast to eliminate the burns on the tooth surface and increase residual compressive stress, thereby enhancing the gear's contact fatigue strength and bending fatigue strength.

The working conditions of the shearer walk gear are harsh, thus the shearer walk gear is one of the weakest parts in the shearer. In order to improve its work life, the electro-slag remelted steel material 18Cr2Ni4WE was used to make the shearer walk gear. The electro-slag remelting greatly reduces the harmful content of non-metallic materials (these ingredients are the causes of quenching crack and fatigue crack), increases the purity of materials, and maximizes material performance. As the gear modulus was large and there was no standard hob, the gear tooth was machined twice, the first machining cut using NC wire cutting, leaving 2–3 mm allowance. The second machining was precisely machined to its place using a processing center. In particular, in the last processes, the amount of feed and cutting speed should be strictly controlled to avoid obvious cutting marks (machining marks are the stress concentration source of gear's tooth; currently fracturing of the shearer walk gear is often caused by these marks). To reduce the gear tooth's early failure due to stress concentration, it should be treated by shot-blast after heat treatment.

High quality medium carbon alloy steel was used to cast the shearer's guiding sliding shoe. At rough machining, the shoe was hardened and tempered to improve its substrate mechanical properties. The high quality wear-resistance material was selected to heap weld the guiding surface, then, the surface was machined using a special machine to reduce the surface roughness and friction force.

The trial production of other components also strictly followed the product standard and were checked to avoid installing non-confirming products in the prototype shearer, and can warrant the reliability of the shearer manufactured.

## 4.3 Rear scraper conveyor for LLTCC coal face

In order to meet the requirements of coal production of 1000 Mtpa at the No. 8105 face in Tashan coal mine, with the consideration of the effects of other uncertain factors, the calculation shows that the total transportation capacity of the front and rear scraper conveyors is 3500 t/h. Considering a cutting and caving ratio of 1:3, the individual transportation capacity of the front and rear scraper conveyors should be greater than 2625 t/h. Taking the uncertainty of caving quantity and some allowances in transportation capacity into consideration, the capacity of the rear scraper conveyor was determined as 3000 t/h.

Because of the specific environment in the underground mine and the matching characteristics of the scraper conveyor, shearer and hydraulic support, there are many constraints on many structural parameters of the scraper conveyor including the width of the pan and other important structural parameters. Balancing between economic and technical contexts, the pan width of the rear scraper conveyor was determined as 1200 mm. Its coal transport section is shown in Fig. 53.

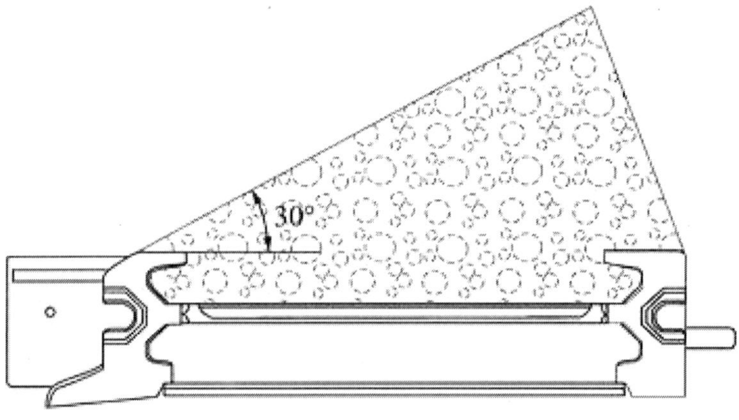


**Figure 53.** Cross-section of coal transportation at rear scraper conveyor

Calculation of chain speed of scraper *V*:

$$V = n/2iZp/60\lambda \tag{17}$$

where *n* is the motor speed, 149 $min^{-1}$; *i* is the reduce deceleration ratio, 28.43; *Z* is the tooth number of driving sprocket, 7; *P* is the chain pitch of 48 × 154, 0.152 m; *λ* is the slip ratio of coupler, 0.95. Substitute the parameters into Eq. (17), get:

$$V = 1491/28.43 \times 2 \times 7 \times 0.152/60 \times 0.95 \approx 1.77 \text{ m/s}$$

Calculate the hourly capacity of coal transportation *Q*:

$$Q = 3600\ VA\rho \tag{18}$$

where *V* is 1.77 m/s; *A* is the cross-section of loads as to rear conveyor, because the top of the cross-section is open, based on the coals rest angle of 30°, the calculated coal transportation area $A = 0.63$ $m^2$; *ρ* is the loose coal density, 0.85–1.0 $t/m^3$, select 0.9 $t/m^3$. Substitute the data into Eq. (18), get: $Q = 3600 \times 1.77 \times 0.63 \times 0.9 \approx 3613$ t/h > 3000 t/h,meet the requirements.

Based on a conveying capacity of 3000 t/h and a chain speed of 1.77 m/s, and the installed power of 2000 kW, the theoretical power consumption utilization was analyzed under the conditions of face lengths of 300, 250 and 207 m respectively (the actual length at the No. 8105 face in Tashan coal mine). The calculation results showed that: when the face length is 300 m, and face dip is 0°, the power utilization reaches up to 94.3 %, power margin is small, which is only used in a flat or downhill face. When the face length is 250 m (or the actual face length at No. 8105 face is 207 m), and the face dip is 0°, the power utilization is 78.6 % and 65 %, respectively, showing a large margin. Therefore, a total power of 2 × 1000 kW can meet the requirement of transport capacity of 3000 t/h.

In order to warrant the non-fracture of the scraper chain, the safety coefficient of the chain was calculated. When the total power is 2000 kW, scraper chain speed is 1.77 m/s and the broken load of scraper chain is 3290 kN, the safety coefficient of scraper chain should reach 1.72 to satisfy the requirements of safe coal transportation.

Based on the analysis discussed, SGZ1200/2 × 1000 large load rear scraper conveyor was selected for the LLTCC face to extract the ultra-thick coal seam at Tashan coal mine. The installed power is 2 × 1000 kW, and transportation capacity exceeds 3000 t/h. The transportation distance meets the length requirement at the No. 8105 face.

In a LLTCC mining operation, the rear scraper conveyor should have reasonable technical parameters and structure; also, the key components should have high reliability. These key elements include a heavy-duty high-strength chain drive system, speed-adjustable soft start device, integrated monitoring transmission system of transmission device, heavy-loaded 1000 kW planetary retarder, high reliability long life high-strength coal transportation trough, high strength compact end discharge frame and automatic retractable tail with electro-hydraulic control, etc.

With the development of 48 × 152 compact high-strength round chain and link chain for the mine, as well as the high-strength forged scraper, the optimization of the meshing characteristics of the chain transmission system and the adaptability and chain tension, along with the development of along life 48 × 152 drive sprocket and component, a heavy-duty high-strength chain transmission system was successfully developed.

By studying the matching ability of controlled adjustable speed soft start device-valve-controlled hydraulic coupler and motor load characteristics, a rational coupler cavity has been designed and the fluid dynamics was optimized. In addition, an electro-hydraulic control technology for the coupler has been developed. A large power valve-controlled hydraulic coupler has been developed with intellectual property rights.

A comprehensive monitoring integrated transmission system has been developed. It consists of central monitoring equipment (upper equipment) and site monitoring equipment (lower equipment), which achieves a state monitoring and control on the transmission device of the rear scraper conveyor, and enhances the operation monitoring capacity of the large power rear scraper conveyor.

Through a combination method of theoretical analysis, three dimensional modelling, mechanical analysis and simulation, virtual prototyping, dynamic testing, bench testing, and industrial trial, a 1000 kW retarder for the mine has been developed.

Through the study on the bending angle design of the middle pan, and the connection method of U-shaped port of middle pan, in addition to the large amount of research and testing on the choice of materials, welding processes and equipment, and machining technology, a high-reliability, long-life coal pan has been developed.

Through the strength design on the end discharge head frame, the connection design of the head frame and joint parts, the connection design of the head frame and transition pan was improved. A high strength, compact end discharge head frame has been developed.

With the analysis on the operating conditions of the scraper conveyor chain, and the calculation on the adjustment required by conveyor tail and the calculation of traction force of the extension mechanism, an automatic retractable conveyor tail electro-hydraulic control system and retractable extension tail frame has been developed. Furthermore, an electro-hydraulic automatic control retractable conveyor tail has been developed.

Through the research and development of the key technologies and components above, the overall reliability of the rear scraper conveyor has been improved to warrant safe, efficient and stable operation.

## 4.4 Large-capacity and long distance gateroad belt conveyor

In order to achieve the transportation of both the coals extracted by the shearer and the coals extracted by top coal caving from the LLTCC operations, the technologies on a large-capacity long-distance gateroad belt conveyor has been investigated.

A CST soft drive system was used, in light loads or heave loads condition, the dynamic process of the loaded belt conveyor's soft start/soft stop can effectively be controlled to achieve a balance of power among various drives.

Based on the variation of tensile force during the start, stop and operation of belt conveyor, a tension technology and equipment of high accuracy and large tensioning stroke has been developed. It can quickly respond and automatically adjust tension and tensioning stroke with the tension variation of the belt conveyor. During normal operations, the tensile force is 0.9–1.1 times of the rated tensile force, during start and stop, the tensile force is 1.3–1.4 times of the rated tensile force, and during the shift of conveyor tail, the equipment can quickly respond and guarantee non-skid. The working principle is: based on the conveyor's start-up and loading, with the feedback of tension sensor signal, the PLC controller and fuel tank can automatically adjust the output of tensile force to avoid slipping between belts and drive pulley, lower the safety factor selected for the belt, and ensure the normal operation of the belt conveyor. Installed with an automatic moved conveyor tail, the automatic tensioning can be achieved when the conveyor tail is automatically moved, thus to a certain extent, the downtime rate of the belt conveyor and the downtime rate of the three face machine can be reduced.

A new high-efficiency belt storage device was developed; the belt can be folded into six layers and stored with a length of 200 m. A belt storage system of multi-layer winding has been developed, which enables an automatic belt central alignment to overcome the deviation of conveyor belts in storage and the tensioning truck's off track.

A low speed large torque hydraulic motor and electro-hydraulic proportional control valves were used to develop a large-torque belt-speed controllable high efficiency hydraulic belt winding device, which significantly reduces the time on belt winding, is easy in operation, and reliable in working.

A high-speed low-friction larger-diameter roller was developed. Using labyrinth seals with special structure and oxidation resistance, water-resistance grease sealing method, the service life of the high-speed large-diameter roller is significantly increased.

Using dynamic analysis software, the system was analyzed to determine a reasonable starting and braking curve. An advanced PLC programmable controller was developed. In addition, an advanced program-controlled automatic monitoring system was developed, which can conduct the operations of data collection, processing, storage, transmission, fault detection, reach and feed, etc. It can meet the requirements of the conveyor's controllable soft start and braking, power balance, automatic tensioning and self-movement of conveyor tail, as well as various functions, such as protection, communication and signal contact. In addition, it can monitor the various protection and safety devices, conveyor belt tension, the temperature of the driving drum and roller bearing, the measurement of throughput, etc.

Through the studies presented, a large-capacity, long-distance belt conveyor has been developed, as shown in Fig. 54. Its main technical parameters are as follows: transportation distance: 2800 m; transportation capacity: 3500 t/h; lifting height: 35 m; belt width: 1400 mm; installed power: 1680 (3 × 500) kW; belt speed: ≥4.5 m/s; stored belt length: ≥120 m.

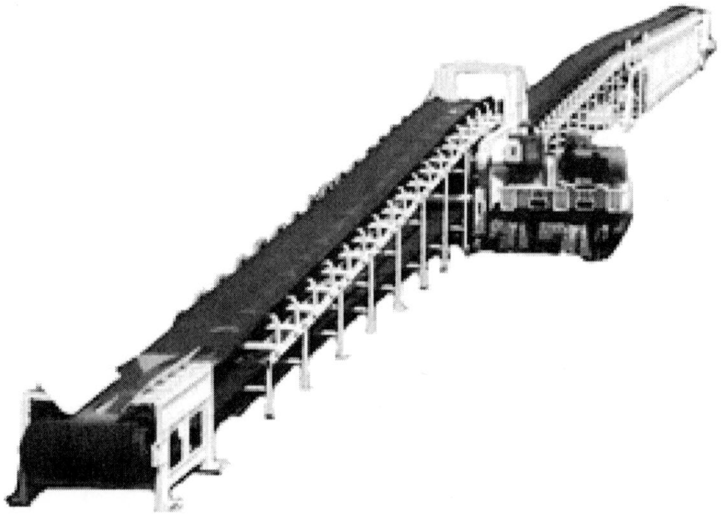

**Figure 54.** The large-capacity, long-distance belt conveyor

## 4.5 Large tonnage shield hauler

The tonnage of hydraulic support for the working face in thick and ultra-thick coal seam is very large. In order to improve the efficiency of coal mining, it requires a fast relocation of coal face equipment. Therefore, a heavy-duty frame shield hauler—WC55Y shield hauler was developed, as shown in Fig. 55. The vehicle is powered by diesel, the carrying capacity is 55 t, and is an efficient equipment for a quick relocation of coalface. If equipped with a hopper, it also can be used as a multifunctional underground transport vehicle.

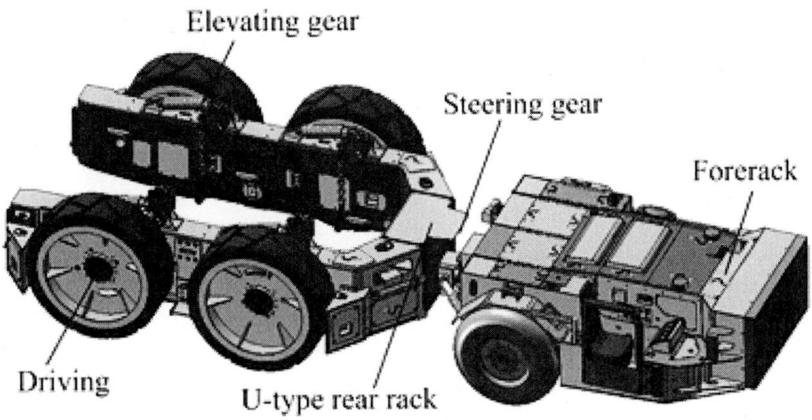


**Figure 55.** WC55Y shield hauler

A V-type six-cylinder diesel engine explosion-proof equipment was used in the WC55Y shield hauler. Based on the requirements of explosion-proofing, the explosion-proof device must be set up in engine intake and exhaust systems, which will increase the resistances of engine's intake and exhaust, reducing engine efficiency, worsen the harmful emissions, and increase the pollution in underground. The difficulty in this project is how to optimize the inlet and outlet structures to minimize its effect on engine performance and reduce the emissions of harmful gases. In terms of the engine's explosion-proofing, the following four key technologies have been developed:

(1)In the explosion-proof diesel engine, exhaust turbocharged water–air cooling technology was used. Forced water circulation technology was used to solve the high temperature problem with the supercharger surface. Compared to natural air intake, the air intake increases 30 %, and lays a foundation for increasing efficiency and reducing emission.

(2)Using theoretical analysis and test methods, the fuel injection control was optimized. The oil injection method of low-speed in the early stages, high-speed in the middle stages and reduced speed in later stages was used to effectively control the emission of NOx, PT, etc.

(3)Intake resistance is an important factor affecting engine power. The intake spark arrestor is a key component of the air intake system in explosion-proofing the diesel engine, which directly affects engine performance. Through the experiment, after the installation of the air inlet device on the diesel engine, the losses of power and torque is up to 14 %. To improve the flow characteristics of the diesel engine intake, the original structure had been optimized. With a comparative analysis of eddy current resistance loss at inlet/outlet section in different intake spark arrestors, an inclined windward surface end grid plate was designed to substantially reduce inlet resistance.

(4)A constant pressure low resistance exhaust gas treatment device was designed. Using a water bath type cylindrical structure, the exhaust resistance was reduced by 5 %.

For the WC55Y shield hauler, a moving speed brake was developed, which integrates a planetary speed retarder and a large torque wetted multi-disc safe brake. Traditional brake concentrates on the high-speed end of wheel-side retarder, and is small in dimension. However, under a larger braking torque and repeated braking, the system generates large amount of heat and consistently fails. The working condition of the shield hauler is harsh. In the aspect of driveless axle hydraulic-driven design, there have been no successful braking studies anywhere in the world. Fully enclosed, high torque and large brake power, small in size, and high efficiency heat dissipation are the difficulties in the study. Meanwhile, the road underground is potholed, thus during the movement of heavy-loaded vehicles, the wheel-side retarder will withstand a greater shock load, and therefore must have enough strength. Otherwise, it will cause failures in the retarder's bearing, such as broken parts. In response to these technical bottlenecks, a “modular integrated technology” was used to design a new planetary gear of wetted multiple-disc brake. Also, an integrated motor-cartridge wheel drive and brake retarder was invented. It is a wheel-side planetary retarder, and integrates all brake functions. The brake was designed as a fully closed wetted-type multi-disc brake with spring braking and hydraulic release. Through the spline, friction tablets and steel tablets are coupled with fixed parts and turned parts respectively. Through the motor input, retarder part input torque, delivered via a two level planetary deceleration device, the torque will be transmitted to the wheels. The brake cavity and retarder cavity are completely insulated by a pair of high reliable floating seals to avoid the interference of two different functions. The braking torque of the integrated brake-retarder is greater than 60,000 N m, thermal equilibrium temperature is less than 90 C° under long term braking, and the average life of the friction disc is greater than 5000 h. Furthermore, it is safe, reliable, has good pollution resistance, and increases operational safety.

The main performance indicators of the WC55Y shield hauler developed are: rated load 55 t, minimum ground clearance 300 mm, full load speed 0–12 km/h and climbing ability 12°, engine rated power after explosion-proof 220 kW, turning radius 2800 mm (inside) and 7000 mm (outside). The WC55Y shield hauler was used in the relocation of the LLTCC coalface at 14–20 m thick ultra-thick coal seam in the Tashan coal mine to successfully solve the relocation problem of large-tonnage hydraulic support at a LLTCC coalface.

# 5 BOLT SUPPORT TECHNOLOGY OF LARGE CROSS-SECTION ROADWAY IN ULTRA-THICK COAL SEAM

## 5.1 Deformation and failure characteristics of the surrounding rocks of coal roadway with a large cross-section in ultra-thick coal seam

The roadways for a LLTCC coalface include headgate, tailgate, top return airway and open-off cut. These roadways are responsible for equipment installation, transportation, ventilation, gas exhaust, personnel passage, etc. A safe, efficient coalface depends on roadway stability and smooth flow. Roadway support is a key to the LLTCC mining operation.

The roadway of a LLTCC coal face has following characteristics:

(1)The headgate, tailgate and open-off cut are developed along the coal seam. The roof is top coals with an average thickness of 12.9 m. Compared to rock, the coal seam is relatively soft, fractured, and thick. The top coal is easily subsided and even caved, which significantly increases the difficulty of roadway support.

(2)Because the power of mining equipment is large, and face production is high, a very large cross-section of the roadway is required. The tailgate and the headgate have a same cross-section with a width of 5.5 m wide, a height of 3.9 m and a size of 21.45 m$^2$. The open-off cut span is up to 10 m. The increase of roadway width can result in significant bending subsidence in the roof, and large height roadway can cause coal wall buckling and even spalling, which significantly affects the stability of the surrounding rock of the roadway, and brings great difficulties to roadway support.

(3)The tailgate suffers the side-abutment pressure caused by the previous longwal gob and the and the front abutment pressure caused by the current longwall panel. In addition, due to the distinct characteristics of ground pressure at a LLTCC coalface, the mining effect on the tailgate is very strong, resulting in serious damage of the surrounding rocks.

## 5.2 Bolt support mechanism of large cross-section coal roadway

Roadway support with bolt and cable has become one of the main methods at coal mines in China. In this project, bolts and cables were used to support the large cross-section coal roadway. However, the surrounding rock of the roadway in the coal seam is soft and fractured. Traditional bolt supporting failed to suppress the large deformation of the roadway due to the high mining-induced stresses. Bolt supporting mechanism for coal roadways should be investigated to provide a theoretical basis for support design.

Many studies have been conducted to investigate the support mechanism of bolt and cable support on coal roadways (Jia and Huang 2005; Zhang et al. 2006; Ma and Zhang 2008; Zhang and Yang 2010) in China. In recent years, it has been recognized that the prestress of rock bolts plays an important role in bolt support (Kang et al. 2007a, b, 2008; Wang et al. 2008; Zhang et al. 2010), such as the binding effect it plays on the layer separation, slippage, and join crack opening of the surrounding rock surface layer, and maintaining the integrity of the surrounding rock. The studies improve the bolting effect, in particular, providing an effective theoretical guidance for complicated roadway support.

Based on the deformation characteristics of large cross-section coal roadway in ultra-thick coal seam, a full coal roadway supporting mechanism is proposed.

(1)The deformation of surrounding rock in a full coal roadway consists of two parts: one is the dilatancy deformation including the separation of coal and rock, sliding, fissures opening, and new cracks at their structural plane; the second is the elastic deformation of surrounding rock and the plastic deformation before its peak strength, and a full deformation of anchorage zone. A reasonable full coal seam roadway support should greatly improve the stiffness and strength of supporting system at initial support, effectively controlling the dilatancy deformation of the surrounding rock, and maintaining the integrity of top coals. At the same time, the supporting system should have sufficient elongation and allow a second deformation to release high stress.

(2)The prestresses of bolts and anchors play a decisive role in roadway support. It is crucial for support design to determine reasonable prestresses according to coal roadway conditions, and enabling prestresses to effectively spread.

(3)The anchor cable in a full coal seam roadway plays its role in two main aspects: one is to connect the bearing structure formed by bolting in top coal with deep surrounding rock in order to improve the stability of load bearing structures; the other is that the large prestresses of anchor cables and the compressive zone of bolts form a skeleton mesh structure to actively support surrounding rock.

(4)In a full coal seam roadway, high prestress powerful bolt and anchor cables should be used to become the single necessary support during the service life of the roadway, avoiding second roadway support and roadway maintenance.

## 5.3 Material of high strength bolt and cable

The yield strength of a traditional thread steel bolt is 335–500 MPa, and the tensile strength is 470–650 MPa, which is applicable to the roadway with normal conditions. For a roadway under complex geological and geotechnical conditions, a higher strength and sufficient elongation steel should be used for bolts and anchor cables in order to achieve high prestress, high strength and high elongation.

In this project, with the cooperation of other steel mills, strong steel for bolts and cables has been developed. The key technology and difficulties in developing this type of steel is to greatly improve the bolt strength, and simultaneously, maintain sufficient elongation and impact toughness of the bolt to prevent bolt fracture and breaking under impact loads, bending and shear loads. Starting from steel-making, a special bolt steel formula was formulated, e.g., adding elements of V, Nb and Ti in the steel to alter the mechanical properties of steel. In addition, an appropriate rolling process was used to manufacture the bolt in accordance with its technical specifications. Table 23 lists two kinds of anchor bolt steel developed with high strength, high elongation, and high impact toughness. The yield strength of the two types of boltreaches 570 and 650 MPa respectively, and the tensile strength reaches 745 MPa and 805 MPa respectively. The elongation is 26 % and 22 % respectively, and their shock absorbing energy is more than 40 J.

**Table 23.** High strength bolt steel

| Strength level (MPa) | Yield (MPa) | Tensile strength (MPa) | Shock absorb energy (J) | Elongation (%) |
|---|---|---|---|---|
| 500 | 570 | 745 | 89.0 | 26.0 |
| 600 | 650 | 805 | 42.6 | 22.0 |

## 5.4 Cable material with large tonnage and high elongation

The anchor cable steel strand widely used in Chinese coal mines is composed of seven wires (Fig. 56a), with a diameter of 15.2 or 17.8 mm. Its application in underground coal mines showed the following disadvantages: the cable diameter is small and doesn't match borehole diameter, thus, significantly affects anchorage force, and is prone to the anchor end sliding. Due to its small breaking load, cable fractures often occur. Because of its low elongation, it cannot adapt to the large deformation of the surrounding rock. Due to its low prestress, it is poor in controlling the separation of rock layers.

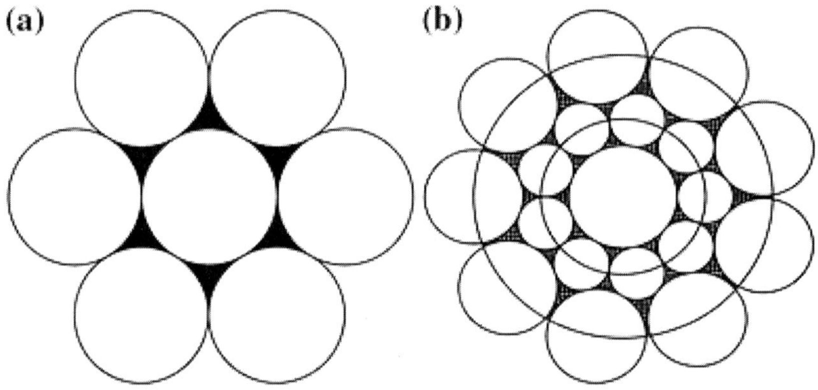


**Figure 56.** Anchor cable structure. **a** 1 × 7 structure, **b** 1 × 19 structure

To solve the problems discussed above, a large diameter, high tonnage strong anchor cable series was developed with a diameter of 18–22 mm, and a capacity of 400–550 kN. The technological approaches used are as follows: (1) changing cable body structure. Using new type of 19 wires (Fig. 56b) to replace the original seven wires, the cable body structure is more reasonable, and the anchor cable elongation has been significantly improved; (2) increasing the diameter of anchor cable body. The cable diameter was increased from 15.2 to 18, 20 and 22 mm to improve the cable body's broken force, and match the cable diameter and drilling diameter. The anchor cable with a diameter of 22 mm has a breaking load of greater than 600 kN, and an elongation of 7 %. The comparison of different mechanical properties of anchor cable steel strand wires are shown in Table 24.

**Table 24.** Mechanical properties of different anchor cable strand wires

| Structure of steel strand wires | Diameter (mm) | Cross-section ($mm^2$) | Tensile strength (MPa) | Breaking load (kN) | Elongation (%) |
|---|---|---|---|---|---|
| 1 × 7 | 15.2 | 140 | 1860 | 260 | 3.5 |
| | 17.8 | 191 | 1860 | 355 | 4.0 |
| | 19.0 | 218 | 1860 | 406 | 4.5 |
| 1 × 19 | 18 | 215.5 | 1897 | 409 | 6.8 |
| | 20 | 262.4 | 1862 | 489 | – |
| | 22 | 321.6 | 1887 | 607 | 7.0 |

## 5.5 Equipment for applying high prestress on bolt

As mentioned previously, the prestress of rock bolts is one of the key parameters for bolting, and plays a decisive role on the effect of anchor support. The previous studies show that the anchor prestress should reach a level of 30 %–50 % of anchor yield strength. According to the conversion relationship, the bolts' tightening torque should be 300–500 N m. To reach such a high prestress, the existing single bolting machines in China cannot meet such a requirement. It is necessary to develop a suitable bolt tightening tool to significantly increase the anchor cable's prestress.

In terms of the equipment for bolting, there are two main methods for increasing bolt's prestress (Kang and Wang 2007): one is to increase the bolt-nut tightening torque; the second is to use a bolt tensioning device, which is similar to imposing large prestresses on anchor bolts. The methods for improving bolt-nut tightening torque include: (1) high torque jumbolter. With a high torque jumbolter, it can not only increase the bolt tightening torque, but also achieve an integration of bolt installation to improve installation speed. For instance, the torque of the jumbolter used with continuous miner can reach more than 300 N m. The rated torque of a single jumbolter in China is not greater than 150 N m, and unable to meet the requirement of high tightening torque of the bolt. (2) Torque multiplier. In order to improve the installation torque of the jumbolter, a torque multiplier can be used on the jumbolter to multiply the nut tightening torque when installing bolt. (3) Torque wrench. Using a large torque preload wrench to tighten the bolts and nuts is an effective way to improve the prestress of anchor bolts.

Based on the jumbolter used in large cross-section coal roadway, and the operation conditions, torque multiplier was selected to improve the prestress of anchor bolts. The bolt torque multiplier developed has an input torque of 100–150 N m and an output torque of 500–600 N m. With a single jumbolter match, the maximum torque magnification is approximately six times, which meets the high prestressing requirement of the bolts.

## 5.6 Stress characteristics of the surrounding rock in a full seam roadway and numerical simulation of the combined support with bolt and cable

In order to better understand the distribution characteristics of variation of surrounding rock in a large cross-section full coal roadway, as well as the support mechanism and main effect factors of anchor bolts and cables, a numerical analysis using FLAC$^{3D}$ was performed based on the data from the No. 5105 return airway of the No. 8105 coalface at Tashan coal mine The stress characteristics of the surrounding rock in a large cross-section coal roadway with different top coal thicknesses, the influence of different roadway layout locations, different roadway width-height ratios, different ground stresses, and different pre-tight forces of anchor bolts and cables were evaluated.

### 5.6.1 Simulation approach

The No. 5105 return air roadway was developed along the seam floor, its cross-section is in a rectangular shape with a width of 5.5 m, a height of 3.9 m. Ground stress data measured are shown in Table 2, vertical stress is 11.44 MPa, the maximum horizontal principal stress is 12.90 MPa, and the minimum horizontal principal stress is 7.24 MPa.

In the numerical simulation, the FLAC$^{3D}$ built-in cable structure element was used to simulate the rock bolts and cables. The bolts have anelastic modulus of 200 GPa, a yield strength of 600 MPa, a tensile strength of 800 MPa. The rock bolts are 2.4 m long and 22 mm in diameter. The cables have an elastic modulus of 195 GPa a length of 8.3 m, a diameter of mm, and a capacity of 600 kN. The Mohr–Coulomb constitutive model was used to describe the coal-rock body. Based on the results from the laboratory tests, the physical and mechanical parameters of coal and rock seams in the calculation are shown in Table 25.

**Table 25.** Physical and mechanical parameters of coal and rock seams in a numerical model

| Lithology | Density (kg/m$^3$) | Volume modulus (GPa) | Shear modulus (Pa) | Cohesion (MPa) | Friction angle (°) | Tensile strength (MPa) |
|---|---|---|---|---|---|---|
| Sandstone | 2650 | 25.3 | 18.2 | 22 | 44 | 1.6 |
| Coal | 1500 | 6.5 | 3.9 | 7.9 | 36 | 0.6 |
| Sandy mudstone | 2600 | 8.85 | 5.8 | 9.2 | 41 | 0.8 |

Combining the geological conditions at the No. 5105 roadway in Tashan coal mine, based on the combined support of ancho bolts and anchor cables in coal roadway, multiple plans were compared in the simulations in this study:

(1)When the horizontal principal stress is 12.90 MPa, the vertical stress is 11.44 MPa, and the roadway was developed along the seam floor, the effect of different top-coal thicknesses on the stress distribution of the surrounding rock. Top-coal thicknesses were 0, 5, 10, 15, 20, and 25 m respectively.

(2)When the horizontal principal stress is 12.90 MPa, the vertical stress is 11.44 MPa, and the coal thickness is 15.72 m, the effect of different positions of the roadway layout on the stress distribution of surrounding rock. In a vertical direction, the roadway was laid out along the roof and along the floor. When the coal-pillar widths in the horizontal direction were 10, 20, 30, and 40 m, the effect after the extraction of two adjacent coalfaces on the stress distribution of surrounding rock of roadway.

(3)When the horizontal principal stress is 12.90 MPa, and the vertical stress is 11.44 MPa, the effect of different width-height ratios on the stress distribution of the surrounding rock of the roadway. The height-width ratios in a full coal seam gateway are 1, 0.75 and 0.5.

(4)When the coal thickness is 16.8 m, the roadway was developed along the seam floor, the effect of different ground stresses on the stress distribution of the surrounding rock of the roadway. Different combinations of stress are shown in Table 26.

**Table 26.** Different ground stress combinations in the numerical simulation

| Different ground stress combinations | Horizontal stress (MPa) | Vertical stress (MPa) | Lateral pressure coefficient |
|---|---|---|---|
| Combination 1 | 10 | 10 | 1 |
| Combination 2 | 20 | 10 | 2 |
| Combination 3 | 10 | 20 | 0.5 |

(5)The effect of different preloads of bolts and cables on the spread of stress in coal (regardless of in situ rock stress). Under the condition of the cable's prestress as 100, 150, and 200 kN, the bolt preloads are 60, 80 and 100 kN, respectively.

### 5.6.2 Effect of top-coal thickness on the stress distribution of surrounding rock of full coal roadway

In Fig. 57a, because the roadway's roof and floor are rock, and the two walls are coal, the stress concentration zones after roadway development are located at the four corners of the roadway in the roof and floor rock strata, the maximum compressed stress reaches 22 MPa. As the rock strengths of roof and floor are relative high, it enables pressure to be uniformly transferred to the coal wall bodies of the roadway to reduce the compressed stress in the coal bodies of the roadway's two sides, and reduce roadway deformation. As shown from Fig. 57b–f, with the increase of top coal thickness, the distribution zone of compressed stress in top-coal increases, and the stress in top-coal is less than that in the roadway floor. There is a distinct interface between top-coal and roof. Overall, during roadway excavation, when top-coal thickness is within 10 m, there is a strong correlation between the stress distribution of surrounding rock of roadway and the top-coal thickness. As the top-coal thickness increased, the stress concentration area in the top-coal expanded and the concentration coefficient reduced. With the continual increase of top-coal thickness, there is no appreciable variation in stress distribution of the surrounding rock.

### 5.6.3 Effect of roadway layout positions on the stress distribution of surrounding rock of full coal roadway

The coalface with full coal roadways is usually a coalface with a large mining height. The increase of mining height will have a great impact on the stress distribution in the coal pillar, thus affecting the stress distribution of surrounding rock of the roadway. In Fig. 58a, b, the stress concentration zone generated at two side walls during roadway development overlapped with the stress concentration zone in coal pillar after coal extraction. The maximum stress in the coal pillar reaches 33 MPa. In Fig. 58c, the stress concentration zone in the surrounding rock of roadway during its development is isolated from the stress concentration zone in coal pillars caused by the extraction of two adjacent coalface. However, it still has some impact on the stress distribution of the surrounding rock of the roadway, the maximum compressive stress on the side coal pillar is approximately 30 MPa. In Fig. 58d, due to the further increase of coal pillar width, the effect of the stress of the adjacent mining face on roadway decreased significantly. The stress concentration zone formed in the surrounding rocks of the roadway during its development is basically separated with the stress concentration zone formed by coalface extraction. The maximum compressive stress of surrounding rocks of the roadway is 27 MPa. Overall, due to the large thickness of coal seams with the coal roadway, after roadway development and adjacent coalface extraction, the stress concentration zone formed in the coal pillar is different to that at thick or thin coal seams. The stress is no longer distributed as standard "arch" or "hump" distribution, but renders approximately triangular distribution.

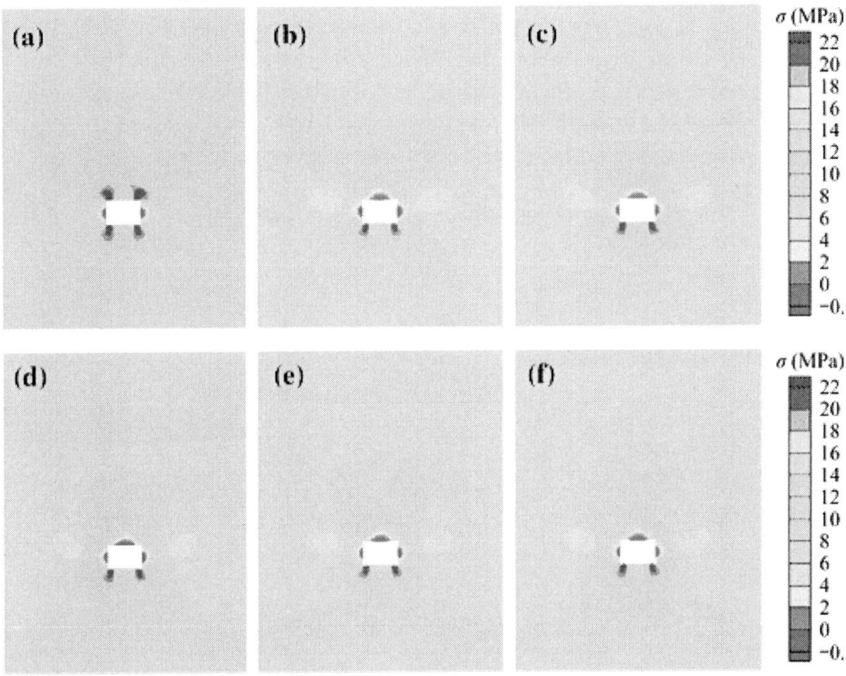


**Figure 57.** Stress distribution of roadway surrounding rock at different top-coal thicknesses. **a** Rock roof **b** top coal 5 m **c** top coal 10 m **d** top coal 15 m **e** top coal 20 m **f** top coal 25 m

A full coal seam roadway has two kinds of vertical arrangements, one is arranged along the floor, the other is arranged along the roof, their stress distributions have a large difference (Fig. 59). When the roadway is arranged along the floor, the stress concentration area is mainly distributed in the two corners of the roadway floor, the maximum stress reaches 22 MPa, and the maximum stress in the top coal of roadway is about 18 MPa. When the roadway is arranged along the roof, the stress state of surrounding rock of the roadway is opposite to that of roadway arranged along the floor, the stress concentration area is mainly distributed on the two corners of the roof, maximum stress is 22 MPa, and the maximum stress of the coal body at the floor is about 18 MPa. Because the stress field distributions of two kinds of arrangements are different, different measures should be taken during the roadway support. When the roadway is arranged along the floor, in addition to the top-coal support, the side walls support should be enhanced or the anchor bolt should be installed at the floor corners to prevent the occurrence of floor heave. When roadway is arranged along the roof, the support on the two corners of the roof should be strengthened, and some measures should be taken to prevent or reduce the occurrence of floor heave.

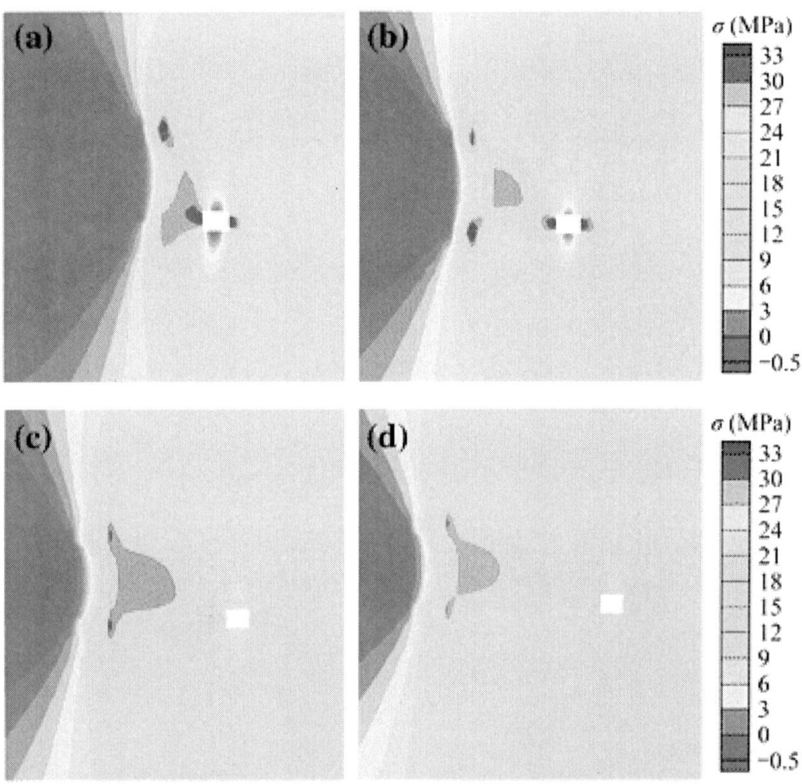


**Figure 58.** Stress distribution of roadway surrounding rock with different coal pillar widths. **a** Coal pillar width 10 m **b** coal pillar width 20 m **c** coal pillar width 30 m **d** coal pillar width 40 m

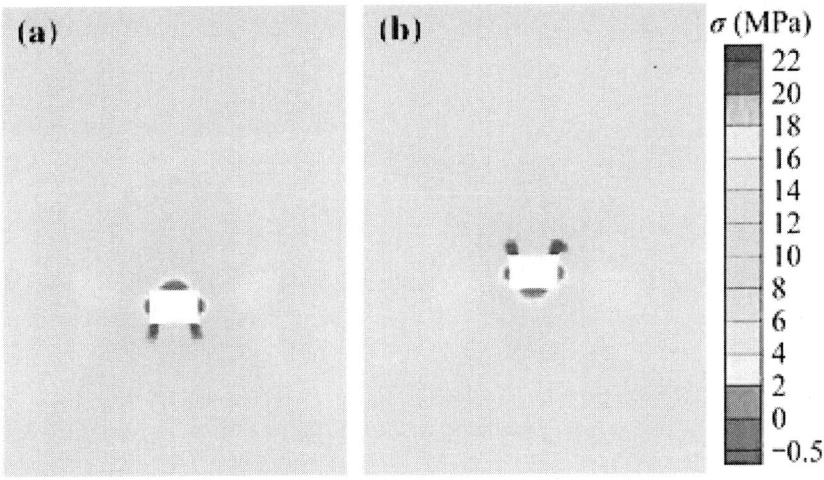


**Figure 59.** Stress distribution of surrounding rock with different roadway positions. **a** Along floor layout **b** along roof layout

### 5.6.4 Effect of roadway height-width ratio on stress distribution of a full coal roadway

The stress distributions of the surrounding rock of the roadway under different roadway height-width ratios are shown in Fig. 60. With the same roadway height, the wider the roadway tunnel is, the higher the level of stress concentration in the top-coal; the greater the stress concentration area in top-coal, the higher the stress concentration factor. When the roadway's height-width ratio is equal to one, the maximum compressive stress in top-coal is 12 MPa. When roadway's height-width ratio is 0.75, the maximum compressive stress in top-coal is 16 MPa. When roadway's height-width ratio is 0.75, the maximum compressive stress in top-coal is 16 MPa, but the compressive stress concentration area increases significantly. When the roadway's height-width ratios are different, the stress distributions formed in the floor during roadway development are significantly different. When the height-width ratio is equal to one, the stress concentration zone in the floor shows an "inverted arch" distribution. When the height-width ratio is 0.75, the stress distribution zone shows an "inverted hump" shape distribution. When the height-width ratio is 0.5, an irregular stress distribution in the floor occurs, but the range increases significantly. Based on the maximum stress values in the floor, with the increase in roadway's width, the maximum stress values follow a downward trend.

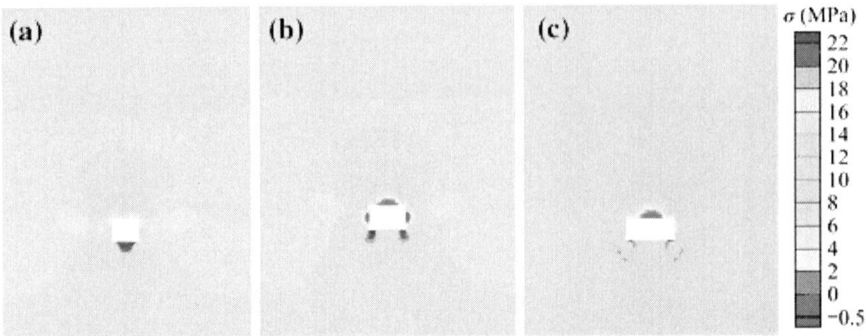


**Figure 60.** Stress distribution with different roadway's height-width ratios. **a** Height-width ratio 1 **b**height-width ratio 0.75 **c** height-width ratio 0.5

### 5.6.5 Effect of ground stress on stress distribution of surrounding rock of a full coal roadway

The stress field distributions of surrounding rock of a full coal roadway under different ground stress conditions are shown in Fig. 61. The stress distribution of the surrounding rock of the roadway after roadway development is correlated to rock strength. When the horizontal and vertical stresses are the same, the stresses in the top-coal and side coal walls are basically the same, their values are relatively low, about 15 MPa. High stress areas are mainly in the floor with high rock strength, the maximum stress is about 21 MPa. When the horizontal stress is twice of vertical stress, the stress concentration areas are mainly in the top coal and the floor rock. In particular, due to the high rock strength in the floor, its stress and stress concentration area are significantly larger than that in top coal, the maximum stress value is up to 33 MPa. When the vertical stress is twice of horizontal stress, the maximum compressive stress of surrounding rock of roadway is approximately 30 MPa, and the stress concentration area shows an arc-shaped symmetrical distribution at two side walls of the roadway.

### 5.6.6 Effect of different bolt prestress on the stress distribution of surrounding rock of a full coal roadway

The increase of compressive stress in the anchorage zone and the range extension of compressive stress are the keys to improving the supporting effect. As shown in Fig. 62a, in the anchor bolt and anchor cable joint support, when anchor bolt pre-tight torque is 200 N m, a prestress overlap zone can be formed in the anchor bolt anchorage zone, but cannot cover the

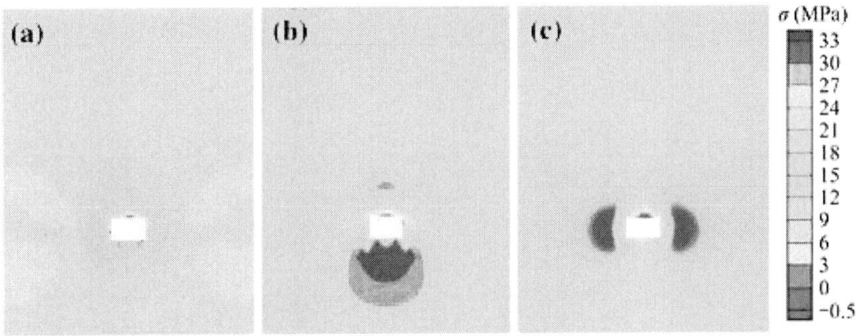


**Figure 61.** Stress distribution of surrounding rock with different ground stress. **a** Combination 1 **b**combination 2 **c** combination 3

area between roof and anchor bolt at two side coal walls. The maximum compressive stress near anchor bolt in the coal body is about for 0.55 MPa, the compressive stress between anchor bolts is approximately 0.25 MPa. When the anchor bolt's pre-tight torque is 300 N m, with the increase of anchor bolt's pre-tight force, the anchor bolt's prestress spread range increases at roadway roof and two side coal walls, and in roadway's top coal, the spread zones can basically join and form one large zone. However, the anchor bolt's prestress spread zone is still small, and cannot cover the whole coal wall. The compressive stress between top coal and the roadway walls anchor bolt increases to around 0.4 MPa. When bolt's tightening torque increases up to 400 N m, the effect of the bolt's prestress spread within bolting range between the roof and two walls of the roadway is good. It covers the entire range of anchor zone, and the compressive stress value between bolts in the coal increases to about 0.5 MPa. Because of the lower prestress of the anchorage cable, the cable's prestress cannot spread to its anchoring range, thus, the overlapping effect of the bolt's prestress and cable's prestress is not obvious.

Compared to Fig. 62a, b shows that with the increase of the cable's prestress, there is a significant increase of prestress spread in the area along the cable length in the roadway's top coal and perpendicular to the direction of cable length. Nevertheless, in terms of the compressive stress in coal body formed by the bolt and cable's prestress, under the impact of the increase of cable's prestress and the superposition effect of the bolt's prestress, the maximum compressive stress close to the cable in the coal body reaches 0.88 MPa. When the bolt's tightening torque is 200, and 300 N m, the distribution of compressive stress formed in the coal body by cables and bolts is not uniform, the compressible stress between two bolts farther away from cables is 0.48 MPa. When the bolt's tightening torque is 400 N m, the effect of prestress spread formed in top coal by cables and bolts is improved to some extent. The compressible stress between two bolts farther away from cables is approximately 0.64 MPa.

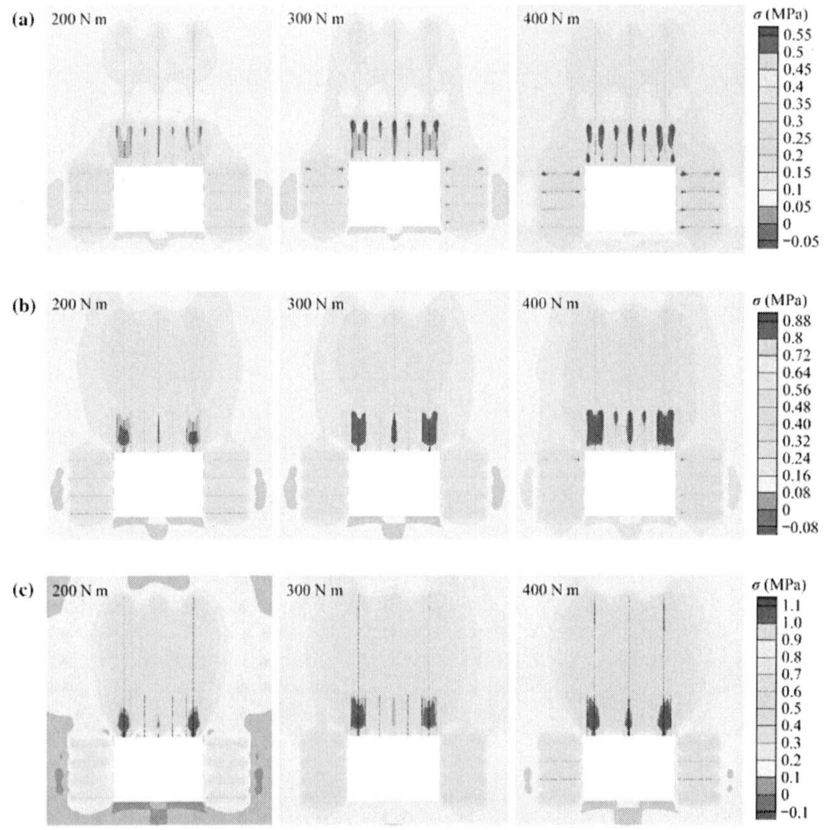


**Figure 62.** Stress distribution of surrounding rock with different combinations of bolt and cable. **a**Cable prestress 100 kN **b** cable prestress 150 kN **c** cable prestress 200 kN

As shown in Fig. 62c, when the cable's pre-tight force increases to 200 kN, the cable plays a major role in prestress spread in the coal body, the range of prestress spread basically covers the entire cable anchoring zone, and the maximum compressive stress formed in coal body is 1.1 MPa. The bolt's pre-tight force mainly affects the compressive stress distribution in the coal body, as the increase of bolt tightening torque, there is a distinct increase of compressive stress spread formed in the coal body and the stress values.

Figure 63 shows the compressive stress distribution on the surface of the roadway under the support of the combination of rock bolts and cables with a pre-tightening force of 400 and 150 kN, respectively. The compressive stress zones on the roadway surface formed by bolts and cables' combined support are interconnected and superimposed. The compressive stress of top coal at the bolt tray reached 2.8 MPa, at cable tray reached 7.7 MPa, the bolt's prestress and cable's prestress basically spread to the entire surface of top coal to form an effective stress arch, and improve the stress state of the surrounding rock of the roadway.

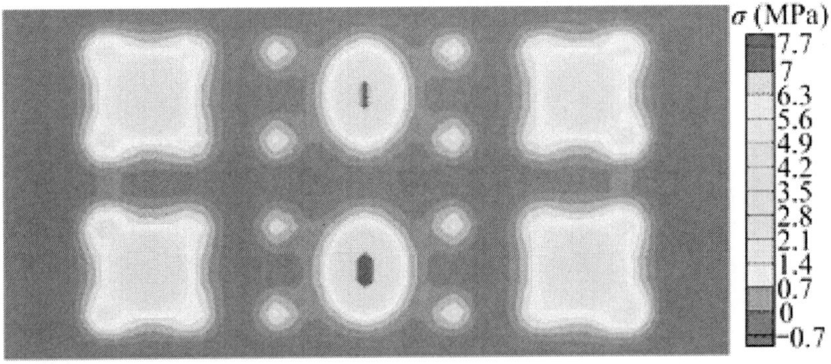


**Figure 63.** Stress distribution on the surface of top coal with the bolt and cable combined support

## 5.7 Support design of a large cross-section full coal roadway

Based on the numerical simulation results and lessons learned, a high strength bolt and cable combined support system was determined for the No. 5105 roadway at the No. 8105 coalface in Tashan coal mine. A BHRB600 bolt was selected with a diameter of 22 mm and length of 2.4 m left-lateral no longitudinal reinforcement steel rebar, extended with resin, and the bolt's tightening torque is not less than 400 N m. A 4 mm thick W steel belt and diamond-shaped metal mesh were used to protect the roof and side walls of the roadway. The roof bolt spacing was 800 mm, and the row spacing was 800 mm. Roof cable's diameter was $\phi$22 mm with 1 × 19 strands high strength low relaxation prestressed steel wires, and its length is 8300 mm. Using one K2335 and two Z2360 low viscosity resin cartridge, the cable was anchored, the anchorage length is 1500 mm. With every two rows of bolts, three cable anchors were installed, the row spacing is 1600 mm, and cable spacing is 2000 mm, and all cables were vertically installed into the roof. The cable anchor's pre-tightening force was 100–150 kN. Figure 64 shows the layout of roadway support.

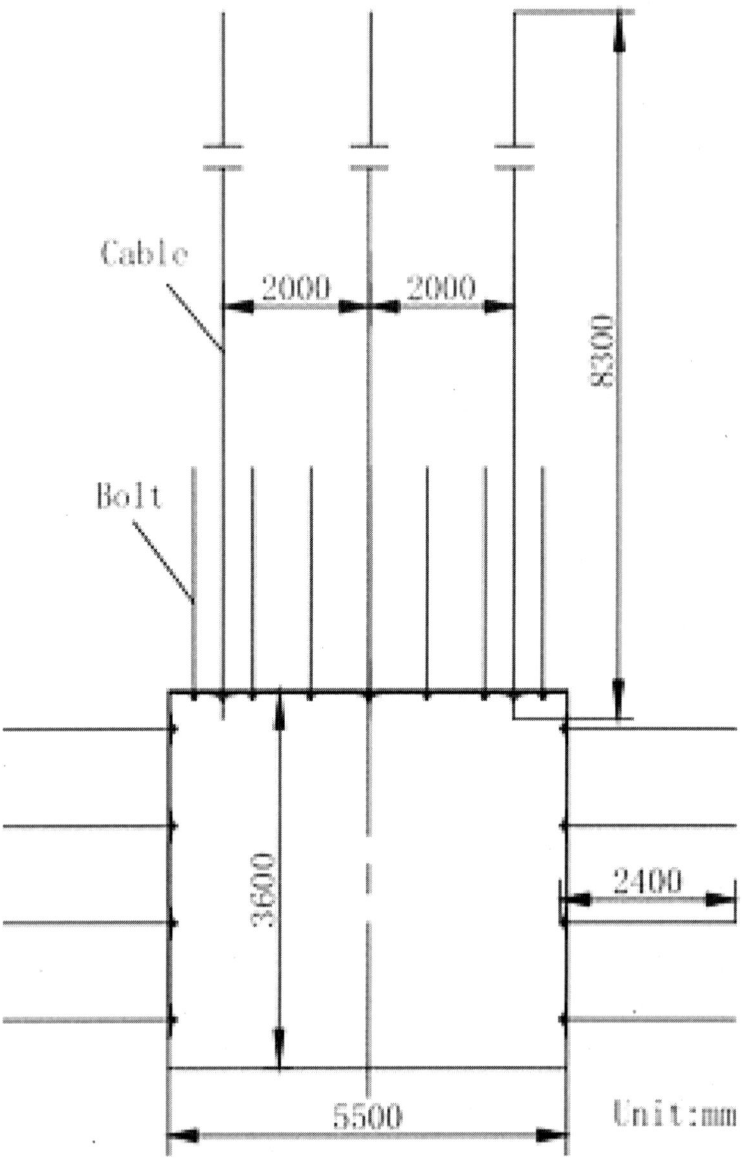


**Figure 64.** Layout of roadway support

# 6 SAFETY TECHNOLOGIES FOR THE LLTCC COAL MINING OPERATION

## 6.1 Gas control technologies for the LLTCC coalface

### 6.1.1 Characteristics of gas distribution at the LLTCC coalface

At the coal seam 3–5 in Tashan coal mine, the original gas pressure varies 0.14–0.17 MPa, the gas content in the coal seam varies 1.60–1.97 $m^3/t$ and the average is 1.78 $m^3/t$. The coal seam permeability coefficient varies 171.71–428.80 $m^2/(MPa^2\ d)$, and the gas flow per hundred meters in the borehole varies 0.015–0.0212 ($m^3$/min hm); the gas discharge attenuation coefficient in the borehole varies between 0.602 and 0.7427 $d^{-1}$. The residual coal gas amount at the coal seam 3–5 is 1.17 $m^3/t$. The coal seams are spontaneous combustion-prone coal seams, and the shortest period of the occurrence of spontaneous combustion is 60 days; the coal seams have a tendency for coal dust explosion hazards and the explosion index is 37 %.

With the analysis of field tests, the gas emission and distribution in a LLTCC coalface have four characteristics:

(1)Low gas storage, high gas emission. Under the influence of large thickness of coal seam and high mining intensity, the LLTCC mining operation in ultra-thick coal seam shows a "low gas storage, high absolute gas emission" feature. At the coal seam 3-5, the original gas pressure was only 0.14–0.17 MPa, gas content in the coal seam was 1.6–1.97 $m^3/t$, and an average was only 1.78 $m^3/t$, however, the absolute gas emissions in the working face exceeded 40 $m^3$/min, and the highest absolute gas emission was up to 65 $m^3$/min.

(2)Unbalanced gas emission. The gas emission sources at the LLTCC coalface in Tashan mine can be divided into three parts, one is the gas at the top position of the goaf including the gas in the upper adjacent layer; the second is the gas in the deep part of the goaf including the gas of the lower adjacent layer; the third is the gas from coal extraction and caving operation carried by the airflow leakage in the working face. The gas emission in the three sources discussed above will be affected by face pressure, upper roof caving and top coal caving, and present the characteristics of imbalance, and the uneven emission coefficient might reach 1.8.

(3)Large gas emission in goaf. Local gas emission in goaf showed that the gas emission often exceeded the gas limit at the zone between the 110th support and upper corner of the coalface; at the window of top coal caving and the gap between supports, the measured gas concentration reached 2 %–3 %, sometimes even higher. At U-type ventilation coalface, the gas concentration seriously exceeded the gas limit in the upper corner of the working face. Without taking any measures in the upper corner, the gas emission concentration often exceeded 5 %. In the 10 % tail region of the coalface, the gas emission accounted for 90 % of the gas emission.

(4)The gas concentration distribution in the coalface showed a nonlinear relationship with the distance from the monitoring station. Figure 65 shows the gas concentration distribution along the vertical direction and face advance direction at the LLTCC coalface. The gas concentration distribution on the vertical face in the goaf showed an increase trend from bottom to top, increasing 2.3 % every 5 m; From the tailgate to internal displacement 32 m, the gas distribution showed an increasing trendency within the same elevation. From the support at the working face to the deep goaf, and within a 200 m range, the gas concentration distribution showed a ladder-type distribution. Within a 0–60 m range from the support to the goaf, the gas concentration increased from 1.5 % to 2.8 %; within a 60–160 m range in the goaf, the gas concentration increased from 3.6 % to 4.6 %; within a 160–200 m range in the goaf, the gas concentration increased from 5.7 % to 6.1 %, and basically coincided with the spontaneous combustion "three-zone".

### 6.1.2 Gas control technologies at the LLTCC coalface

Based on the characteristics of gas occurrence, a "mainly in strengthening gas drainage in goaf, complemented with the optimization of ventilation system in the working face" approach was used to develop a gas drainage roadway in roof-based comprehensive control technology for the LLTCC coalface. A three-step integrated program was developed: the first step was to use seals to block the gas at the upper and lower corners, and wind curtains to induce and dilute the gas for controlling the gas limit at the upper corner of the coalface at the early mining stage; the second step was to establish a large flow gas drainage system, including high-position pre-buried vertical tube, upper corner drainage tube and coalface ventilation system optimization; the third step was to developed a high drainage roadway in the roof, and use the closed roof high drainage roadway to drain the gas in the goaf. The gas drainage and mining at the No. 8105 coalface in Tashan coal mine is shown in Fig. 66.

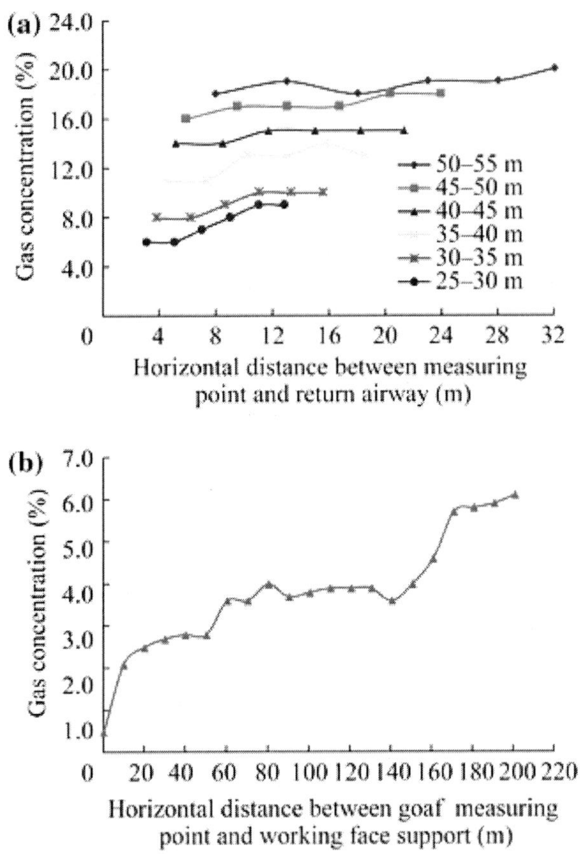


**Figure 65.** Gas concentration distribution along the directions of vertical height in the goaf and face advance. **a** Along the direction of roof height **b** along the direction of face advance

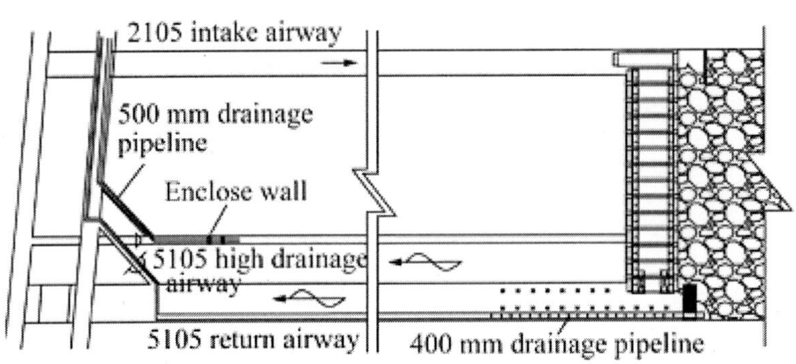


**Figure 66.** Gas drainage at the No. 8105 working face

## 6.2 Fire prevention technologies for LLTCC coalface

### 6.2.1 Large flow mobile nitrogen generator mounted on rubber tire vehicle underground

The nitrogen injection method was used to prevent fire at LLTCC coalface in ultra-thick coal seams. Therefore, a large flow mobile nitrogen generator mounted on rubber tire vehicle in the underground was developed. Figures 67, 68 and 69 show the units of large flow pressure swing adsorption nitrogen generator in the manufacturing process. Figure 70 shows the nitrogen plant in a field test.

The large flow mobile nitrogen generator mounted on rubber tire vehicle has following technical characteristics:

(1)Comparing and taking from the coarse and fine particle combined adsorption tower filling method in the US, the same method in Europe, the "blizzard" type adsorption tower absorption method, and the vibration desktop type filling method were used to develop a carbon molecular sieve filling method with the combination of vibration desktop type filling and coarse and fine grain filling, which greatly improved the service life of the molecular sieve;

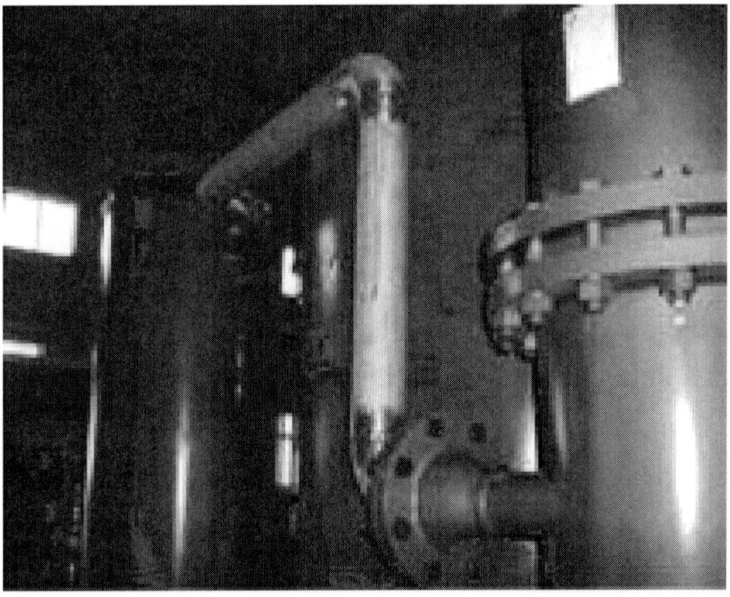

**Figure 67.** Nitrogen generator in making

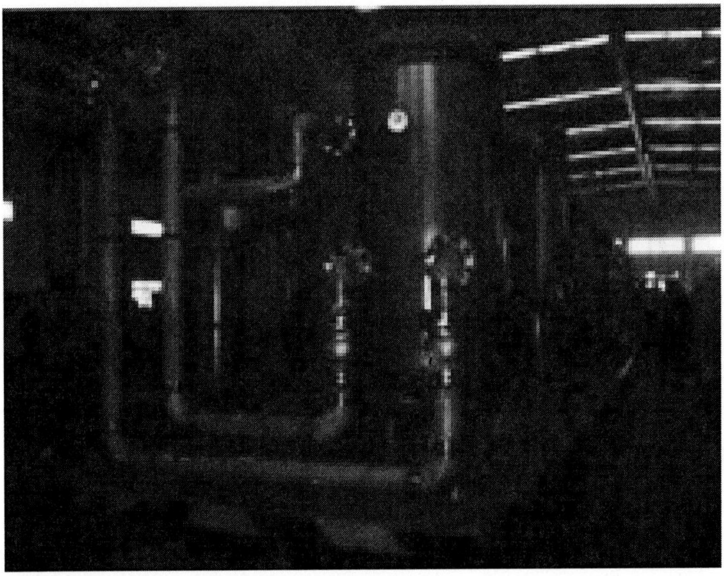

**Figure 68.** Nitrogen generator in assembling

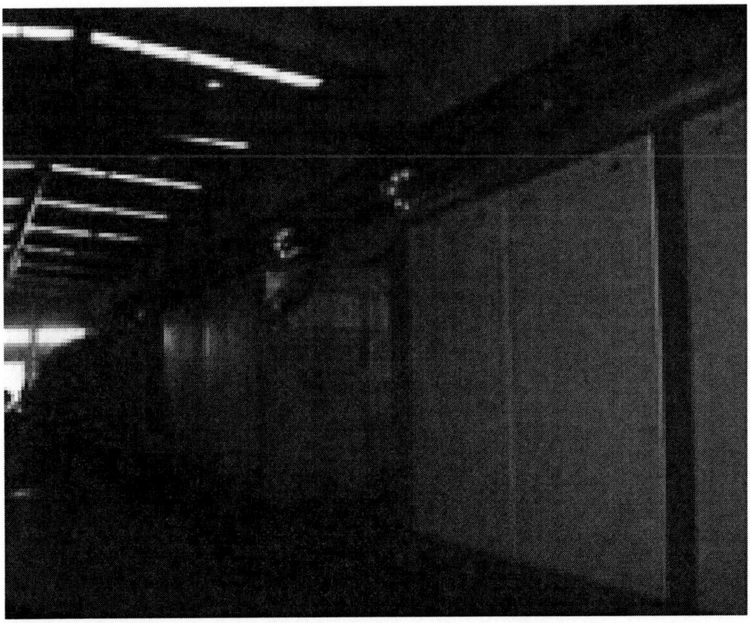

**Figure 69.** Nitrogen generator after assembly

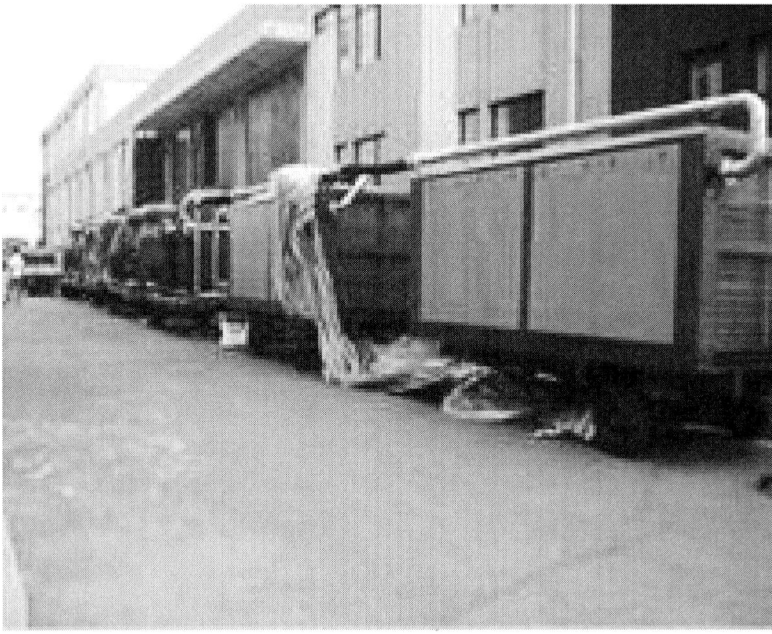

**Figure 70.** Nitrogen generator at site test

(2)The recirculation calculation formula of minimum industrial pressure swing adsorption tower $\omega_2$ (minimum) $\approx 1.15\omega_0(t_a/t_p)(p_3/P_0)$ was used to replace the calculation formula of the minimum regeneration cleaning amount required by the continuous adsorption process $\omega_2$ (minimum) $\approx \omega_0(t_a/t_p)(p_{j0}/P_{j3})(p_{j3} - P_{j3})/p_0$ ($\omega_2$is the Minimum cleaning quality flow rate of regeneration, kg/s; $\omega_0$ is the initial gas mass flow rate, kg/s; $t_a$ is the limiting adsorption time, s; $t_p$ is the holding regeneration time, s; $p_3$ is the export airflow pressure, Pa; $p_0$ is the initial pressure entrance airflow, Pa), thus, the minimum amount of regeneration recirculation was determined. Combined with the control recirculation valve of the PLC controller, by reverse blowing with the inlet direction, the fast and high efficient generation of nitrogen with the carbon molecular sieve device was achieved to increase the nitrogen amount generated by the nitrogen generator, as well as the nitrogen purity. In addition, it was possible to reduce the size of the nitrogen generator, and make the nitrogen generator more in line with the underground environment;

(3)The activated carbon filtering method was used with the combination of C, T and A three-stage fine filtrations. The activated carbon was used to remove large particles of water and oil in the compressed air, to prevent the absorption and break by the carbon molecular sieve. Using C, T, and A three-stage fine filtrations, the particles of water, oil and dust greater than 0.1 μm in compressed air will be removed to avoid large particle impurities not deposing to adsorption bed, reduce the adsorption bed resistance except maintaining the service life of the adsorbent. Furthermore, the nitrogen generator can work in a high nitrogen purity situation for a long time, ensuring that the molecular sieve service life can be extended and the efficiency of carbon molecular sieve can be improved;

(4)A dual PLC control automatic control system was developed. With the control of a dual control system, the unstable system problem caused by the interference of variable-pressure absorption in the same of twin towers was avoided during the operation of the four adsorption towers.

### 6.2.2 Study on the process and properties of large flow nitrogen generator

With a full consideration of the speed effect of the pressure swing adsorption tower, the size effect of adsorption bed and the adsorption equilibrium of carbon molecular sieve, the pressure swing adsorption tower was designed and the tower was filled with the vibration bench filling method and the coarse–fine combination filling method. Selecting the suitable pressure swing adsorption process, through a control system, the pressure swing adsorption nitrogen-making process was controlled, to ensure the time of pressure swing adsorption, and the time of adsorbent regeneration. Using product gas reverse blowing regeneration technologies, the nitrogen generation capacity of pressure swing adsorption and nitrogen purity were improved, and the nitrogen purity reached the requirement of ≥98 %. With the methods of activated carbon filters, and C, T and A three-stage fine filtration, the particles of water, oil and dust greater than 0.1 μm in compressed air was removed to ensure the service life of the adsorbent while reducing the adsorption bed resistance, and maintain the generation of high purity nitrogen.

Based on research and the comparison on the method of other existing models of pressure swing absorption molecular sieve nitrogen generator, through a small scale laboratory test, a comparison on the different processes, different adsorption media was conducted to determine the best process. The process is as follows: air compression—air buffer (and preliminary water removal)—activated carbon filter (removal of most of the water, and oil in compressed air)—fine filter (removal of the particles of water, and oil and dust greater than 0.1 μm in compressed air in)—pressurized adsorption (nitrogen generation)—pressure release—even pressure regeneration (reverse blowing process)—product nitrogen. In the compressed air system, two 250 kW screw-type air compressors were used to compress air, and the two sets of PLC controllers were used to control the pressure swing adsorption process. They ensure the smooth completion of adsorption and desorption process of the pressure swing adsorption nitrogen generating apparatus. After a 24 h continuous operation test, with the condition of nitrogen purity was greater than 98 %, the nitrogen flow rate was greater than 2000 $m^3$/h.

### 6.2.3 Development of fast curing stackable sealing material

The sealing on the upper corner of the coalface is an effective method for reducing the risk of spontaneous combustion in the goaf. However, in Tashan mine, the cross-section of intake and air return roadways are all up to 20 $m^2$. The use of traditional means, i.e. fly ash and yellow mud, would result in heavy workloads and high cost, which affects the normal transportation in the mine. Therefore, a fast curing stackable sealing material was developed.

Fast curing stackable sealing material is a polymer composite with multi-component, multi-usage, and solid gel combination, and is composed of a polymer compound, foaming agents, catalysts, flame retardants and other components. The feeding sequence for making the sealing material is: A material → B material → water-cement-sand mixture → curing agent. At the same time, the sealing material was quickly mixed to a uniform status, then pressurized and sprayed. The volume of the sealing material would instantly expand to (10–30) times of its original volume to achieve fast sealing. This material does not contain formaldehyde, is nontoxic, odorless, and non-corrosive. During the reaction expansion process, the sealing material can fill the space and cracks in coal and rock, and has a strong bonding property. It can bond coal (rock) body, concrete, and other materials to form one solid body. It has a certain level of pressure resistance and shear resistance strength. It has good flexibility, is shockproof and pressure resistant, has strong elastic resilience after compression, with no cracking after curing, and no shedding. It has insulation properties, including heat insulation and flame retardant properties, suitable for filling at different locations in an underground coal mine.

The response time of rapid curing stackable material is 5–60 s adjustable at (23 ± 2) °C. The foam index is 10–30 times adjustable. The flame retardant: oxygen index is not less than 32, vertical and horizontal combustion level is V0. The content of heavy metals (Pb) is less than 0.90 mg/kg (assessment value 90 mg/kg).

# 7 TEST IN UNDERGROUND COAL MINE AND RESULT ANALYSIS

## 7.1 Parameters of working face and equipment

At the No. 8105 LLTCC coalface in Tashan coal mine, the face length is 207 m, the maximum cutting height is 5.0 m, and the cutting depth is 0.8 m. The installed capacity for the working face is 10 Mtpa. Based on the technical parameters and performance of fully mechanized coal mining equipment in China, the main technical parameters of the fully mechanized coalface equipment are determined as shown in Table 27.

**Table 27.** Equipment for the coalface

| No. | Equipment name | Main parameters of equipment | Reference type |
|---|---|---|---|
| 1 | Hydraulic support | Height:2800–5200 mm; center distance: 1750 mm; support intensity: >1.35 MPa | ZF15000/28/52 |
| 2 | Shearer | Cutting power: 2 × 750 kW; cutting height: 2.7–5.0 m; cutting depth: 800 mm; AC electric traction; voltage: 3300 V | MG750/1915-GWD |
| 3 | Front scraper conveyor | Length: 220 m; power: 2 × 855 kW; voltage: 3300 V; transportation capacity: 2500 t/h | SGZ1000/2 × 855 |
| 4 | Rear scraper conveyor | Length:220 m; power:2 × 1000 kW; voltage: 3300 V; transportation capacity: 3000 t/h | SGZ1200/2 × 1000 |
| 4 | Stage loader | Transportation capacity: 3500 t/h; power: 450 kW; voltage: 3300 V | PF6/1542 |
| 5 | Crasher | Crashing capacity: 4250 t/h; power: 400 kW;voltage: 3300 V | SK1118 |
| 6 | Emulsion pump | Working pressure: 31.5 MPa, Rated flow rate: 400 L/min; motor power: 250 kW, voltage: 3300 V, fluid box: 2, volume: 2500 L | BRW400/31.5 |
| 7 | Spray pump | Working pressure: 12.5 MPa, Rated flow rate: 500 L/min.motor power: 132 kW, voltage: 3300 V, fluid box: 1,volume: 3000 L | BPW500/12.5 |

In April 2010, the combined trial operation on surface of the complete equipment developed was conducted at Tashan coalmine (Fig. 71). From October to December in the same year, an underground industrial trial was completed.

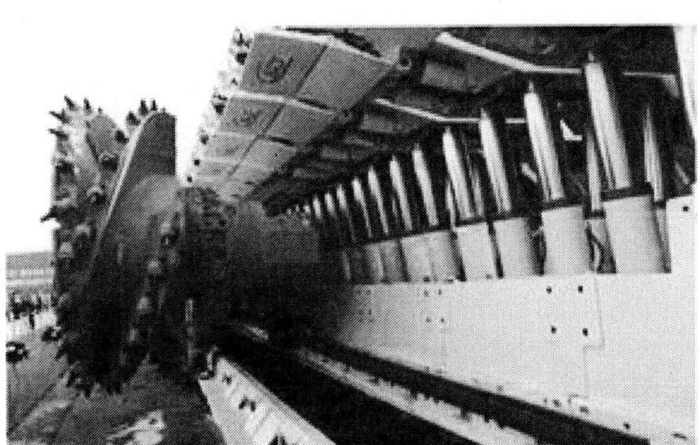

**Figure 71.** Combined trial operation on the surface of complete equipment for the working face

## 7.2 Operation of trial equipment and production

During the period of the industrial trial at the No. 8105 face from October to December 2010, the statistics of production downtime caused by major equipment accidents are shown in Table 28. From October to December 2010, the production downtime caused by shearer accidents was 31 h and 5 min, the shearer usage rate was 98.45 %, and its performance was stable. The production downtime caused by hydraulic support failure was zero, its working resistance varied within a 9000–13,000 kN range, and overall the support was in good condition. The production downtime caused by scraper conveyor failure was 17 h and 15 min with an usage rate of 98.95 %. The production downtime caused by belt conveyor accidents was 13 h and 55 min, with an usage rate of 99.15 %. The production downtime caused by power system accident was 6 h and 35 min, failure-free rate was 99.61 %.

**Table 28.** Statistics of production downtime caused by major equipment failure during the industrial trial period from October to December 2010

| Time | Shearer | Hydraulic support | Scraper conveyor | Belt conveyor | Power supply system |
|---|---|---|---|---|---|
| October 2010 | 22 h 35 min | 0 | 0 | 8 h 30 min | 2 h 35 min |
| November 2010 | 4 h | 0 | 15 h 50 min | 5 h 10 min | 4 h |
| December 2010 | 4 h 30 min | 0 | 1 h 25 min | 15 min | 0 |
| Total | 31 h 5 min | 0 | 17 h 15 min | 13 h 55 min | 6 h 35 min |

In October 2010, the production downtime caused by cumulative electrical accidents during the production period was about 57 h and 40 min. Based on four shifts with six hours each shift in the working face, the usage rate was 89.3 %. In November 2010, the production downtime caused by cumulative electrical accidents during the production period was about 53 h and 50 min, the usage rate was 91.3 %. In December 2010, the production downtime caused by cumulative electrical accidents during the production period was about 7 h and 10 min, the usage rate was 95.7 %. In the industrial test period from October 2010 to December 2011, average usage rate of equipment in use was 92.1 %.

During the industrial test period from October to December 2010 at No. 8105 coalface, the cumulative face advance was 472.5 m, average daily advance was 5 m, maximum daily advance was 8 m; the cumulative coal production was 2.723 Mt, the average daily production was 30,300 t, maximum daily production was 38,000 t; average manpower efficiency was 364.5 t/worker. In three consecutive months during the industrial test, average monthly production reached more than 900,000 t, coal recovery rate at the working face reached 89.9 %. In 2011, the average monthly coal production was 904,000 t, the cumulative coal production for the year was 10.849 mt, achieving the goal of producing 10 Mtpa. The production statistics for the industrial test at the No. 8105 coalface from October to December 2010 is listed in Table 29.

**Table 29.** Production statistics at No. 8105 coalface during the industrial test period from October to December 2010

| Time | Number of working days | Cutting height average/ maximum (m) | Face advance (m) | Production (t) | Average/maximum monthly production (t) | Average daily production (t) | Average manpower efficiency (t/worker) | Coal recovery (%) | Equipment usage (%) |
|---|---|---|---|---|---|---|---|---|---|
| October 2010 | 30 | 4.5/5.0 | 147.75 | 901,732 | 907527/916785 | 30057.8 | 362.2 | 88.9 | 92.1 |
| November 2010 | 30 | | 152.25 | 904,065 | | 30135.5 | 363 | | |
| December 2010 | 30 | | 172.5 | 916,785 | | 30559.5 | 368.2 | | |
| Total | 90 | 4.5/5.0 | 472.5 | 2,722,582 | 907527/916785 | 30250.9 | 364.5 | 88.9 | 92.1 |

## 7.3 Analysis of roadway support

During the excavation and support in the No. 5105 roadway, the deformation of the surrounding rock of the roadway was monitored, see Fig. 72a. The wall-to-wall convergence and the roof-to-floor convergence during the roadway excavation period was 25 mm and 16.6 mm, respectively. The support effect during the excavation period is shown in Fig. 73. In general, the deformation was small during roadway excavation period, and the effect of roadway support was good.

After the coal extraction at the No. 8105 coalface, under the influence of coal extraction, there were some variations in stress distribution of the surrounding rock in the roadway. The stress concentration occurred in coal and rock body in front of the coalface and in the surrounding rock of the roadway, resulting in the deformation of surrounding rocks in the roadway. The roadway surface displacement was monitored in the No. 5105 roadway within a 100 m range in front of the No. 8105 coalface, the monitoring results are shown in Fig. 72b. As can be seen from the figure, there was no change for the roadway surface displacement exceeding 78 m from the coalface, the roadway deformation affected by the coalface abutment pressure appeared from a location 78 m in front of the coalface. Within 78–66 m range in front of the coalface, large deformations occurred at the same time in the roof and two walls. Subsequently, the deformation increased as the coalface advanced slowly. Within 36 m range from coalface, with the advance of the coalface, the deformation began to dramatically increase. In the location of the monitoring station 5 m away from the coalface, the two side walls of the roadway moved closer by 280 mm, the roof and floor closer by 210 mm. However, in general there was no obvious damage to the surrounding rock of the roadway during the coal extraction period, the amount of deformation was small, and the transportation and ventilation requirements was fully able to be met.

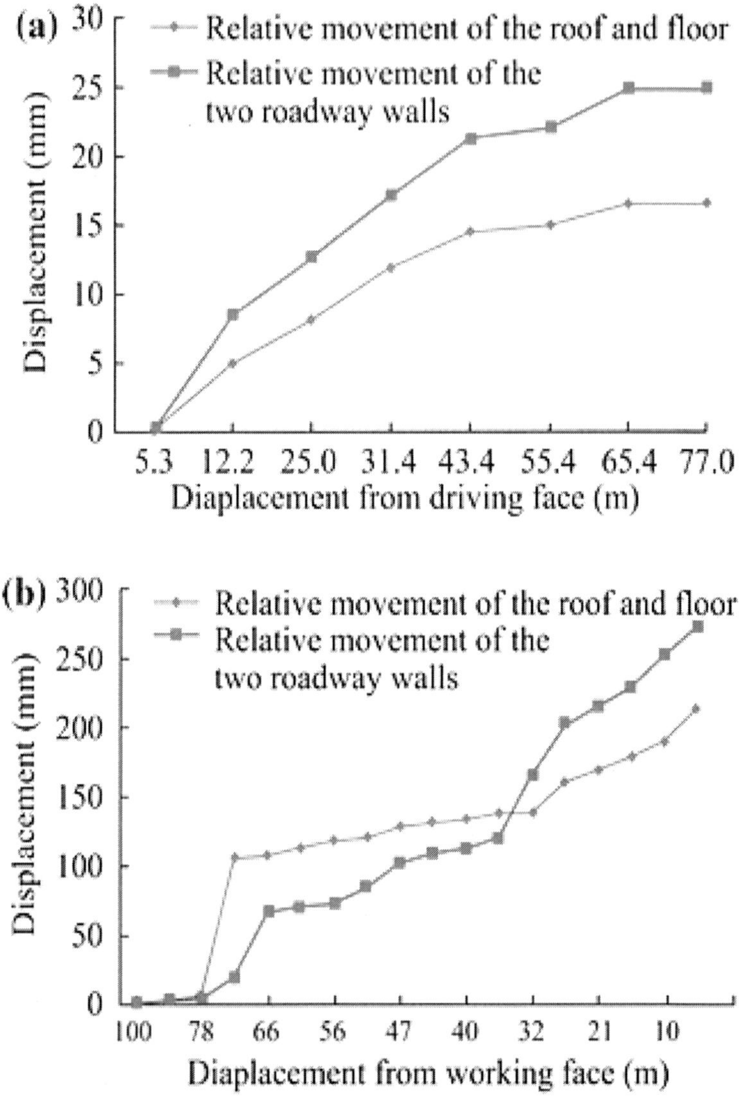


**Figure 72.** Displacement curve of the roadway surface. **a** During roadway development **b** during coalface operation

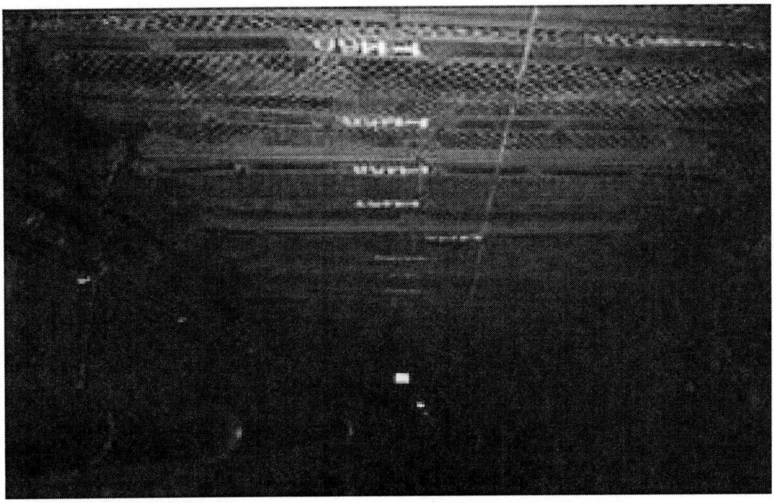

**Figure 73.** Roadway support at the No. 5105 roadway

## 7.4 Analysis on gas control

On the 9th of November 2010, the No. 8105 coalface and roof drainage roadway were connected. After the connection, a 2BEC80 gas drainage pump was used to drain the gas, the gas concentrations were maintained between 1.5 % and 2.2 % in the high drainage roadway, between 0.2 % and 0.3 % at the upper corner of working face, between 0.2 % and 0.3 % at the tail of the rear scraper conveyor, and between 0.15 % and 0.25 % in the return air. Thus, the gas management at the coalface achieved very good results.

The gas emissions at the coalface were monitored before the coalface extraction, from coalface extraction to the initial caving of the upper roof, to first gas drainage at the upper corner of coalface, during the gas drainage at the upper corner of coalface, and from the gas drainage at the upper corner of the coalface to the gas drainage in return airway and high drainage roadway. The monitoring curve of absolute gas emission volumes are shown in Fig. 74.

Figure 75 shows the gas concentration variations at the upper corner of the coalface, the coalface and in the return air since the extraction of the No. 8105 coalface. As can be seen from the diagram, coalface gas emission rates gradually increased, the volume of gas drainage increased, while the gas concentration at the upper corner of the coalface, in the coalface and the return air gradually leveled off, and achieved a zero gas overlimit.

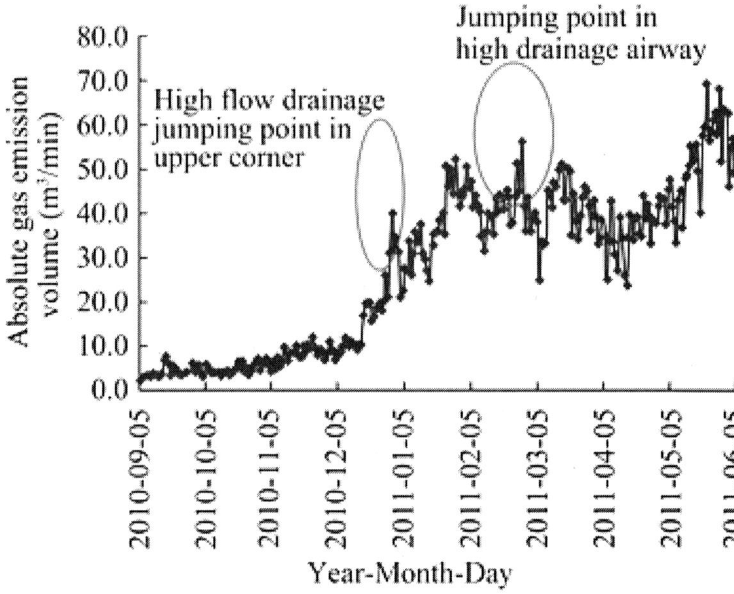


**Figure 74.** Monitoring curve of absolute gas emission volume

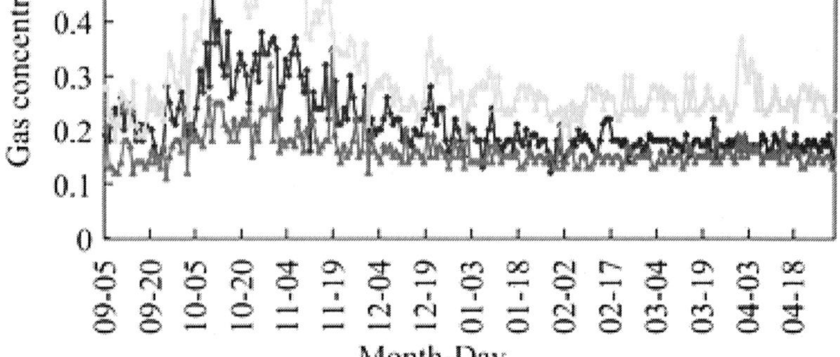


**Figure 75.** Variation curves of gas concentration at the upper corner of coalface, coalface and in return air after coal extraction

Site monitoring results showed that: the technology of roof high roadway drainage combined with other drainage can significantly reduce the gas concentration at the return air corner of the goaf, control the gas emission from the goaf to the coalface, play a role of "split-flow" of gas flow, and reduce the gas concentration in the goaf. The effect for preventing the gas accumulation at the upper corner of the coalface was significant. The drainage rate in the goaf reached 40 % of total gas emission in the goaf, achieving a zero overlimit, and ensuring a safe and smooth face advance. The gas control achieved a satisfactory result.

## 7.5 Analysis on fire prevention using nitrogen injection

Based on air quantity tests at different measuring points in the coalface, the amount of air leakage in the goaf was determined. With the installation of a bundle tube in the goaf and the connection of the bundle tube in the goaf with the main bundle tube monitoring system in the mine, the gas in the goaf was analyzed automatically. In addition, the airflow in the goaf was simulated in 3D to analyses the oxygen concentration in the goaf. Thus, a "three-zone" distribution was found in the goaf. Based on the finding, the nitrogen injection method and the amount of nitrogen injection were given at different face advance speeds.

Based on the actual mining conditions at the No. 8105 LLTCC coalface in Tashan mine, the nitrogen injection parameters were optimized, and the relevant nitrogen injection process and methods were developed. After calculation, an additional 3890 $m^3/h$ nitrogen injection was required in addition to original 2500 $m^3/h$, to enable oxygen concentration at the spontaneous combustion zone to drop to an average of 7 %. Pipe nitrogen injection technology was used for fire prevention. The first nitrogen injection pipe along the goaf at the intake side of the coalface was buried. When the pipe was buried at a certain depth into the goaf, nitrogen injection commenced. Subsequently, a second nitrogen pipe was buried into the goaf (the shift interval of the nitrogen injection nozzle was 50 m). When the second nitrogen injection pipe was buried and started nitrogen injection into the spontaneous combustion zone in the goaf, the first pipeline of nitrogen injection stopped, and a new pipe was buried again for nitrogen injection. The process was repeated until the coalface extraction was completed.

The nitrogen injection method was determined based on fire prediction, in the case of nitrogen injection quantity of 2500 $m^3/h$, and coalface advance speed of 1.4 m/d, a continuous nitrogen injection method must be used. When the advance speed is less than 1.4 m/d or if the coalface has stopped, the amount of nitrogen injection must be increased. When the coalface has stopped working for more than 68 days, the nitrogen injection quantity should be not less than 6390 $m^3/h$; when the face advance speed is greater than 1.4 m/d, it would be appropriate to reduce the amount of nitrogen injection. Using the methods presented above, the occurrence of fire in LLTCC coalface can be prevented to achieve safe mining operation.

# 8 APPLICATION AND BENEFITS

The following problems are present in coal mining in China: one is that the capacity in maintaining safety in mining is relatively low; the second is that technology and equipment, technical management, and the technical innovation level are not at a high level; the third is that the waste of resources is relatively serious; the fourth is that the added-value and technological-content of products are relatively low; the fifth is that the centralization of business is relatively low.

The technologies and equipment for LLTCC coal mining operation in ultra-thick coal seam have achieved a safe and high efficiency extraction of the coal seam with a thickness of 14–20 m. The technologies and equipment developed have effectively increased the coalface production rate and top-coal recovery. The large mining height shock-resistance top-coal caving hydraulic support and the electrohydraulic control technology developed for top-coal caving greatly improved top-coal caving and discharge speed, reduced labor intensity, and increased coalface productivity. The anchor bolt support technology and material developed for the support of large cross-section full coal roadway significantly improved the effects of roadway support, and ensured the roadway is stable and unblocked. The gas control and fire prevention technology and equipment ensured safe coal production.

After adopting the technology and equipment developed, the investment on equipment in Tashan mine was decreased. Compared to the No. 8104 coalface, the investment on equipment at the No. 8105 coalface saved about 100 million yuan.

With the geological and mining conditions at the No. 8105 coalface, compared to the sub-level caving method in ultra-thick coal seam, the technologies and equipment developed enabled coal production at the No. 8105 coalface in Tashan coal mine to be doubled; the economic benefit is significant.

In addition to the Tashan mine in Datong, currently the LLTCC technologies and equipment for ultra-thick coal seam have been used in 32 coal mines in China, including 13 mining areas such as Datong, Pingshuo, Shengdong, Xinjiang, covering 8 provinces or autonomous regions in China, such as Shanxi, Inner Mongolia, Xinjiang, Shaanxi, Shandong, Gansu, Anhui, Liaoning.

Currently, 14 large coal bases have been planned in China including Shendong, Northern Shaanxi, Huanglong, Northern Shanxi, Jinzhong, Jindong,

Luxi, Lianghuai, Jinzhong, Henan, Yungui, Eastern Inner Mongolia (northeast), Ningdong, and Xinjiang, where thick and ultra-thick coal seams are predominantly mined. The main coal seams in the coal mines with 10 Mtpa capacities each currently under construction are mainly thick or ultra-thick coal seams. The coal mines built with a capacity of 10 Mtpa each mainly extract the coal seams with thickness of 6–20 m, the seams above 6 m account for 50 %, such as Halagou, Shigetai, Daliuta, Buliantai, Yujialiang, Shangwan in Shengdong coalfield, Yangchangwan in Ningdong coalfield, Huangling No. 2 mine in Huangling coalfield, Anjialing mine in Pingshuo coalfield, Dafosi mine in Binchang coalfield and Sihe coalmine in Jincheng coalfield. With the construction of large-scale coal production bases in China in the future, LLTCC coal mining technologies and equipment provide technological support for the safe, high efficiency and high recovery coal production in these mines. The technologies and equipment developed will drive the upgrading of existing mechanized caving technology and equipment. The research results will be widely used and the products will have great business potential.

At the same time, the development of technologies and equipment strongly promote the development of coal mining methods and related theories, and lead the progress of coal mining technologies. It enables the capability of manufacturing the complete set of the LLTCC coal mining equipment in China, driving the development of machine processing technology, electromechanical integration technology, and automation and information technology. It curbs the occurrence of roof, gas, and fire accidents, safeguard coal mine practitioners' personal safety, improves underground mine working environment, ensures coal mine safety, efficient, integrated production, improves the efficiency of coal mining and energy supply, and provides reliable energy security for China's sustained, healthy and stable economic development.

## 9 CONCLUSIONS

With the study and development of the LLTCC coal mining technologies and equipment for over 10 years, the following main conclusions are obtained:

(1)In terms of coal seams with a thickness of 14–20 m, the LLTCC coal mining method has been proposed, which increases the coal cut height to 5 m, coal caving height to 15 m, and the total mining height to 20 m. The effect of different coal caving intervals and top-coal caving patterns on top-coal recovery has been investigated, which concludes that the recovery rate can be improved in long wall caving by applying the caving patterns of one-cut-one-caving and discharge in multi-round and multiple windows sequence alternately.

(2)A "cantilever beam-articulated beam" model has been established for the overlying strata at the LLTCC coal mining face. Based on the model, the working resistance of the LLTCC hydraulic support has been determined. Furthermore, the law of top coal and roof movement at the LLTCC coalface has been obtained. In front of face coal wall, the main characteristics of top coal and roof movement are mainly horizontal compressive deformation under abutment pressure; in the rear of the face coal wall, the characteristics of roof movement are mainly fractures and subsidence, the characteristics of top coal movement are mainly vertical caving movements caused by roof fractures and subsidence. The speed of horizontal deformation of the top coal and roof in front of the face coal wall under abutment pressure is much smaller than that of the vertical subsidence of the top coal and roof after fracture at the rear of the face coal wall.

(3)Comprehensive spalling prevention and control technologies have been proposed, including controlling the coalface advance speed, increasing the initial support force, and improving the ability of wall protection. These technologies reduce coal wall spalling and maintain the normal advance of the coalface.

(4)A large-diameter double telescopic shock-resistance prop and a 1000 $min^{-1}$ large flow safety valve quick unloading device have been developed, which improve the shock-resistance of hydraulic support; an articulated front beam and high reliable telescopic beam with a secondary wall protection structure have been developed, which overcomes the wall spalling problem at LLTCC coalfaces; and a strong disturbance-type top coal discharge device with high efficiency and high top coal recovery has been developed, which improves coal recovery. On the basis of the developments presented above, a 5.2 m cutting height LLTCC hydraulic support has been developed.

(5)A high efficiency and high reliability electric traction shearer has been developed, its specifications are: coal cutting height 2.8–5.5 m, total installed power 1945 kW, coal cutting power 750 kW, maximum haulage speed 15–25 m/min, and maximum traction force 2 × 570 kN. An analysis method of the shearer reliability has been established. Furthermore, a new control system and walking system for the shearer has been developed, and the new material of ranging arm shell body and the performance of drum tooth have been optimized to improve the reliability of the shearer.

(6)A large-capacity SGZ1200/2 × 1000 rear scraper conveyor has been developed with installed power of 2 × 1000 kW, and transportation capacity of more than 3000 t/h. The transportation distance meets the requirements of the No. 8105 coalface in Tashan mine. In addition, some key accessories, including the heavy-load and high-strength chain transmission system of the scraper conveyor, controllable speed-adjustable soft start device, the integrated monitoring transmission system of transmission device, heavy-load 1000 kW planetary retarder, high-reliability and long-life coal pan, high strength and compact type end unloading headframe, and electrohydraulic control automatic telescopic conveyor tail, have been investigated to improve the performance of the LLTCC rear scraper conveyor.

(7)Various devices have been invented in the project, including a height adjustable ring chain lifting device, a new high efficient air inlet flame arrester and exhaust processing box, and an integrated motor plug type wheel side drive and brake retarder. A WC55Y support hauler with a load of 55 tons has been developed, achieving a safe, high efficiency, non-demolition, "point-to-point" transportation of the LLTCC hydraulic support, and improves the efficiency of LLTCC coalface relocation.

(8)The stress distribution of surrounding rock of large cross-section coal roadway is significantly influenced by the in situ stress and the rock strength. Under the same stress conditions, the higher coal and rock mass strength, the higher the stress magnitude of surrounding rock after the roadway excavation. The support effect of rock bolts on the roadway is mainly to generate compressive stress zones through the prestress force of bolts, and form a prestress loading structure with cables and other supporting structures, thus to strengthen the surrounding rock of the roadway, and constrain the separation, sliding, and opening of fracture in the surrounding rock, and subsequently maintain the integrity and stability of the roadway surrounding rock.

(9)A special bolt steel formula has been developed, which changes the steel mechanical properties. With suitable rolling method, a high strength (500–600 MPa), high elongation bolt material has been developed. Using new 19 structure wires instead of 7 structure wires, a large elongation, powerful cable bolt has been developed. Also, a bolt torque multiplier has been developed, which enables the output torque of bolt driller to be amplified 6 times, and solves the problems of rock bolt prestressing.

(10)In terms of the characteristics of "low gas reserve, high gas emission" in the LLTCC coalface, comprehensive gas control technology, using mainly the roof high drainage roadway, has been developed. The gas drainage amount from the goaf accounts for 40 % of the total gas emission in the goaf, achieving gas zero overlimit; a large flow underground mobile nitrogen generator has been developed to solve the fire prevention problems at the 10 Mtpa LLTCC coalface and guarantees safe coal mining.

(11)The key technologies and equipment for LLTCC coal mining operation has been successfully evaluated at the No. 8105 coalface of the Tashan coal mine. The underground test demonstrated that the match of "shield, shearer and scraper conveyor" is rational, average usage of face equipment reaches 92.1 %, face coal recovery reaches 88.9 %, the cumulative coal production was 10.849 Mtpa in 2011, achieving the target of 10 Mtpa for a LLTCC coalface in China, and safe and high efficiency coal mining in an ultra-thick coal seam.

## REFERENCES


1. Alehossein H, Poulsen BA (2010) Stress analysis of long wall top coal caving. Intern J Rock Mech Min Sci 47(1):30–41
2. Altounyan P, Taljaard D (2001) Developments in controlling the roof in South African coal mines—a smarter approach. International conference on coal research. South African Institute of Mining and Metallurgy, pp 33–40
3. Buddery PS, Oldroyd DC (1992) Development of a roof and floor classification applicable to collieries. Proceedings of the Eurock '92 conference. Thomas Telford, London, pp 197–202
4. Cao SG, Liu CY (1997) Study on the stiffness of the immediate roof of longwall face. Ground Press Strata Control 4:16–19
5. Cao SG, Qian MG, Liu CY, Miao XX (1998) New research about support and surrounding rock relationship in working face. J China Coal Soc 23(6):575–579
6. Cao SG, Qian MG, Liu CY (1999) Mechanical characteristics of the immediate roof in working face and working resistance of supports. Mining Science and Technology'99. vol 8, pp 309–312
7. Chen Y, Yu L, Lan TW (2010) Numerical simulation research on surrounding rock activities in shallow coal seam face. 2010 International symposium on safety science and technology. Science Press USA Inc, pp 1618–1622
8. Cheng SP (2008) Research on surface movement rules off full-mechanized caving mining with large mining height in mountain area. Coal Min Technol 13(4):37–39
9. Deng GZ (1994) Characteristics of movement and rupture of the roofs during longwall top coal caving process. Ground Press Strata Control 2:23–26
10. Duan WS, Gao XC, Dou J (2008) Law of movement and fracture of overlying strata of fully-mechanized top-coal caving face in the hard and thick coal seam. J Xi'an Univ Sci Technol 28(2):211–214

11. Fan YC, Kang LJ, Kang YH (2003) Fully mechanized longwall top coal caving mining technology. China Coal Industry Publishing House, Beijing

12. Fang XQ (2002) Study on stability of support-surrounding rocks and it's control in fully-mechanized top-coal caving face. Doctor's Thesis: China University of Mining and Technology

13. Fu YG (2008) Study about mining height fully-mechanized coal winning caving face gas governing technology. Coal 17(12):9–12

14. Hou W, Jiang FX, Wang CW, Feng ZQ, Wang DZ (2009) Pressure control in sub-level long face surrounded by three sides minedAreas of C-shaped stratas patial structure. J China Coal Soc 34(3):310–314

15. Hu W (1995) Roof control and selection of drawing roof-coal stope. J Xiangtan Mine Inst 10(4):7–13

16. Huang K (2002) Mechanical system of chock-roof and stability of soft coal longwall face during top caving process. Doctor's Thesis: China University of Mining & Technology (Beijing)

17. Jia AL, Huang X (2005) Research on bolt support system for full seam gateway in high stressed thick seam. Coal Sci Technol 33(7):45–48

18. Jia XR, Zhai YD, Yang SS (1998) Structure of roof rocks in sub-level caving face and calculation of roof weighting. J China Coal Soc 23(4):366–370

19. Jiang FX (1995) Structure patterns and roof-chock relationship in longwall top coal caving. Coal Mine Mod 1:33–35

20. Jiang FX (2006) View point of spatial structures of overlying strataand its application in coal mine. J Min Saf Eng 23(1):30–33

21. Jin ZM, Wei JP, Song XM, Xue Y, Niu Y (2002) Test Study on The top cracking process of large coal sample. Proceedings of the '99 international symposium on mining science and technology, Beijing, pp 405–408

22. Kang LJ (1990) Rupture characteristics and the interaction between roof and chocks in gently-inclined thick coal seams using longwall top caving methods. Master's Thesis: China Coal Research Institute

23. Kang LJ (1995) Study on top coal stress in caving mining. Proceeding of the international mining Tech'95 symposium. Beijing, pp 18–25

24. Kang LJ (1996) Ground pressure characteristics in longwall top coal caving work face for gently-inclined seam coal seams. Coal Sci Technol 24(11):39–42

25. Kang LJ (1998) Limiting effect of strain-softening character of the top coal on loads exerted on the powered supports in a fully mechanized sub-level caving face. J China of Coal Soc 23(2):140–143

26. Kang LJ (1999) Mechanical coupling relationship between roof and chock in longwall top coal caving method.Coal. Min Technol 4(12):69–71

27. Kang LJ, Qi QX (1998) Discrete element modelling of longwall top coving process. Coal Min Technol 3(2):3–6

28. Kang HP, Wang JH (2007) Rock bolting theory and complete technology for coal roadways. China Coal Industry Publishing House, Beijing, pp 83–86

29. Kang LJ, Shi YW, Yao JG (1991) Interaction between chock and roof in longwall top coal caving for gently-inclined coal seam. Ground Press Strata Control 1:19–24

30. Kang LJ, Wu G, Zhang YJ (1997) Top coal movement characteristics during longwall top caving process in the Yanquansikuang coal mine. Coal Sci Technol 25(9):13–16

31. Kang LJ, Zheng XZ, Feng ZC (1998) Investigation on the ground pressure characteristics of the tailgate driven alongside the #10 longwall gob in the Nantun coal mine. Coal Sci Technol 26(7):41–45

32. Kang LJ, Liu JH, Ceng HF, Wang LX (1999) Study on the behavior and controlling method for hard roof strata of seam No. 4 in Wang ping Colliery. Coal. Min Technol 1:69–71

33. Kang TH, Chai ZY, Li YB, Ge YY, Zhang HB, Liu RR (2007a) Study on physical simulation of full-seam mining for a 20 m very thick and medium hard seam by sub-level caving mining with high bottom cutting Height. Chin J Rock Mech Eng 26(5):1065–1072

34. Kang HP, Wang JH, Lin J (2007b) High pre-tensioned stress and intensive bolting system and its application in deep roadways. J China Coal Soc 32(12):1233–1238

35. Kang HP, Jiang TM, Gao FQ (2008) Design for pre-tensioned rock bolting parameters. J China Coal Soc 33(7):721–726

36. Kong LH, Jiang FX, Liu J, Yie GX, Wang CW, Song GD (2009) High-precision microseismic monitoring system to reasonable width of segment coal pillar in extra-thick coal seam fully mechanized top-coal caving mining. J China Coal Soc 34(7):871–874

37. Kong LH, Jiang FX, Yang SH, Song JW, Wang CW (2010a) Movement of roof strata in extra-thick coal seams in top-coal caving mining based

on a high precision micro-seismic monitoring system. J Univ Sci Technol Beijing 32(5):552–558

38. Kong LH, Jiang FX, Liu J, Wang CW (2010b) Relationship between support and strata in extra-thick coal seam fully-mechanized sublevel caving mining based on high precision microseismic monitoring technology. Chin J Geotech Eng 32(3):401–406

39. Kong LH, Jiang FX, Wang CW (2010c) Study of reasonable working resistance of support in fully-mechanized sublevel caving face in extra-thick coal seam. Chin J Rock Mech Eng 29(11):2312–2318

40. Li MZ, Liu KM, Zeng MS (2006) Full seam cutting and caving mining technology in and its development prospect. Coal Mining Technology 11(5):28–29, 43

41. Li L, Xu G (2009) Researchon supporting density of powered support for full-mechanized caving ming in Shuiliandong colliery. Coal Min Technol 14(5):86–88

42. Liu CY (1996) Mechanical characteristics of immediate roof and chock-roof relationship in longall mining face. Doctor's Thesis, China University of Mining & Thechnology

43. Liu J (2008a) Microseismic monitoring in longwall top coal caving for an extra-thick coal seam. Min Saf Environ Prot 35(1):44–46

44. Liu KG (2008b) Studying about mining hight fully-mechanized coal winning caving the roof activity. Coal 17(6):9–11

45. Liu QM (2010) Research on space effect of face length of fulimechanized caving mining with large mining height. Coal Min Technol 15(3):27–29

46. Liu CY, Huang BX (2009) Technical parameters of drawing and coal-gangue field movements of a fully mechanized large mining height top coal caving working face. Min Sci Technol 19(5):549–555

47. Liu CY, Qian MG, Cao SG, Miao XX (1997) Influencing mechanism of immediate roof on the relation between supports in the workings and surrounding rocks. J China Coal Soc 22(5):471–476

48. Liu CY, Wan ZJ, Cao SG (2002) The deformation destroying interaction regulation of immediate roof and top-coal in long wall sublevel caving face. Proceedings in mining science and safety technology. Science Press, Beijing, pp 105–109

49. Liu YD, Zhang DS, Wang HS (2006) Simulation analysis of coal mining with top-coal caving under hard-and-thick strata. J China Univ Min Technol 16(2):110–114

50. Lu XS, Zhao XL (2006) XU XD, Xue SJ. Kit technique research about fully-mechanized coal winning equipment. Coal 15(6):6–7

51. Ma QH (2005) Study of the overlying strata "O" letter type spatial structures of long wall and correlate rock pressure. Doctor's Thesis: Shandong University of Science and Technology

52. Ma JY, Zhang ZQ (2008) Research on coal roadway supported by bolting with mesh. J Taiyuan Univ Technol 39(5):233–235

53. Mao DB, Yao JG (2010) Adaptability of long wall top coal caving with high cutting height. J China Coal Soc 35(11):1837–1841

54. Meng QK (2007) Fully mechanized high cutting height and caving mining technology and hydraulic powered support selection in Wobei mine. Coal Sci Technol 35(8):53–54

55. Meng D, Shen J, Zhao Y (2010) Determination of the hydraulic supporting resistance based on a simplified structural system. Metal Mine 10:24–28

56. Miao SJ, Lai XP (2011) Top coal flows in an excavation disturbed zone of high section top coal caving of an extremely steep and thick seam. Min Sci Technol (China) 21(1):99–105

57. Nan H, Xu T, Wei ZD (2008) Application of RFPA 2D in sublevel caving mining extra-thick coal seams. Materials Sci Forum 575:1246–1251

58. Qian MG, Shi PW (2003) Coal mine pressure and roof control. China Coal Industry Publishing House, Beijing

59. Qian MG, He FL, Miao XX (1966) The system of strata control around long wall face in China. Mining Science & Technology, pp 15–18

60. Qian MG, Miao XX, He FL, Liu CY (1996) Coupling mechanics of chock and roof in longwall mining face. J China Coal Soc 21(1):40–44

61. Ren RH (2005) Surface movement regularity of super-wide mining face with top-coal caving. J China Univ Min Technol 15(1):68–71

62. Shi H (2005) Study and applications ability of hard and massive overlying stratain fully mechanized sub level caving face. Doctor's Thesis: Shandong University of Science and Technology

63. Shi YW, Chen SJ (1993) Ground control of floor in retreating mining face. China Coal Industry Industry Publishing House, Beijing

64. Shi H, Jiang FX (2004) Mechanical analysis of rupture regularity of hand and massive overlying strata of longwall face. Chin J Rock Mech Eng 23(18):3066–3069

65. Shi H, Jiang FX (2005) Study on relationship between roof stability and recovery ratio of top coal at first weight period in fully-mechanized sublevel caving face. Chin J Geotech Eng 27(4):414–417

66. Shi YW, Ning Y, Qi QX (1993) Ground control and optimum parameters in longwall top coal caving technologies. China University of Mining & Technology Press, Xuzhou

67. Shi H, Jiang FX, Wang HJ (2005) Study on relationship between roof stability and top coal's recovery ratio burning cyclic weighting in fully-mechanized sublevel caving face. Chin J Rock Mech Eng 24(23):4233–4238

68. Shi HM, Du JW, Li ZQ (2009) Mining height long caving mining stope pressure control technology. Coal 18(11):14–16

69. Song JW, Gao RP, Wang AW (2010) Science and Technology of West China 20(9):6–10

70. Su H (2008) Stability analysis and ground control of coal measures during longwall top coal caving process China. Coal 34(2):35–36

71. Wang JC (2005) Fully mechanized longwall top coal caving technology in China and discussion on issues of further development. Coal Sci Technol 33(1):14–17

72. Wang JH (2006a) Present status and development tendency of fully mechanized coal mining technology and equipment with high cutting height in China. Coal Sci Technol 34(1):4–7

73. Wang HJ (2006b) Resarch on the movement and control of "O"letter type overlying milti-strata spatull structures of face surrounded by mined areas. Doctor's Thesis: Shandong University of Science and Technology

74. Wang JC (2009) Theories and technologies for mining thick coal seams. Metallurgical Industry Press, Beijing

75. Wang GF (2010a) Top-caving powered support and fully-mechanized caving technology. China Coal Industry Publishing House, Beijing

76. Wang M (2010b) Study on the laws of strata behavior in the top-coal caving of fully mechanized mining. Master's Thesis: Taiyuan University of Technology

77. Wang JH (2011) Present status and prospects of modernized mining technology and equipment in China coal mine. Coal Sci Technol 39(1):1–5

78. Wang JH (2013a) Key technology of complete equipment for fully-mechanized top coal caving face with large mining height in extra-thick seam. Coal Sci Technol 41(9):1–5

79. Wang JH (2013b) Key technology for fully-mechanized top coal caving with large mining height in extra-thick coal seam. J China Coal Soc 38(12):2089–2098

80. Wang ZF, Li QS, Yang LP, Liu J (2001) Research to ensure the height of displacement caving zone in overlying strata at Xiashijie coal mine combined working face. Coal 16(1):1–3SciNet

81. Wang JS, Chai ZY, Kang TH, Li YB (2007) Numerical simulation of full seam mining for a 20 m very thick and medium hard seam by fully mechanized sublevel caving. J Taiyuan Univ Technol 38(2):175–178

82. Wang JH, Kang HP, Gao FQ (2008) Numerical simulation on load-transfer mechanisms and stress distribution characteristics of cable bolts. J China Coal Soc 33(1):1–6

83. Wang GF, Pang YH, Liu JF (2012) Determination and influence of cutting height of coal by top coal caving method with great mining height in extra thick coal seam. J China Coal Soc 37(11):1777–1782

84. Wu J (1998) Reviews on the longwall top coal caving technologies in the past 15 years. Proceedings of the 3rd Longwall Top Coal Caving Theory and Application Conference

85. Wu YP (2008) Research on full mechanized caving mining technology in extremely thick and complicated coal seam. Coal Min Technol 13(1):18–20

86. Wu J, Fu Q (1998) Current situation and prospect of top coal caving technology in China. J China Univ Min Technol 8(2):108–112

87. Wu J, Yan SH (1995) Basic concepts of determining resistance of face support with fully mechanized mining and top coal caving. Mine pressure and roof management 3(4):69–71SciNet

88. Wu J, Zhang Y (2001) The new concept of relationship between support and surrounding-rock in longwall top-coal caving faces. J China Coal Soc 26(4):350–356

89. Xie GX (2005) Mechanical characteristics of fully mechanized top-coal caving face and surrounding rock stress shell. J China Soc 30(3):303–313

90. Xie GX (2006) Influence of mining thickness on mechanical characteristics of working face and surrounding rock stress shell. J China Coal Soc 31(1):6–10

91. Xie GX, Luo Y (2005) Study on the Countermeasures against methane outburst of mining multiple upper protective layers in coal seams C luster. J Coal Sci Eng 11(1):31–35SciNet

92. Xie YS, Zhao YS (2009a) Numerical simulation of the top coal caving process using the discrete element method. Intern J Rock Mech Min Sci 46(6):983–991

93. Xie YS, Zhao YS (2009b) Technique of top coal caving with vibration. Procedia Earth Planet Sci 1(1):219–226

94. Xie GX, Chang JC, Yang K (2006a) Investigation on the stress field characteristic of top coal at FMTC faces under the influence of caving thickness. J Coal Sci Eng 13(2):123–125

95. Xie GX, Yang K, Liu QM (2006b) Study on distribution laws of stress in inclined coal pillar for fully-mechanized top-coal caving face. Chin J Rock Mech Eng 25(3):545–549

96. Xie GX, Yang K, Chang JC (2007a) Study on distribution characterics of 3D stress and thickness effects of coal-seam in unsymmetrical disposal and fully-mechanized top-coal caving. Chin J Rock Mech Eng 26(4):775–779

97. Xie GX, Yang K, Hua XZ (2007b) Influence of mining velocity on mechanical characteristics of surrounding rock in fully mechanized top-coal caving face. Chin J Geotech Eng 29(7):963–967

98. Xie GX, Chang JC, Yang K (2009) Investigations into stress shell characteristics of surrounding rock in fully mechanized top-coal caving face. Intern J Rock Mech Min Sci 46(1):172–181

99. Xing SJ, Wang JZ, Zhao YB (2009) Development and application of top coal caving hydraulic supports with large mining height. China Coal 35(4):81–83

100. Yan SH (2008) Research on side and roof falling mechanism and control approaches in caving mining with large mining height. Coal Min Technol 13(4):5–8

101. Yan SH (2009) Theory study on the load on support of long wall with top coal caving with great mining height in extra thick coal seam. J China Coal Soc 34(5):590–593

102. Yan SH, Fu Q (2003) Movement characteristics of the strata above the coal seam under longwall top coal caving. China Coal Industry Publishing House, Beijing

103. Yan SH, Yin XW (2008) Discussing about the main theoretical problems of long wall with top coal caving. J China Coal Soc 33(5):481–484

104. Yan SH, Jia GS, Liu XL (1996) Analysis of mechanism of overlying strata structure transmitting toward upper position in top coal caving. Mine Press Roof Manag 3:3–5

105. Yan SH, Yin XW, Xu HJ, Xu G, Liu QM, Yu L (2011) Roof structure of short cantilever-articulated rock beam and calculation of support resistance in full-mechanized face with large mining height. J China Coal Soc 36(11):1816–1820

106. Yang JL (2007) Stability and ground control of coal measures during longwall top coal caving process.China. Coal 33(11):37–39

107. Yang PJ (2009) Research on the relationship between two-leg sublevel caving shield support and surrounding rocks and adaptability. Doctor's Thesis: China University of Mining and Technology

108. Yasitli NE, Unver B (2005) 3D numerical modeling of long wall mining with top-coal caving. Intern J Rock Mech Min Sci 42(2):219–235

109. Yin XW, Yan SH, An Y (2008) Characters of the rib spalling in fully mechanized caving face with great mining height. J Min Saf Eng 25(2):222–225

110. Yu L, Fan ZZ, Xu G (2011) Study on the structure characteristics and ground pressure behavior of overlying strata with shallow buried coal seam. Adv Mater Res 255–260:3780–3785

111. Yu L, Yan SH, Liu QM (2012) Determination of support working resistance of top coal caving in extra thick coal seam. J China Coal Soc 37(5):737–742

112. Zhang DL (1995) Stability and ground control of coal measures in longwall top coal caving. Doctor's thesis: China University of Mining & Technology

113. Zhang DL (1999) Ground control in longwall top coal caving. China Coal Industry Publishing House, Beijing

114. Zhang HJ, Liu QM (2008) Research on the fuzzy clustering of comprehensive support working resistance. China Min Mag 17(10):93–98

115. Zhang CW, Yang WB (2010) Technology of supporting deep full-seam coal roadway with high stress. Coal Min Technol 15(4):63–64

116. Zhang BS, Kang LX, Yang SS (2006) Numerical simulation on roof separation and deformation of full seam roadway with stratified roof and large section. J Min Saf Eng 23(3):264–267

117. Zhang Z, Kang HP, Wang JH (2010) Pre-tensioned stress coordination function analysis of bolt-cable anchor support in coal roadway. J China Coal Soc 35(6):881–886

118. Zhang JG, Zhao ZQ, Gao Y (2011) Research on top coal caving technique in steep and extra-thick coal seam. Procedia Earth Planet Sci 2:145–149

119. Zhou ZL, Su H (2008) Support technologies for longwall top coal caving face ends. Coal 17(6):18–20

120. Zhu LF, Yan SH (2011) Numerical simulation of top-coal movement rule in fully-mechanized caving mining with large mining height. Coal Min Technol 16(1):11–13

# Chapter 5

# Coal Bursts in the Deep Longwall Mines of The United States

**Christopher Mark**

*U.S. Mine Safety and Health Administration, Pittsburgh, PA, USA*

## ABSTRACT

Coal bursts involve the sudden, violent ejection of coal or rock into the mine workings. They are a particular hazard because they typically occur without warning. During the past 2 years three US coal miners were killed in two coal bursts, following a 6-year period during which there were zero burst fatalities. This paper puts the US experience in the context of worldwide research into coal bursts. It focuses on two major longwall mining coalfields which have struggled with bursts for decades. The Utah experience displays many of the "classic" burst characteristics, including deep cover, strong roof and floor rock, and a direct association between bursts and mining activity. In Colorado, the longwalls of the North Fork Valley (NFV) also work at great depth, but their roof and floor strengths are moderate, and most bursts have occurred during entry development or in headgates, bleeders, or other outby locations. The NFV bursts also are more likely to be associated with geologic structures and large magnitude seismic events. The paper provides a detailed case history to illustrate the experience in each of these coalfields. The paper closes with a brief discussion of how US longwalls have managed the burst risk.

**Keywords:** Underground mining Coal Burst Longwall Strata control

# 1 INTRODUCTION

Coal bursts involve the sudden, violent ejection of coal or rock into the mine workings (Figs. 1,2). They are almost always accompanied by a loud noise, like an explosion, and ground vibration. Bursts are a particular hazard for miners because they typically occur without warning. Despite decades of research, the sources and mechanics of bursts are imperfectly understood, and the means to predict and control them remain elusive.

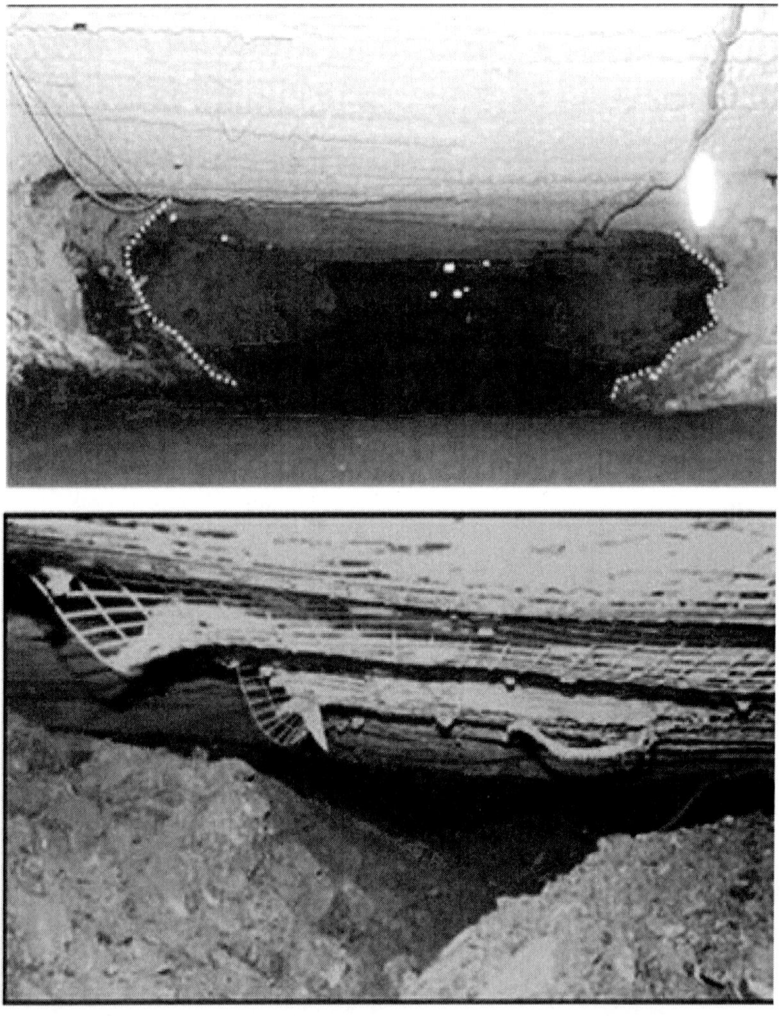

**Figure 1.**Effect of a coal burst on roadway (the *top* shows the roadway before the burst, and the*bottom* is after the burst)

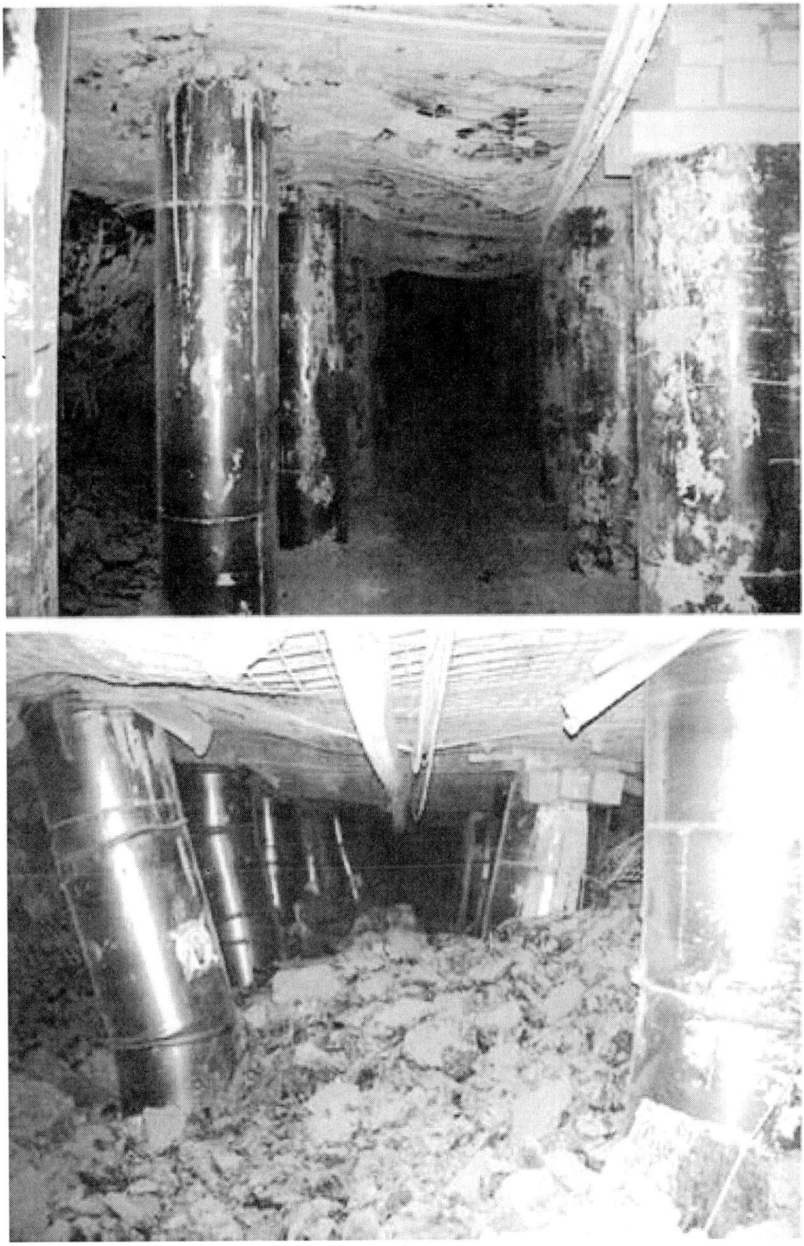

**Figure 2.** Effect of a coal burst on a longwall tailgate

High stress is a universal feature of burst-prone conditions. The overburden depth is responsible for the overall level of stress, but pillar design, multiple seam interactions, and/or mining activity can concentrate stresses in distinct locations.

Geologic factors also contribute. The presence of strong, massive sandstone near the seam has often been noted where bursts have occurred (Bräuner 1994; Maleki 1995; Iannacchione and Zelanko 1995; Agapito and Goodrich 2000). In the Utah coalfields of the western US, for example, miners refer to "bump sandwich" geology where the coal seam is slotted between massive sandstone roof and floor. In Germany, a study that compared rock cores from 35 areas that experienced bursts with cores from 400 burst-free areas found that the burst risk was significant when there was either a 4.5-m-thick "package" of strong sandstone in the first 10 m above the mining horizon, or a 2-m-thick "package" within the first 4.5 m of the floor (Baltz and Hucke 2008).

Near seam geology does not wholly determine the burst risk, however. Other geologic factors that have been identified as contributing to a heightened burst risk include the following:

(1)Rapid changes in the depth of cover (Holland 1958; Maleki 1995; Maleki et al. 1999)

(2)Sandstone channels that concentrate load (Hoelle 2008; Agapito and Goodrich 2000; Maleki et al. 2011)

(3)Seam rolling and pitching (Iannacchione and Zelanko 1995; Maleki et al. 2011)

(4)Faults (Holland 1958; Holub 1997; Agapito and Goodrich 2000; Alber et al. 2008; Swanson et al. 2008)

As long ago as the early 1930s, coal bursts were classified into two types according to their apparent cause (Rice 1935). "Pressure bursts" were thought to originate in the seam itself and were associated with high stress and direct mining activity. Typical pressure bursts occur while a continuous miner is extracting a pillar or a longwall shearer is cutting the tailgate corner of the face.

"Shock bursts", on the other hand, were thought to be caused by "the breaking of a thick, massive, rigid strata at a considerable distance above the coal bed, causing a great, hammerlike blow to be given to the immediate roof of the mine opening, (transmitting) a shock wave to the coal pillar or pillars" (Rice 1935). These events could occur on off shifts, outby the face, in bleeder pillars, or other unexpected times and locations. Today, we understand that the sudden, dynamic failure in the overlying (or underlying) strata releases elastic energy in the form of seismic waves. The failures include sudden downward movements of the rock above the worked-out areas, shear slip motion on faults or fractures in the overburden, or some combination of these two mechanisms (Pankow et al. 2008). Shear slip motion can occur on newly-created fractures, or on reactivated pre-existing faults (Swanson et al. 2008; Alber et al.2008). The seismic energy released by such events can cause damage both underground and on the surface.

The "shock burst" phenomenon is well known internationally, both in hard rock mines and in burst-prone coalfields. For several decades, the deep South African gold mines have been aware that mining too near a fault can trigger a major rock burst. Researchers at the Australian Centre for Geomechanics (ACG) have developed a quantitative rock burst risk control method that includes the following elements (Potvin 2009):

(1)Identifying sources of seismic energy, including faults and other geologic or mining structures

(2)Estimating the maximum likely seismic energy release from each individual seismic source

(3)Assessing the largest potential ground motion (peak particle velocity) in the mine as a function of the magnitude of the event and the distance of the mine workings from the event

(4)Assessing the potential damage to the mine resulting from the ground motions, and modifying the mine plan as necessary to control the risk

The ACG approach relies on the availability of seismic source locations obtained from high quality, three-dimensional seismic monitoring systems. Such systems have been employed in some burst-prone European coalfields. In Czechoslovakia, for example, researchers have been able to study the relationship between the magnitude and location of seismic events and the extent of damage underground. In one instance, extensive damage resulted from a seismic magnitude ($M$) event, where $M = 2.8$, that was located more than 100 m away from the workings (Holub et al. 2011). On the other hand, even very large events may have little impact on the mine if they occur well above the workings. During one 5-year period in Poland, there were 15 large mining-induced events with $M$ ranging from 2.2 to 4.0 (Mutke and Stec 1997). Only 6 of these had any significant effect underground. Seam level "mining tremors", on the other hand, are often too small to register on a regional seismic network, but they can result in serious injury if a miner is in the vicinity (Mutke and Stec 1997).

It is evident that a wide range of causes can result in coal bursts. The volume of coal involved in bursts also covers a wide spectrum, from a few chunks of coal up to a whole array of pillars. The common link between all these events appears to be the failure mechanism of the coal itself. In general, coal is able to carry high vertical stress (or more precisely, maximum principal stress (sigma 1)) only when it also carries large confining stresses (or minimum principal stress (sigma 3)). If the vertical load is increased under these conditions, failure usually takes the form of non-violent yielding. A coal burst, on the other hand, apparently results when the confining stress is suddenly reduced. Research by Babcock and Bickel (1984) indicated that a wide variety of coals can be induced to fail violently by this "loss of confinement" mechanism. The loss of confinement can either be the result of mining activity, or of the ground shaking that accompanies an off-seam seismic energy release (a mining-induced earthquake).

One factor that does not seem to be strongly correlated with bump proneness is the character of the coal. Iannacchione and Zelanko (1995) noted that bursts have occurred in at least 25 different US coalbeds, varying from strong, blocky seams to very friable ones like the Pocahontas No. 3 and No. 4. Extensive German laboratory studies using large-scale specimens have also concluded that nearly all bituminous coals can burst. In these experiments, coal seams ranging in unconfined, compressive strength from 5 MPa to 50 MPa have all been shown to be burst-prone (Bräuner 1994).

## 2 COAL BURSTS IN THE US

The long history of coal bursts in the US has been well-documented. Iannacchione and Zelanko (1995) analyzed a database of 172 bursts that had occurred between 1936 and 1993. These bursts had resulted in a total of 87 fatalities and 163 injuries. Reflecting the mining technology in use during this period, 61 % of the events occurred during pillar recovery operations, and 25 % during longwall mining. The remaining 14 % occurred during development.

Three main coalfields have accounted for the vast majority of bursts. Iannacchione and Zelanko reported that 65 % of the bursts in their database occurred in the Central Appalachian coalfields of West Virginia, Virginia, and Kentucky. Most of the rest occurred in Colorado (17 %) or Utah (15 %). Bursts occurred at more than 50 different mines during this period. Iannacchione and Zelanko found that nearly all bursts occurred at depths greater than 300 m, and most were greater than 400 m.

A database of coal bursts that occurred during the period 1994–2013 was recently developed. It includes a total of 140 events that were reported to MSHA.[1] An additional 13 events involved roof "thumps", but since they did not result in violent ejection of coal or rock they were not included in the total.[2]

Four of the 140 events in the new database resulted in a total of five fatalities, two on longwalls, and three during two pillar recovery events. Note that the Crandall Canyon mine disaster which claimed six lives is not included in the database. That event was unique and can be best described as a catastrophic, mine-wide, pillar system failure. The area that collapsed at Crandall Canyon was enormous, encompassing 20 rows of pillars over approximately one square kilometer. It has more in common with the massive pillar collapses described by Mark et al. (1997) and Zipf (1992) than with a typical coal burst.[3]

Figure 3 shows that since the 1980's there has been a generally declining trend in the number of reported bursts. Some of this improvement can be attributed to changes in mining methods and geologic environments. Longwall mining has largely replaced pillar recovery in the western US, and much less coal is being mined from the burst prone Pocahontas coalfields of Virginia and West Virginia. On the other hand, longwalls work deeper seams today than they did 30 years ago, and multiple seam interactions are much more prevalent. Therefore it seems evident that much of the improvement must be due to the better mining practices, some of which will be discussed further on.

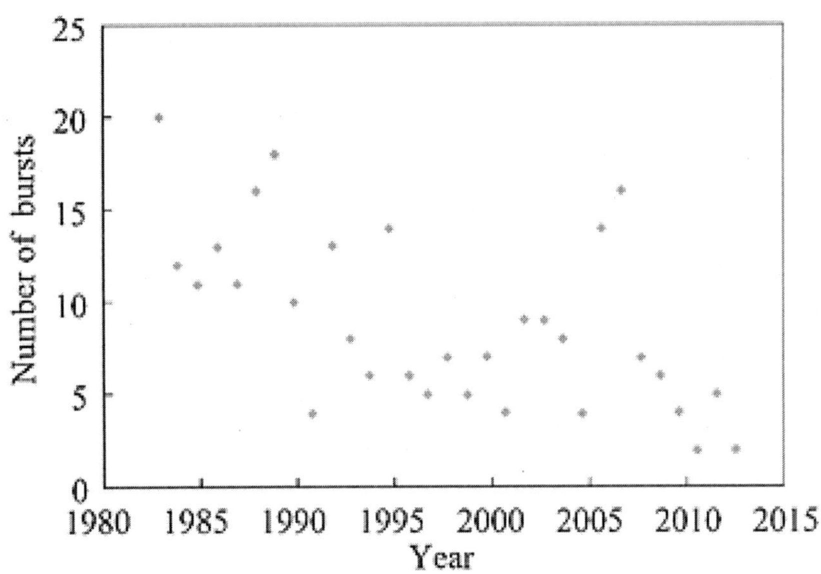


**Figure 3.** Number of coal bursts reported to MSHA, 1983–2013

Figure 4 shows that during the past 20 years Utah mines have accounted for the largest number of bursts, followed by Colorado. Virginia and West Virginia only recorded one burst each, though together those two states had accounted for 54 % of the bursts during the earlier period analyzed by Iannacchione and Zelanko (1995). Unfortunately, in 2014 a coal burst killed two West Virginia miners. Most coal mining in Central Appalachia is conducted by room-and-pillar methods, though the experience of one burst prone longwall has been described in detail by Hoelle (2008).

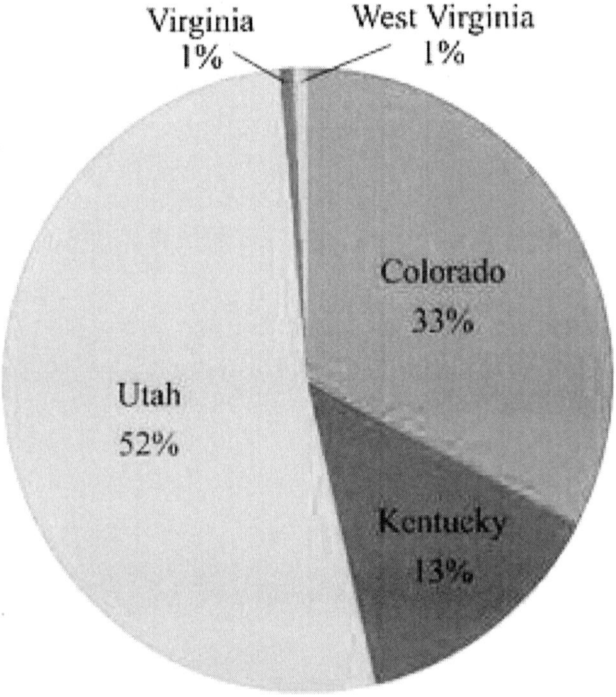


**Figure 4.** Coal bursts reported to MSHA, by state, 1994–2013

Figure 5 shows that 41 % of the bursts during the past 20 years have occurred on the longwall face. Another 20 % affected the tailgate entry at the corner of the longwall face, and 12 % occurred during retreat mining. All of these locations are subject to very high stresses, and they are directly affected by mining activity, and so might be considered likely locations for bursts. On the other hand, 14 % of the bursts occurred during entry development, and another 13 % affected pillars in the headgate, bleeder, or other outby locations.

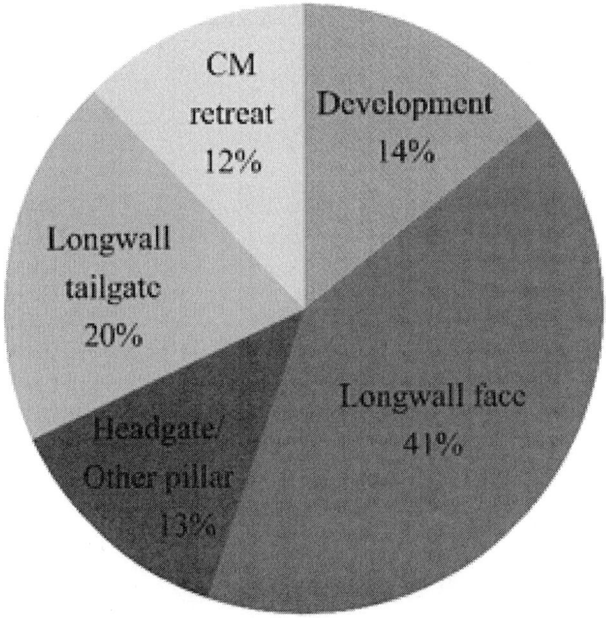


**Figure 5.** Coal bursts reported to MSHA, by location in the mine, 1994–2013

There are also some significant regional trends. In Utah, 76 % of the total 68 events occurred on the longwall face, and another 10 % occurred either in the longwall tailgate or during pillar recovery. Similarly, in Central Appalachia, 81 % of the 21 reported bursts occurred on the longwall face, tailgate, or pillar line. In Colorado, on the other hand, nearly half of the bursts occurred during entry development or in the headgate, bleeder, or other outby location. And although 40 of the 46 Colorado events took place in longwall mines, only two occurred on a longwall face.

## 2.1 Utah experience

The coalfields of Utah are located in the mountainous central region of the state (Fig. 6). The minable coal seams crop out of plateau escarpments, giving rise to rapid increases in cover depths. Typical mining depths of 450–900 m are among the very deepest in the US. The strata are characterized by numerous thick and strong sandstone and siltstone beds, with rock strengths reaching 130 MPa.

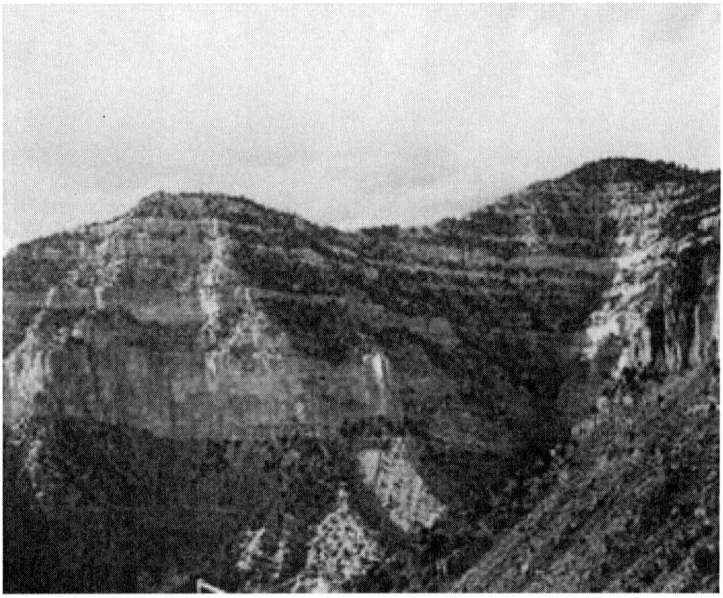

**Figure 6.** Mountainous terrain in the Utah coalfields. Note the thick, cliff-forming sandstone units

The first coal bursts were recorded in Utah almost 100 years ago. They were typically associated with pillar recovery under deep cover. However, Peperakis (1958) noted that severe bumps at the Sunnyside Mine in Utah had occurred in virgin development a long distance away from active workings, and were attributed to geologic faults.

Bursts were one reason why Sunnyside was one of the early longwall pioneers in the US. Through a lengthy process during which many gateroad configurations were trialed, Sunnyside engineers developed a two-entry, yield pillar system that virtually eliminated pillar bursts. The yield pillars were typically 9 m wide in 2.5–3 m thick seams (DeMarco et al. 1995). Mining engineers also learned to avoid "critical" pillars which are too large to yield non-violently yet too small to support large abutment loads. The width-to-height ratios of such burst-prone, critical pillars normally exceeded 4 or 5 (DeMarco et al. 1995). Longwall face bursts continued to be a problem however, typically once the cover depth exceeded 450 m.

Seismicity induced by mining operations in Utah has also been extensively studied. The University of Utah operates a regional seismic system which recorded 148 mining induced events with Local Magnitude $M_L > 2.5$, including 18 with $M_L > 3.0$, between 1978 and 2000 (Arabasz and Pechmann 2001). Of the larger events, three were judged to have shear–slip mechanisms, while

13 had possible collapse-type mechanisms. Few of these large events coincided with longwall bursts underground. The largest mining induced event ever recorded in Utah was the $M = 4.2$ shear-slip event that was located 150 m above face of the second panel the Willow Creek mine. This event was large enough to cause rock falls that closed a railroad and major highway, but it resulted in only minor damage in the vicinity of the longwall (Ellenberger and Heasley 2000).

Case history Mine A was located in the Book Cliffs region of central Utah (MSHA 1996). The massive Kenilworth sandstone formation lies 6–12 m above the seam, and the strata between it and the seam includes other strong siltstones and sandstones with typical strengths of about 100 MPa. Another massive sandstone, the Aberdeen, lies directly beneath the seam. The seam dip was 6–12 degrees, so each successive panel was about 40 m deeper than the previous one. Some mining had been conducted in a coal seam lying approximately 85 m above Mine A, but there were no noticeable stress transfers.

Longwall mining began in 1995. Panels were developed 225 m wide in the 3 m thick seam. A three-entry yield pillar system, with entries on 15 by 36 m centers, separated the first longwall panel from the second. The cover above the tailgate of the second panel was about 480 m.

As the second panel retreated, "bounces" consisting of sudden forceful vibrations became increasingly common on the tailgate end of the panel. Five of these events resulted in broken shearer torque shafts.

A major coal burst occurred when the panel had been retreated 225 m. The shearer had just begun the double-cut at the tailgate that began the return pass towards the headgate. Approximately 30 m of the face blew out, propelling coal across the conveyor and into the shields, and causing fatal injuries to the shearer operator. Floor, roof, and rib damage from the burst was also visible for 45 m along the tailgate entry. This event registered $M = 2.2$ on the regional seismic network (UUUS 2014).

In the wake of this incident, the remainder of the second panel was abandoned. A new tailgate was driven for the third panel, leaving the remainder of the second panel as an interpanel barrier pillar protecting the third panel tailgate from abutment loads arising from the first panel. Subsequent panels were also developed with the interpanel barrier design, leaving solid pillars up to 180 m wide between adjoining panels. Two independent sets of two-entry yield pillar gates were driven for each new panel.

Almost 10 years after the first fatal burst, the seventh longwall panel was being retreated at Mine A under almost 840 m of cover (MSHA 2006). Bounces were common along the longwall face, ranging from thumps in the roof or floor to coal being blown from the face. These events occurred all along the longwall face, but were most common near the headgate and tailgate entries. “Bounce procedures” were in place to protect the workers by limiting access to the face when the shearer was near the gate entries and specifying that shearer operators should position themselves behind the 8 m long deflector shields mounted above the shearer. The deflector shields were hinged off the shearer frame to be lowered or raised to accommodate mining clearance. In addition, expanded metal guards were attached to the armored face conveyor periodically along the walkway, and sheets of conveyor belting were suspended from the bottom of shield canopies along the walkway.

Despite these precautions, a fatal bounce killed a shearer operator located approximately 15 m from the headgate corner as the shearer was double-cutting towards the headgate (Fig. 7). The burst extended approximately 15 m along the face, with the largest cavity about 1 m deep directly in front of the victim. This event measured $M = 1.2$ on the seismic network. Mine A closed not long afterward, because the burst hazard could not be effectively managed at the even greater depths above the remaining reserves.

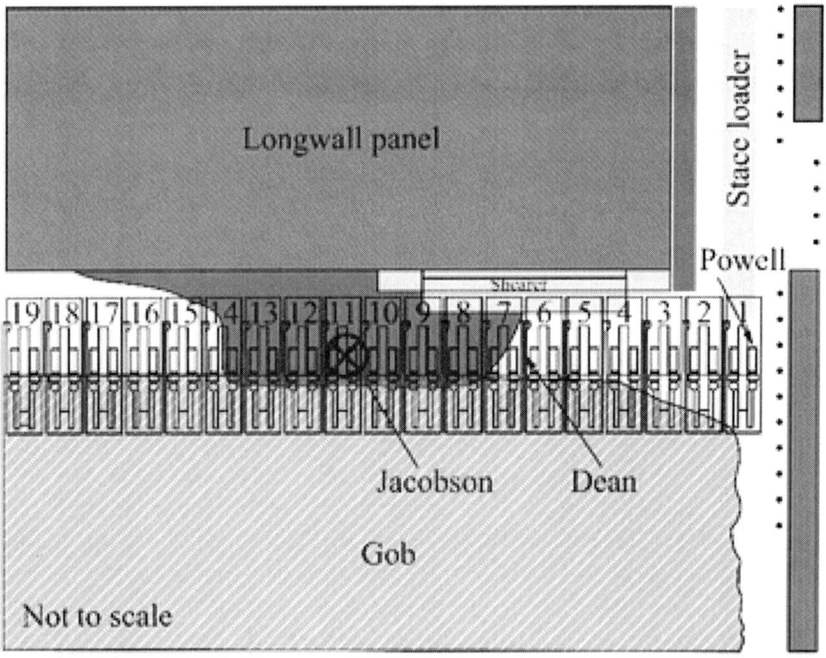


**Figure 7.** Sketch of the second burst accident scene at Utah Mine A (MSHA 2006)

The experience at Mine A demonstrated both the advantages and limitations of the two Utah longwall pillar design techniques. While the yield pillar system used on the first two panels typically performs well at depths up 600 m or so, it concentrates the load on the tailgate corner of the longwall face, and this can make it unworkable at greater depths. After the interpanel barrier method was introduced at Mine A, it was adopted at several other Utah longwalls (Gilbride and Hardy 2004). In some cases, rather than leave a full barrier, these mines elected to make mid-panel moves around the area of deepest cover, thus providing a local interpanel barrier for the next panel (Maleki 2006).

The interpanel barrier effectively protects the tailgate corner from the influence of previous panels, but at greater depths the single-panel stresses on the longwall face reach the same levels as were present with abutment loads and yield pillars. This limitation led one major Utah operator to announce in 2008 that it would write off reserves at depths exceeding 900 m as unmineable (Foy 2008).

## 2.2 Colorado experience

While coal bursts have occurred in several different coalfields in central and western Colorado, in recent years the problems have focused on operations in the North Fork Valley (NFV) of the Gunnison River. The NFV is an area of extremely mountainous topography where drift mines can encounter depths of cover that exceed 600 m. Past mining also gives rise to multiple seam interactions in some areas.

The geology of the NFV differs from Utah in that the immediate roof of the most common mining horizons is of weak to moderate strength. Usually composed of interbedded siltstone, fossiliferous shale, and thin layers of sandstone, Coal Mine Roof Rating (CMRR) values typically range between 40 and 60, with typical UCS values of 50–80 MPa (Maleki et al. 2006; Stewart et al. 2006). The immediate floor usually contains a considerable thickness of coal. Massive sandstone units, with strengths exceeding 100 MPa, are typically found about 15 m beneath the mineable seams (Maleki et al. 2009). Faulting and joint zones are present throughout the coalfield, and active tectonism continues to occur in the region today (Swanson et al. 2008).

Case history Mine B began longwall mining in 2002 (Mark et al. 2012). In 2004, a series of three bursts occurred in the tailgate of the active longwall face as it was passing over underlying works at greater than 450 m of overburden. A fourth event occurred the following year in the adjacent panel tailgate in the absence of underlying workings. A fifth burst occurred 3 years later beneath some of the deepest overburden encountered up to that time (540 m). No multiple seam interaction was present in this instance. The pillars in this district were developed on 33 by 60 m centers, and maintained Analysis of Longwall Pillar Stability (ALPS) stability factor (SF) of less than 0.6.

Late in 2009, the mine began longwalling in a new district, with depths of cover that consistently exceeded 600 m. The pillars were significantly larger than any that had been used at the mine in the past, with three entries driven on 57 m centers, and they maintained an ALPS SF of 1.12 (bleeder loading) even at a depth of 680 m. The first panel (panel D-1 in Fig. 8) was extracted without serious incident, but, midway through the D-2 panel in 2011, a powerful burst that registered $M = 3.1$ caused extensive pillar failure and floor heave over a 3 ha area of tailgate pillars. Ventilation was also severely affected, and the panel was abandoned.

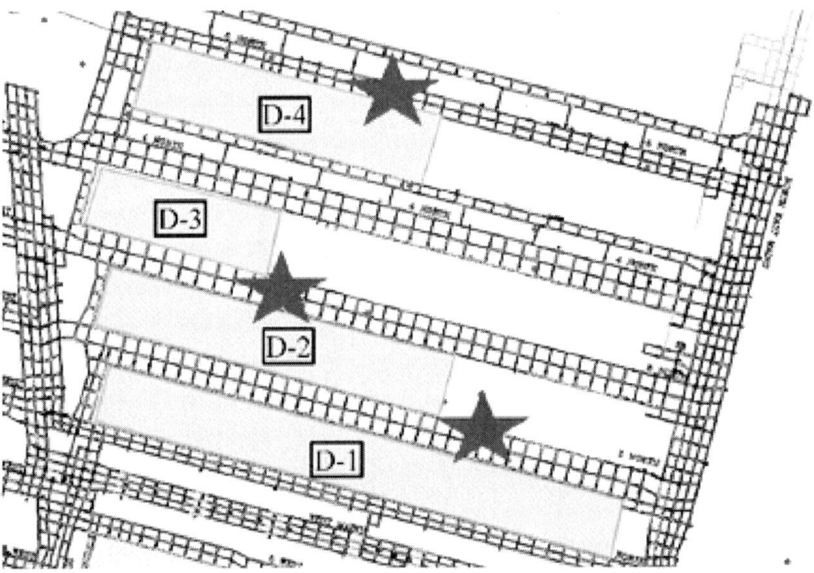


**Figure 8.** Map of Colorado Case History Mine B, showing the locations of the bursts discussed in the texts (*red stars*)

The burst in the D-1 tailgate was centered at least 150 m outby the tailgate corner, so it is unlikely that front abutment stresses were a significant contributing factor. The burst did occur within the linear projection of a densely jointed and slickensided joint zone that had been identified in the mains more than 1000 m away several years before. It was one of a series of joint zones that were arrayed with roughly constant spacing across the mine reserve, exhibiting an approximate N 70°E trend.

Another of these other structural features was associated with a burst that resulted in an injury during the development of the headgate for the D-3 panel. This feature was cause for concern because it crossed the tailgate of the D-3 panel at about mid-panel. When another large tailgate burst occurred during the mining of the D-3 panel, however, it was well in by this zone. While not as destructive as the burst that occurred on the D-2 panel, it destroyed 1.6 ha of tailgate pillars and again forced the abandonment of the panel. This event was recorded as $M = 3.2$.

A new gateroad was developed in order to leave an additional 75 m interpanel barrier to isolate the D-4 panel from the D-3 panel. Mining had advanced approximately 400 m in the D-4 panel, and the face was beneath almost 800 m of cover, when the largest burst yet, with $M = 3.4$, destroyed 4 ha of *headgate* pillars in by the face. Ventilation was again severely affected. Several weeks later, before the face could be recovered, a heating event developed in the gob. Ultimately the face was abandoned and the mine was sealed.

Case history Mine B illustrates some of the typical key characteristics of NFV bursts, which make the area somewhat unique among burst-prone coalfields around the world:

(1)The immediate roof and floor seldom consists of strong, massive rock, but typically consists of relatively thin beds of moderate strength or even weak material.

(2)While the incidence of bursts clearly increases with depth, with almost all occurring at depths greater than 450 m, often the bursts do not occur beneath the maximum cover in an area.

(3)Most bursts are apparently not directly triggered by coal-cutting activities, and many occur in areas of lower mining stress such as headgates or development sections.

(4)In many cases, the pillar designs were sufficiently robust that they would have been expected to provide adequate support to the overburden.

(5)The bursts often have a greater effect on the floor than they do the pillar ribs.

(6)The bursts are often associated with known geologic structures, particularly low-angle faults and zones of high-density jointing that exhibit little to no displacement.

(7)The bursts are often associated with large seismic events.

Taken together, these characteristics imply that the most significant bursts in the NFV are largely of what Rice (1935) would have called the “shock bump” variety. In other words, they appear to be driven by large seismic energy releases occurring at some distance from the coal seam, often apparently from the massive sandstones below.

# 3 MANAGEMENT OF COAL BURSTS

Managing the risk of coal bursts begins with an evaluation of the factors that increase the likelihood of bursts. These include the depth of cover, the presence of past mining above or below, the roof and floor geology, and the presence of faults and other geologic factors. A past history of bursts is one of the most powerful indicators of burst risk during any type of mining. Major bursts have often been preceded by smaller ones. Often these "precursors" have occurred at the same stage in the mining process as the subsequent large event (for example, in the same location on the longwall face). Also, once a mine has experienced bursts, later situations with similar geology and mining methods should also be considered high risk.

Once zones at elevated risk of bursts are identified, the next step is to determine appropriate control techniques to employ within each one. According to risk management principles, the most effective way to reduce a risk is to eliminate it entirely (Iannacchione et al. 2008). In the context of burst control, this would be achieved by not mining at all in the areas of greatest risk.

Where the risk is not great enough to indicate complete avoidance, mining may be limited to development only. For example, in a mountainous area, the main entries might be developed beneath the ridgeline where the cover is deepest.

Pillar design is the primary engineering control for minimizing the risks of pillar failure and coal bursts during retreat mining under deep cover. In longwall mines, three types of pillar design have been used to reduce the risk of coal bursts (Fig. 9). Operational techniques used by longwall mines to reduce the burst risk include reducing the depth of the web, reducing the the speed of the shearer, uni-directional cutting, and/or avoiding double cuts at the gate ends.

Administrative controls can be used to limit the exposure of miners to the areas of highest burst risk (Varley and Whyatt 2008). They can include:

(1)Allowing only the minimum number of persons required to extract the coal into the areas where coal is being mined.

(2)Positioning remote-control equipment operators as far from the active mining as practical (depending on radio signal range and visibility constraints).

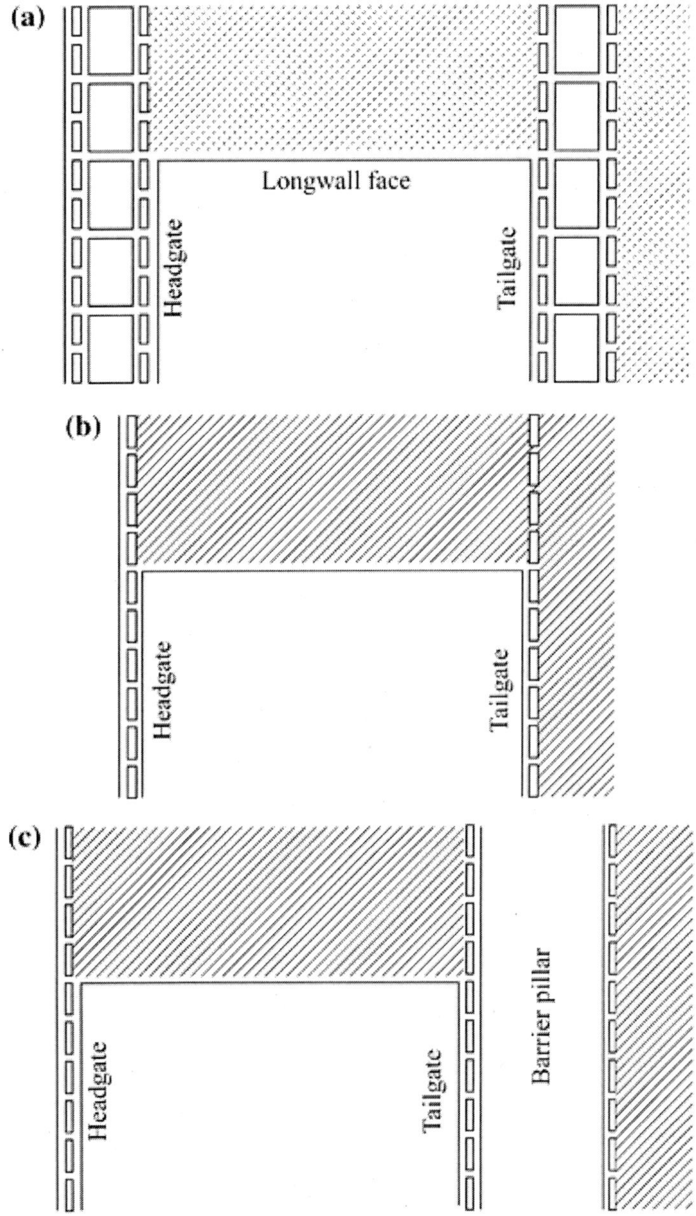


**Figure 9.** Longwall pillar configurations used in the US to control coal bursts. **a** "Conventional" four-entry design using a large abutment pillar flanked by two smaller pillars; **b** a two-entry yield pillar design; **c** an inter-panel barrier design

Physical barriers can be used to protect miners from the full force of a burst event. They can be helpful against small bursts, but are likely incapable of absorbing the energy from the largest events. Examples of physical barriers that have been used on longwalls include conveyor belting secured between the shields and the face conveyor, and metal plate burst protectors installed on shearing machines. Miners can also be provided with personal protective equipment (PPE), such as helmets, face shields, or body armor, though such devices can only protect miners from small events.

The value of administrative controls, physical barriers, and PPE is also compromised if they are not correctly and consistently employed. Therefore, such techniques require worker training and constant management attention.

Destressing techniques, including drilling, water infusion, hydrofracturing, and blasting, have occasionally been used to reduce the burst risk (Varley and Whyatt 2008; Maleki et al. 2011). While some of these techniques are used routinely in German mines (Baltz and Hucke 2008), their performance in the US has been mixed. The difficulties of identifying optimum distressing times and ability to assess the effectiveness of each destressing attempt, the limited time available for face destressing (to avoid production delays) and adverse drilling conditions reduced the overall success of the efforts. Hydrofracturing is perhaps the most promising technique for modern high-production longwalls (Hoelle 2008).

Underground observations and monitoring are critical components of a burst risk management program. Mining crews should be trained to observe coal burst warning signs, particularly the occurrence of small bursts, which are often the best indication that an area is becoming more burst prone. A record-keeping system should be maintained, and management processes developed to ensure that warning signs receive appropriate responses.

## 4 CONCLUSIONS

Coal bursts remain a significant hazard for miners in the US and around the world. While coal bursts cannot be predicted in advance, the risk can be estimated through careful evaluation of those factors known to be associated with coal bursts. Understanding the different characteristics of coal bursts in specific coalfields is also critical to the risk evaluation.

## FOOTNOTES

1 In the US, coal mines must report to MSHA any "coal or rock outburst that causes withdrawal of miners or which disrupts regular mining activity for

more than 1 h" (Code of Federal Regulations, Title 30, Part 50.2). However, there is no special data field which identifies an accident report as a burst. The burst database employed in the present study was constructed by searching MSHA accident report narratives for terms such as "burst", "bump" and "bounce". Only those incidents where the narrative clearly indicated that a burst had occurred were retained in the database.

2 An example of this type of event is given by the following narrative, which describes an event that occurred during pillar recovery at a West Virginia mine in 1996: "Employee was helping set timbers on pillar line when the top bumped, rolling a coal rib onto his lower back."

3 The second event that occurred at Crandall Canyon and killed three rescuers *was* a pillar burst, but it has also been excluded because it occurred during the unique circumstances of a mine rescue.

## REFERENCES

1. Agapito JFT, Goodrich RR (2000) Five stress factors conducive to bursts in Utah, USA, coal mines. In: Proceedings of the 19th international conference on ground control in mining. West Virginia University, Morgantown, WV, pp 93–100
2. Alber M, Fritschen R, Bichofff M, Meier T (2008) Rock mechanical investigations of seismic events in a deep longwall coal mine. Int J Rock Mech Min Sci 46(2):408–420
3. Arabasz WJ, Pechmann JC (2001) Seismic characterization of coal-mining seismicity in Utah for CTBT monitoring: report to Lawrence Livermore National Laboratory, LLNL Research Agreement No. B344836, variously paginated, 3 appendices.http://www.seis.utah.edu/Reports/llnl2001/index.shtml
4. Babcock CO, Bickel DL (1984) Constraint: the missing variable in the coal burst problem. In: Proceedings of the 25th U.S. symposium on rock mechanics, Evanston, IL, pp 639–647
5. Baltz R, Hucke A (2008) Rockburst prevention in the German coal industry.. In: Proceedings of the 27th international conference on ground control in mining. West Virginia University, Morgantown, WV, pp 46–50
6. Bräuner G (1994) Rockbursts in coal mines and their prevention. Taylor & Francis, New York, p 152
7. DeMarco MJ, Koehler JR, Maleki H (1995) Gate road design considerations for mitigation of coal bumps in western U.S. longwall

operations. In: Maleki H, Wopat PF, Repsher RC, Tuchman RJ (eds) Proceedings: mechanics and mitigation of violent failure in coal and hard-rock mines. U.S. Department of the Interior, Bureau of Mines, SP 01-95, Spokane, WA, pp 141–165. NTIS No. PB95211967

8. Ellenberger JL, Heasley KA (2000) Coal mine seismicity and bursts: historical case studies and current field activity. In: Proceedings of the 19th international conference on ground control in mining. West Virginia University, Morgantown, WV, pp 112–120

9. Foy P (2008) Utah's deep coal operators face heavy regulation. Associated Press news item, 28 June

10. Gilbride LJ, Hardy MP (2004) Interpanel barriers for deep western U.S. Longwall mining. In: Proceedings of the 23rd international conference on ground control in mining. West Virginia University, Morgantown, WV, pp 35-41

11. Hoelle J (2008) Coal bumps in an Eastern Kentucky coal mine 1989 to 1997. In: Proceedings of the 27th international conference on ground control in mining. West Virginia University, Morgantown, WV, pp 14–19

12. Holland CT (1958) Cause and occurrence of coal mine bumps. Min Eng, 994–1004B

13. Holub K (1997) Predisposition to induced seismicity in some Czech coal mines. Pure Appl Geophys 150(3–4):435–450

14. Holub K, Rušajová J, Holečko J (2011) Particle velocity generated by the rockburst during exploitation of the longwall and its impact on the workings. Int J Rock Mech Min Sci 48(6):942–949

15. Iannacchione AT, Zelanko JC (1995) Occurrence and remediation of coal mine bursts: a historical review. US Department of the Interior, U.S. Bureau of Mines, Special Publication 01-95, pp 27–68

16. Iannacchione AT, Varley FD, Brady TM (2008) The application of major hazard risk assessment (MHRA) to eliminate multiple fatality occurrences in the U.S. minerals industry. U.S. Department of Health and Human Services, Centers for Disease Control and Prevention, National Institute for Occupational Safety and Health, Pittsburgh, PA, DHHS (NIOSH) Publication No. 2009B104, IC 9508

17. Maleki H (1995) An analysis of violent failure in U.S. coal mines: case studies. US Department of the Interior, U.S. Bureau of Mines, Special Publication 01-95, pp 5–26

18. Maleki H (2006) Caving, seismicity, and mine design in four Utah coal mines. In: Proceedings of the 25th international conference on ground

control in mining. West Virginia University, Morgantown, WV, pp 268–276

19. Maleki H, Zahl EG, Dunford JP (1999) A hybrid statistical-analytical method for assessing violent failure in U.S. coal mines. In: Mark C, Heasley K, Iannacchione A, Tuchman R (eds) Proceedings of the second international workshop on coal pillar mechanics and design. NIOSH, Pittsburgh, pp 139–144

20. Maleki H, Stewart C, Hunt G (2006) Subsidence characteristics at Bowie Mines, Colorado. In: Proceedings of the golden rocks 2006, 41st US symposium on rock mechanics. American Rock Mechanics Associationm, Alexandria, VA, doc ID 06–932

21. Maleki H, Stewart C, Stone R, Abshire J (2009) Practical application of numerical modeling for the study of sudden floor heave failure mechanisms. In: Proceedings of the international workshop on numerical modeling for underground mine excavation design. NIOSH, Pittsburgh, PA, pp 89–100

22. Maleki H, Rigby S, McKenzie J, Faddies T (2011) Historic mine designs and operational practices used in deep mines for controlling coal bumps. In: Proceedings of the 45th US rock mechanics/geomechanics symposium. American Rock Mechanics Association, Alexandria, VA, doc ID 11–276

23. Mark C, Chase F, Zipf RK, Jr (1997) Preventing massive pillar collapses in coal mines. In: New technology for ground control in retreat mining, NIOSH IC 9446, pp 35–48

24. Mark C, Phillipson SE, Tyrna P, Gauna M (2012) Characteristics of coal bursts in the North Fork Valley of the Gunnison River, Colorado. In: Proceedings of the 30th international conference on ground control in mining. West Virginia University, Morgantown, WV, pp 1–12

25. MSHA (1996) Coal mine fatal accident report, fall of face.http://www.msha.gov/FATALS/1996/FTL96C33.HTM. Accessed 14 Nov 1996

26. MSHA (2006) Coal mine fatal accident report, fall of face.http://www.msha.gov/FATALS/2006/FTL06c16.asp. Accessed 29 Jan 2006

27. Mutke G, Stec K (1997) Seismicity in the upper Silesian Coal Basin, Poland: strong regional seismic events. Geophys J Int 168(2):757–768

28. Pankow K, McCarter M C, Arabasz W, Burlacu R (2008) Coal mining seismicity in Utah—improving spatial resolution using double-difference relocations. In: Proceedings of the 27th international

conference on ground control in mining. West Virginia University, Morgantown, WV, pp 91–97

29. Peperakis J (1958) Mountain bumps at the Sunnyside mines. Min Eng 211:982–986

30. Potvin Y (2009) Strategies and tactics to control seismic risks in mines. J S Afr Inst Min Metall 109(3):177–186

31. Rice GS (1935). Bumps in coal mine of the Cumberland Field, Kentucky and Virginia: causes and remedy. US Bureau of Mines RI 3267

32. Stewart C, Hunt G, Mark C (2006) Geology, ground control and mine planning at Bowie Resources, Paonia, CO. In: Proceedings of the 25th international conference on ground control in mining. West Virginia University, Morgantown, WV, pp 284–290

33. Swanson P, Stewart C, Koontz W (2008) Monitoring coal mine seismicity with an automated wireless digital strong-motion network. In: Proceedings of the 27th international conference on ground control in mining. West Virginia University, Morgantown, WV, pp 79–86

34. UUUS (2014) Catalog of coal bursts in Utah, 1981–2013.http://www.seis.utah.edu/EQCENTER/LISTINGS/Catalogs/UT_81.csv

35. Varley F, Whyatt JK (2008) Work practices to manage bump prone ground. In: Peng SS, Tadolini SC, Mark C, Finfinger GL, Heasley KA, Khair AW, Luo Y (eds) Proceedings of the 27th international conference on ground control in mining. West Virginia University, Morgantown, pp 20–28

36. Zipf RK (1992) Analysis of stable and unstable pillar failure using a local mine stiffness method. In: Iannacchione A, Mark C, Repsher RC, Tuchman R, Jones CC (eds) Proceedings of the first international workshop on coal pillar mechanics and design. USBM IC 9325, Pittsburgh, PA, pp 128–143

# Chapter 6

# The Health Costs of Revised Coal Mining Limits in Northern Bohemia

**Vojtěch Máca * and Jan Melichar**

*Charles University Environment Center, Jose Martiho 2, 160 00 Prague 6, Czech Republic*

## ABSTRACT

Brown coal has been the major source of energy for more than 150 years for the Czech economy, but its role in the coming decades is nowadays the source of heated debate. Many of the recurring discussions address the coal reserves that were set aside in 1991 in order to halt the massive destruction of the landscape and the unprecedented deterioration of the human environment in Northern Bohemia. We study the proposed variants of the revised mining limits using the impact-pathway approach in order to quantify and monetize the health effects of airborne emissions from coal mining and the use of extracted coal for the production of electricity and heat. We find that the dominant health impacts associated with the revision of the limits, estimated to be up to 7 billion euros over the 2015–2050 period, will stem from the use of coal for the production of electricity and heat and that a large part of the impact will be borne by populations outside the Czech Republic.

**Keywords:** coal mining; coal-fired power plant; airborne pollution; impact-pathway approach; external costs

# 1. INTRODUCTION

Brown coal has been the most important of the primary energy sources in the Czech Republic for decades, in particular for electricity generation. Its share among primary sources has been decreasing, however, from 36.6% in 2000 to 28.9% in 2013, although it still accounts for over 40% of gross electricity production. A particular feature of the Czech energy system is the large scale deployment of district heating systems that compete with power plants for available brown coal. It is therefore no doubt that the availability of brown coal is a key issue in current energy policy considerations. The declining annual coal extraction trend is largely determined by diminishing exploitable reserves, but also the generally decreasing quality of coal (lower calorific value, higher sulphur and ash content) also plays a role.

For the last five years the Ministry of Industry and Trade has been working on an update of the 2004 National Energy Policy, a key policy document setting the long-term priorities for the development of the Czech energy sector. In spite of the fact that the first draft was published already in 2010, and a revised version in 2012 and 2014, the update was finally adopted by Czech government only in May 2015. The key priority of the National Energy Policy following the 2015 update ("NEP2015") is "a balanced mix of primary energy sources and sources for electricity generation based on a broad portfolio, the effective use of all available domestic energy sources and maintaining a surplus in the energy system output balance with sufficient reserves" [1].

The NEP2015 foresees an increase in decentralized energy generation and renewables (biomass in the first place), and at the same time a gradual phasing out of coal-fired plants due to outdated technology, lack of compliance with emission limits set by Industrial Emission Directive and a shrinking brown coal supply. In particular, the shrinking reserves of domestic brown coal within the existing mining limits are seen as a potentially major limiting factor.

The main brown coal deposits in the Czech Republic are located in the North Bohemian Brown Coal Basin in the foothills of the Ore Mountains, a natural border with Germany. The mining activities accelerated greatly in the 1950s and 1960s (seeFigure 1), and together with the associated industrial production (electricity and heat generation, oil processing, heavy chemistry, *etc.*) they imposed a huge burden on the people and environment of the region, a part of the infamously renown Black Triangle. It was only in 1991, shortly after the collapse of the Soviet bloc, that the Czech government decided to curtail the opencast mining in the region. A Government Resolution in 1991 imposed mining limits in six mining locations in the North Bohemian Brown Coal Basin. Mining authorities were obliged to modify mining areas and write-off the coal reserves. This has been accomplished in all but two mines—Czechoslovak Army (henceforth "CSA") and Bilina. If the mining limits were revoked at these two mines, about 400 million tonnes of brown coal would become available for future mining.

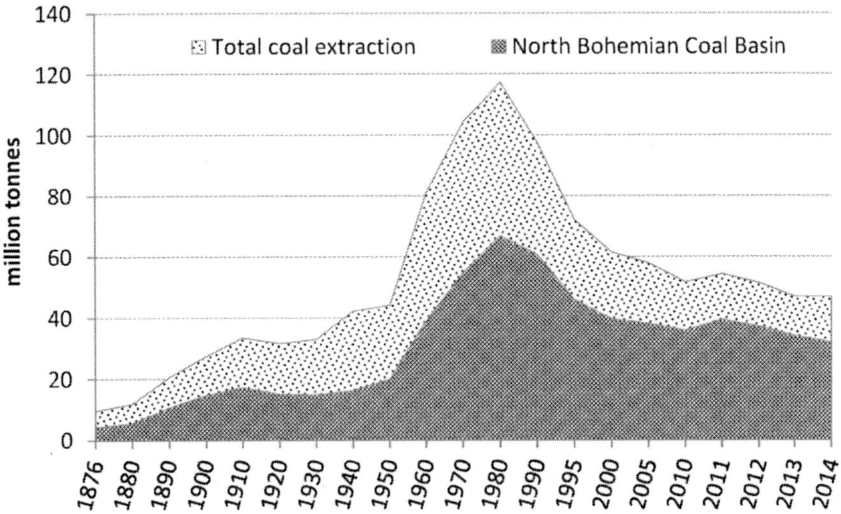


**Figure 1.** Coal mining in the Czech Republic (black, brown coal and lignite).

The mining limits were meant to set "unbreakable spatial borders beyond which mining or energy production activities cannot directly disturb and destroy natural elements that constitute the territorial system of landscape ecological stability, residential structures and infrastructure safeguarding the liveability of the territory and the maximum permissible pressures on key environmental elements—soil, water and air" [2]. The mining limits were to be reflected in the National Energy Policy until 2005, and it was originally anticipated that these would be revisited during the drafting of a new energy policy to see if there were any more environmentally-friendly alternatives to open-cast mining that could possibly be used. Yet, a powerful lobby of mining companies, mining trade unions and the Ministry of Industry and Trade continued to press for the abolition of the coal mining limits in the two mines by drawing a gloomy picture of massive unemployment in the region (and beyond) without the mines and arguing that brown coal is the only abundant domestic energy source and as such would bolster national energy security. In spite of this lobby, the National Energy Policy of 2004 was adopted in a version that kept the limits in place. During the governmental discussions about the recent update of the National Energy Policy, it was repeatedly argued that any decision that may interfere with the mining limits should be preceded by proper analyses of the economic, social and environmental consequences of repealing the limits.

So far, the market has coped well with the declining annual volumes of brown coal being extracted, but concerns about the future of district heating systems and energy security in general poses a challenge to decision-makers. If the coal mining limits are preserved in their current state, it is expected that by 2038 the only brown coal mine to remain in operation would be Vrsany; its reserves can last until around 2060. The overall situation regarding future demand and the supply of domestic brown coal depicting the potential gains from three recently discussed mining limit revision options is illustrated in Figure 2.

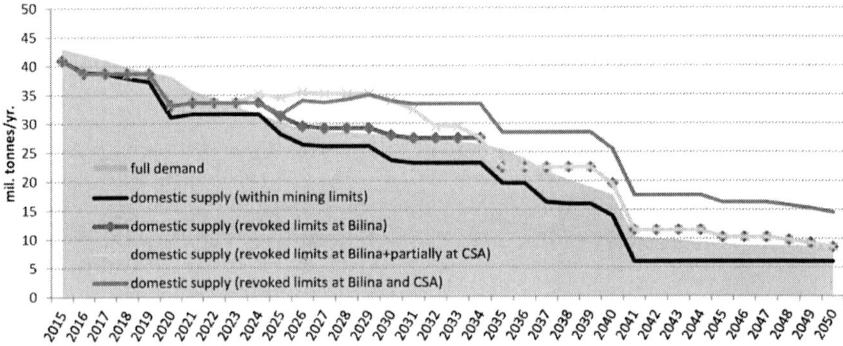


**Figure 2.** Domestic brown coal supply and demand for heat and electricity production under the revised mining limits [3].

The figure suggests that the pace with which the coal reserves within the mining limits will be depleted is greater than the planned gradual decommissioning of the power and heating plants. While questioned by some experts, it provides strong argumentation to Ministry of Industry and Trade to abolish (at least one of) the mining limits, although this is not openly advocated in the NEP2015.

There are two important external drivers, apart from the mining limits, that exert pressure for the gradual abandonment of brown coal mining and its use for energy generation in the not too distant future. The first concerns the EU leaders' commitment to reduce $CO_2$ emissions by 80%–95% by 2050 (compared to 1990) that led the European Commission in early 2015 to announce the Energy Union Package aimed at creating a sustainable, low-carbon and climate-friendly energy system. It claims, *inter alia,* that "we have to move away from an economy driven by fossil fuels, an economy where energy is based on a centralised, supply-side approach" [4]. Clearly, decarbonisation of the economy is one of the five key dimensions of the Energy Union strategy, although the means to achieve this goal are (mostly) old ones—an emission trading scheme, renewable energy targets and direct support schemes.

A second driver, acting through interconnected electricity networks and markets, comes from neighbouring Germany where a massive energy transition package (Energiewende) is being sought. This effort accelerated following the Fukushima nuclear accident in 2011 when 40% of nuclear generating capacity was closed down in Germany almost immediately, with the remaining units to be phased out by 2022. This decline was partly compensated with electricity from coal and as a consequence, brown coal accounted for a 29.5% share in energy sources for electricity production in 2012, the highest figure in a decade, but the share since then has shrank to 28.8% in 2014, according to the German Energy Balances Working Group (AGEB). The role of coal in the energy transition is still under discussion, with some arguing for the need to secure employment in coal mining regions. Yet a recent modelling study by the German Institute for Economic Research (DIW) [5] suggests that the construction of new brown/lignite coal power plants in Germany is not viable either from an economic, technical and environmental perspective. In addition, the study asserts that it is likely that a gradual phasing out of brown coal/lignite from the German electricity system will culminate in 2040–2045 with the closure of the last plants.

Hence, in light of these diverging interests, this article aims to illustrate the extent of the health impacts associated with a policy decision regarding mining limits. Our focus is limited here to the health impacts from airborne emissions related to coal mining and the burning of coal during electricity and heat generation that would be released were the coal reserves beyond the mining limits at coal mines Bilina and CSA to be extracted.

## 2. PREVIOUS RESEARCH

Over recent decades a great deal of environmental cost studies focused on quantifying the environmental and health effects of various energy generation pathways (fuel cycles) have been undertaken to establish monetary values that can be readily incorporated into public (and private) decision-making. A recent review [6] provides a critical methodological review for accounting for the true costs of electricity based on four influential primary costing studies conducted in the United States and the European Union [7,8,9,10,11].

Cost estimates are commonly made by either a damage function approach or an abatement cost approach. The first approach estimates the increase in health and environmental impacts by projecting changes in emissions and exposure to pollutants using a predefined set of exposure-response relationships; a valuation of welfare change due to any suffering from these effects is subsequently provided by specific (unit) values for respective health outcomes. The latter—abatement cost—approach examines the costs of achieving mandated emission limits, using it as a proxy for damage, *i.e.*, assuming that the regulation mandates for the optimal level of pollution. This is essentially a very strong assumption because to establish an optimal level of regulation, an estimation of damage costs would be needed anyway. Consequently, the damage function approach is considered more appropriate if data are available.

A frequently used "shortcut" is the benefit-transfer that adapts engineering, environmental, or economic data from previous studies to a new study (assuming transferability between donor and transfer location and other characteristics). Even primary costing studies rely in some stages on a benefit transfer (e.g., in a valuation of impacts), but benefit-transfer studies commonly use benefit-transfer to skip some of the steps in the damage function approach (e.g., by using average values like euro or dollar per tonne of emission estimates from previous studies). Another example of a shortcut in the damage function approach can be illustrated by the stream of research on the health impacts of one open cast mining method—mountaintop removal (MTR)—in the Appalachian Mountains in the USA, showing that living near active MTR operations is associated with higher risks of cardiovascular, cardiopulmonary, lung, kidney and chronic respiratory diseases [12,13,14], mortality risks from lung, colorectal and bladder cancer and leukaemia [15,16], as well elevated risks of birth defects [17]. In a similar vein, the association between distance from mining activity and mortality from neoplasms was also observed in a study by Fernández-Navarro [18] and colleagues in Spain.

An important distinction among environmental costing studies arises from what activities (and related environmental burdens) preceding and following energy generation are included in the assessment. The two extreme options are to focus either on full life cycle or on generation only, the latter occurring much more frequently. Burtraw and colleagues [6] point out that analyses confined to just the electricity generation phase will underestimate the total burden while full life cycle may be quite complex and resource demanding, and suggest effective compromise by adding selectively those components of the fuel cycle that are likely to contribute significantly to the external cost estimates.

In several national implementations of the European ExternE methodology [11] coal mining was included in the coal fuel cycle assessment. In the German national implementation, the coal fuel cycles assessed include both underground and open pit mining (reference mines were in Ruhrgebiet for hard coal and Garzweiler mine for opencast mining). The latter variant uses electrically driven conveyor belts for transporting coal from the mine to the power plant. The study points to high emissions of particulates from the loading and unloading of coal/lignite (0.2 kg dust per tonne as provided by the German Umweltbundesamt), although these emissions are not taken into account in the impact assessment for their local impact. Discharges of effluents from mining activities are not quantified, although the authors note the potentially significant impacts on groundwater systems. Occupational health effects from brown coal opencast mining are considered to be very similar to average industrial activities (as opposed to underground mining). Other considered impacts include the negative effects of mining on aquatic ecosystems (low pH from sulphur) and the resettlement of local communities on the mine locality. About 95% of public health damage from the lignite fuel cycle, estimated at approx. 1.6 eurocents/kWh, come from power generation, with the remaining 5% from other fuel cycle stages.

The Spanish national implementation considered the coal fuel cycle with open cast coal mining in Puertollano. As in the German case, PM emissions from coal mining are considerable but it is expected that their impact will be low since they are emitted near ground level and are quickly deposited (presumably affecting only mine workers and these effects are accounted for as occupational health impacts). Like the German case, the overwhelming majority of estimated public health damage (2.6 eurocents/kWh) originates from power generation, while occupational health impacts from other fuel cycle stages bring an additional 0.24 eurocents/kWh.

In a Belgian case study, emissions from mining (coal imported from abroad) are taken from the ecoinvent life-cycle database and occupational health impacts were also quantified (although they are considered less important). Conversely, liquid effluents were not quantified, but it is acknowledged that they can play an important role. The results show that non-global warming impacts are by and large dominated by the public health impact from power generation, and especially by the chronic mortality impacts occurring at the regional scale.

A study on the external cost of coal conducted by the Dutch consultancy CE Delft for Greenpeace International [19,20] assessed the impacts on human health from air pollution, climate change damage, and fatalities due to major accidents in mining from a global perspective. Hence, instead of site-specific data they built upon emission factors from national inventories and the Life Cycle Assessment (LCA) database. They find that the overwhelming majority of external costs originates from emissions from coal combustion in power plants, with a central estimate of 365 billion euros, and mining emissions contributing an additional 674 million euros and occupational mining externalities (with part of these assumed to be internalised through insurance) 161 million euros.

Recently, the Health and Environment Alliance (HEAL) published a study on the health impacts of coal-fired power plants in Europe [21], claiming that EU-wide health impacts from coal combustion amount to more than 18,200 premature deaths, 8500 new cases of chronic bronchitis and over 4 million lost working days annually. This totals between 15.5–42.8 billion euros in the EU-27 per year (depending on what valuation metrics were used for premature mortality) or—denominated per kWh—on average between 6.2 and 95 eurocents.

Beyond the EU, Epstein *et al.* [22] addressed the full costs of the coal life cycle in the USA. They account for the external costs of different phases in the coal cycle—mining, transport, combustion—and impact categories, including land disturbance, emissions of air pollutants, carcinogens, mercury and greenhouse gases. The best estimate for externalities related to coal is 17.84 US cents per kWh (low and high estimates 9.42 and 26.89 US cents per kWh, respectively); slightly more than half of these externalities originate from emissions of air pollutants from combustion and a further quarter from the public health burden of communities in the Appalachian region where the mining takes place.

Mahapatra and colleagues [23] analysed the life-cycle environmental impacts of coal-based electricity generation in Ahmedabad in western India. They applied spatially resolved estimates of damage to human health, crops and building materials from coal mining and power plant operations. For source apportionment, the authors opted for the energy balance accounting approach (providing the amount of coal related emissions from the power sector) instead of receptor modelling conventionally used in the impact-pathway approach. Coal mining impacts were calculated as the sum of impacts from mine fires, mine dust emissions, and fugitive (methane) and $CO_2$ emissions. The authors estimated the external costs of mining at around 12 paisa per kWh (approximately 0.27 US cents per kWh) and the overall external costs of electricity generation at around 206.8 paisa per kWh (4.6 US cents per kWh).

Nkambule and Blignaut [24] analysed the external costs of coal mining and transportation to the Kusile power plant near Emelahleni in South Africa. They quantify the external costs to human health (air pollution and accidents) and the environment (climate change, water pollution and consumption, loss of ecosystem services) mostly based on benefit transfer. The external costs are estimated at around 20–40 cents per kWh (*i.e.*, 50%–100% of the average electricity price). Over 90% of the impacts quantified were due to water consumption that was quantified using a benefit transfer from [25], who used the production function approach to derive the opportunity costs of water. In this respect, it is highly specific to local conditions and the estimation of the production function is also rather tentative for its hypothetical setup and mixing different power generation technologies.

Wang *et al.* [26] compared the external costs of power plants fired by coal *versus* biomass in a stylized life cycle approach. The (hard) coal mining part of their external cost quantification accounts for gangue, water contamination, methane emissions and occupational mortality and morbidity, and the quantification of these impacts follows a top-down approach. They find that the coal combustion stage makes a large majority of external costs quantified (0.067 US cents per kWh) compared to coal mining (0.003 US cents per kWh) and other upstream processes.

Any comparison of the published estimates of the externalities of coal should made cautiously. In particular, there are huge differences among various studies in terms of scope and impacts covered, methods used for the quantification of impacts and their monetization [27]. Frequent use of benefit-transfer also hinders the possibility of tracking down particular methodological assumptions and technicalities. In the valuation part, a profound difference results from the choice of metric for mortality valuation. In the US, the value of statistical life (VSL) is conventionally used for valuation of premature deaths, while in Europe (in particular in ExternE methodology since 2003) it is primarily estimated as change in life expectancy leading to Years of Life Lost (YOLLs). This difference is further exacerbated when these estimates are transferred for use in other countries or regions by using different adjustment factors for the local economic conditions (e.g., purchasing power *vs.* exchange rate) as well as when the values are transferred in relation to time. This often explains some relatively surprising results, such as the considerably low external cost estimates in China or India. On the one hand, less stringent emission control technologies are employed in these countries and larger populations tends to be exposed, but on the other hand the monetary valuation of impacts is adjusted for the prevailing economic conditions there.

In spite of these numerous differences, primary costing studies looking beyond the electricity generation phase tend to confirm that airborne (and greenhouse gas) emissions from power generation represent a major portion of estimated external costs. Nkambule and Blignaut's work [24] is an exception to this rule, but their estimates are not consistent with the damage function approach. Occupational impacts may also be important but more so in underground mines and in countries with a lack of or ineffective occupational safety laws.

## 3. METHODS

The approach used here for the quantification of external costs is based on a bottom-up Impact Pathway Approach (IPA) developed in the ExternE project series [10]. IPA allows the evaluation of impacts in a detailed spatial and technology resolution (local and regional meteorological conditions, population density, fuel specification, installed capacity, load hours, *etc.*). This analysis tracks all pollutant pathways from the point where it is emitted to the affected receptors (inhabitants, crops, natural ecosystems, buildings, *etc.*). The relationship between the increase in pollutant concentration and physical impacts on receptors is then determined by means of concentration-response functions (e.g., increase in asthma attacks as a consequence of a higher ambient air concentration of $NO_2$).

The IPA is conceptually compatible with Life Cycle Assessment (LCA), hence a site-specific IPA can principally be conducted for a full LCA (*i.e.*, cradle-to-grave). In spite of this overarching perspective, a large majority of IPA applications encompasses electricity generation in power plants only. Yet the operation part, *i.e.*, electricity production, is linked both to up-stream (transport, mining, construction, *etc.*) and down-stream (electricity transport, waste disposal, decommissioning of power plants, *etc.*) processes.

The choice of impact pathways is largely limited by the ability to establish a relationship between the environmental and/or health impact and the burden that causes that impact and the receptor bearing the burden. Air pollution is arguably the best established domain of environmental impacts (and on human health in particular). In spite of the vast knowledge on both the short and long term health effects of air pollution there are still great uncertainties. One of the most intriguing questions is whether there is sufficient evidence on the differential health effects of particulate matter (beyond differentiation to coarse and fine particles, $PM_{10}$ and $PM_{2.5}$ respectively) according to its components and sources (such as coal or biomass burning, road traffic, secondary particles formed by chemical reactions in the atmosphere). Particulate matter is a complex mixture including black/elemental carbon, secondary inorganic aerosols, and primary and secondary organic aerosols. While it is unlikely that all components have the same health effect potential, the evidence currently available remains insufficient to attribute different health damaging potentials to these components or as an Health Effects Institute's Review Panel of National Particle Component Toxicity (NPACT) Initiative studies stated "it is not likely to easily identify a single culprit PM component or source category (of PM toxicity)" [28]. This is a conclusion also shared by the WHO's Review of evidence on health aspects of air pollution (REVIHAAP) report [29] and recent statement by the UK Committee on the Medical Effects of Air Pollutants [30]. Another intriguing question concerns the direct health effects from $NO_2$ exposure and their additivity to effects attributed to particulate matter. The latest evidence gathered in the REVIHAAP review corroborates the finding that a direct effect remains after adjusting for other pollutants not only for a short-term effect but also for long term effects [29].

Our take on IPA consists of a combination of a local scale modelling of emissions from mining and regional scale modelling of impacts from coal burning in large combustion (heating and) power plants. The dispersion of dust emissions from coal mining, namely $PM_{2.5}$ and $PM_{10}$ fractions, was modelled using the Gaussian dispersion model ATEM (ATEM Ltd., Prague, Czech Republic) (a reference method for dispersion modelling in urban and rural areas pursuant to Czech air quality legislation) with detailed climatic and meteorological data. Annual concentrations of $PM_{2.5}$ and $PM_{10}$ were calculated as contributions from individual pollution sources in the mining area and related (mainly transport) activities. The dispersion of emissions of dust, $PM_{10}$, $PM_{2.5}$, $SO_2$, $NO_x$ ($NO_2$) and non-methane volatile organic compounds (NMVOC) from a set of 32 (33) large combustion plants and imposed health impacts was estimated via an EcoSenseWeb (Institute for Rational Use of Energy, University of Stuttgart, Germany) model, an integrated atmospheric dispersion and exposure assessment model developed in the ExternE project series. In EcoSenseWeb the transport of primary air pollutants on a local scale (100 km × 100 km around the pollution source) is modelled with the Industrial Source Complex Model, a Gaussian plume model, while the formation and deposition of secondary pollutants (secondary inorganic aerosols-sulphates and nitrates, and tropospheric ozone) on a European scale is done with Source-Receptor matrices parameterized with the European Monitoring and Evaluation Programme/Meteorological Synthesizing Centre's (EMEP/MSC-West) Eulerian dispersion model [31].

To accommodate our assessment with recently updated epidemiological evidence on the health risks of air pollution and a recommended set of concentration-response functions by the twin WHO projects REVIHAAP and HRAPIE (Health Risks of Air Pollution In Europe), we use a subset of concentration-response functions that are additive in their effects from the HRAPIE set compiled for the cost-benefit analysis of the EU Clean Air Package [32] instead of the default set of functions contained in EcoSenseWeb. Necessary background data for these updated concentration-response functions such as population age distribution or mortality and morbidity incidences were compiled from WHO, EUROSTAT and World Bank databases for all 64 countries distinguished in the EcoSenseWeb model (52 European, five North African, five Middle Eastern and two Asian post-Soviet countries), with a total population exceeding 1 billion people. In cases where no data were available we input the regional average or neighbouring country data if the latter seemed more appropriate.

The valuation of health impacts is based on a set of unit values updated for a cost-benefit analysis of the EU's Thematic Strategy on Air Pollution [33] with the following modifications—the valuation of mortality is pursued solely using the value of a life year (VOLY) derived by Desaigues *et al.* [34], *i.e.*, the lower range suggested by [33]. For infant mortality, the value used is the middle of the range suggested in [33]. This set of unit monetary values was primarily compiled as EU central values (see Table 1, last column), but as our assessment stretches beyond the EU, we opted to transfer these central values to country-specific values. We note that a convenient alternative would be to take a stance of a Czech decision-maker and value all the impacts based on Czech preferences. Somewhat surprisingly, however, the Czech decision-makers were concerned only with impacts incurred in the Czech Republic, arguing that they have to weight costs and benefits of the revision of mining limits on behalf of their (Czech) electorate. By using country-specific values we aimed to reflect individual preferences (albeit at the country-level only), *i.e.* what the valuation studies notoriously show that the valuation of a health impairment is driven by income/wealth and generally is higher in Western European than in Eastern European countries. This also reflects that the valuation of morbidity entails a loss of productivity and resource costs that differ among countries and (to some extent) in relation to the income level. The country-specific values were calculated by multiplying EU central values by the ratio of country *vs.* EU GDP per capita at purchasing parity power using data from the World Bank, in manner similar to the sensitivity analysis by [19]. Impacts attributed to a particular country were consequently valued using these country-specific values.

In addition, as our assessment stretches over a longer time period it means that economies will evolve as well and this will affect valuation of endpoints. Considerable empirical evidence shows that valuation of health (*i.e.*, willingness-to-pay) rises with income. As future income is unknown, we use as a proxy GDP growth for the 2015–2050 period from the integrated assessment World Induced Technical Change Hybrid (WITCH) model [35,36]. The WITCH model estimated GDP endogenously for 13 regions of the world assuming that economic growth follows the trajectory of greenhouse gas emissions evolving according to the Representative Concentration Pathways (RCP) mitigation scenario 4.5. We use GDP growth predicted for 4 regions, starting at 4.3% per year in Middle Eastern and North African countries, 3.7% in post-Soviet non-EU countries, 2.7% in Eastern European EU countries and 1.6% in Western European countries, and gradually declining to 2.3%, 2.3%, 1.5% and 1.3% in the respective regions at the end of the period. In addition, we use income elasticities of willingness to pay of 0.65, 0.68 and 0.3 for mortality, severe and mild health endpoints, respectively, in line with [37], to translate the assumed income rise to a valuation of health endpoints.

A list of health endpoints that appear in the concentration-response functions used along with their classification into two groups (a limited set consisting of functions quantified against larger epidemiological evidence and an extended set with additional functions) as well as EU central monetary values attributed to these endpoints is shown in Table 1.

**Table 1.** Evaluated health effects from air-borne pollution exposure and their monetary valuation.

| Pollutant | Endpoint | In Limited Set | Monetary Value (€$_{2014}$) |
|---|---|---|---|
| | **Long-Term Exposure** | | |
| $PM_{2.5}$ | Adult mortality (loss of life expectancy, YOLLs) | yes | 65,066 |
| $PM_{10}$ | Post-neonatal infant mortality | no | 2,762,767 |
| $PM_{10}$ | Incidence of chronic bronchitis in adults | no | 60,443 |
| $PM_{10}$ | Prevalence of bronchitis in children | no | 663 |
| | **Short-Term Exposure** | | |
| $PM_{2.5}$ | Restricted activity days | no | 104 |
| $PM_{2.5}$ | Work days lost | no | 147 |
| $PM_{2.5}$ | Hospital admissions, respiratory diseases | yes | 2503 |
| $PM_{2.5}$ | Hospital admissions, cardiovascular diseases | yes | 2503 |
| $PM_{10}$ | Incidence of asthma symptoms in asthmatic children | no | 47 |
| $O_3$ | Adult mortality (YOLLs) | yes | 65,066 |
| $O_3$ | Hospital admissions, respiratory diseases | yes | 2503 |
| $O_3$ | Hospital admissions, cardiovascular diseases | yes | 2503 |
| $O_3$ | Minor restricted activity days | no | 47 |

Note: YOLLs stands for years of life lost. Source: adapted from Holland [32,33].

# 4. DATA AND SCENARIOS

## 4.1. Scenarios

In order to reflect the options and preferences for the use of coal beyond the mining limits at the Bilina and CSA mines, four scenarios were assessed (see also Figure 2 above). The status quo scenario (Variant 1) assumes the mining limits will remain unchanged and mining will be wound down at the Bilina mine by 2037 and at the CSA mine by 2024. In Variant 2 the mining limits are abolished at the Bilina mine only, resulting in continued extraction at this mine beyond 2050, but at the same time mining at the CSA mine will conclude by 2024. In Variant 3 the mining limits are abolished at the Bilina mine and partially at the CSA mine also, resulting in an extension of mining in the latter case by 10 years until 2034. Finally, in Variant 4 the mining limits are completely abolished at both mines and both keep operating beyond 2050.

## 4.2. Emissions from Coal Mining

The dominant sources of emissions from strip mining activities are topsoil (overburden) removal and coal mining with dragline excavators, overburden replacement by conveyors, transportation of coal to a coal preparation plant (using conveyors) and the loading of coal onto railcars and trucks. In all variants considered the overburden is deposited in the mining pit and therefore we do not consider any other impacts from waste disposal although in different settings these might be important.

At the Bilina mine it is expected that two overburden and two coal excavators will be used for the whole period until 2050 and these excavators are modelled as two line sources (they move continually over a year on the mining front). Conveyor belts are located around the southern edge of the mine and will be extended as the mining proceeds westwards and the emissions are estimated based on the length of the belts and the operating hours. Overburden deposition (spoil piles) will move from the eastern side of the mine as the mining proceeds by a corresponding distance westwards. Three "snapshots" (the years 2015, 2035 and 2048) were chosen for detailed modelling of mining activities at the Bilina mine and its impacts on the surrounding area comprising over 93,000 inhabitants. Emissions of dust were modelled upon annual extraction of about 9, 6, 4 million tonnes of coal and 57, 36, 12 million $m^3$ of overburden in 2015, 2035 and 2048, respectively.

At the CSA mine the mining line stretches in a north-easterly direction and the conveyor belts are located on the south-eastern edge of the mine. Similarly as at the Bilina mine, no external deposition of extracted overburden is planned. At the CSA mine, the three "snapshots" chosen for detailed modelling of mining activities are slightly different—corresponding to planned mining in 2015, 2030 and 2050. At this mine, the three mining variants considered differ in the distribution of the affected population, and in the two variants based on a revision of the mining limits a relocation of inhabitants is assumed to take place around 2020—this would affect about 800 inhabitants of Horni Jiretin in the event of a partial abolition of the limits or about 2150 inhabitants of Horni Jiretin and Cernice in the event of a full abolition of the mining limits at the CSA mine. Emissions of dust were modelled for annual extraction of about 3.4, 6 and 6 million tonnes of coal and 34.5, 34.5 and 17 million $m^3$ of overburden in 2015, 2030 and 2050, respectively.

The main characteristics of the current mining activities and related emissions were derived from respective environmental impact assessment (EIA) documentations. Emissions from transfers of both coal and overburden between conveyors are related to the total volume of extracted material and its moisture content; the average moisture was taken from the US EPA AP-42 Compilation of Air Pollutant Emission Factors [38]. Coal expedition is modelled as an area source, including vehicle movements, accounting for both direct exhaust emissions and dust resuspension from vehicle movements. For dust resuspension by wind, a methodology developed for the Usti Regional Authority is used [39]. As not all emissions from mining and related activities enter ambient air (*i.e.*, do not get beyond the mining area) the estimated emissions are factored by reduction coefficients suggested in [39]. The reduction coefficients account for horizontal and vertical distance from the mine edge and days with rain and snow. Estimated $PM_{10}$ emissions from coal mining and related activities amount to about 250 tonnes per year ($PM_{2.5}$ about 75 tonnes per year) at the Bilina mine [40]. At the CSA mine estimated $PM_{10}$ emissions vary—generally depending on the volume of extraction—between 125 tonnes (year 2015) and 223 tonnes (year 2050), and similarly $PM_{2.5}$ emissions vary between 37 and 67 tonnes per year (in 2015 and 2050, respectively) [40].

## 4.3. Emissions from Heat and Power Generation

In a bottom-up approach such as IPA, estimating the health impacts of coal use needs a precise allocation where (in what facility) the coal extracted at the Bilina and/or CSA mine is going to be used. Circumventing a complex energy system optimization, we chose to maintain the current allocation of coal from the two mines and to restrict our assessment to large stationary combustion plants only. The latter limitation is mostly a practical one because modelling emission dispersion from residential coal use was not thought to be feasible in such detail that would correspond to dispersion modelling from large combustion sources. The location of large combustion sources—power plants and combined heating and power plants (along with the location of the two mines)—is shown in Figure 3. In total, 33 sources are considered, 31 are currently in operation and a new power plant in Ledvice (to be set in operation in 2016) and in Pocerady (a future power plant relevant only in the variant relating to the total abolition of mining limits from 2041 onwards). The allocation of coal extracted at the Bilina and CSA mines under respective mining limit variants to these power (and heating) plants was proportional up to their full capacity.

The emissions of dust, $PM_{10}$, $PM_{2.5}$, $SO_2$, $NO_x$ ($NO_2$) and NMVOC for these 33 plants were established for every year until 2050 (or their expected lifetime if prior to 2050) in such a manner that it reflects both their actual emissions and the envisaged tightening of future regulation of large combustion plant (LCP) emissions. Hence for 2015 the emissions were derived from 2014 data obtained from the Emission and Stationary Sources Registry maintained by the Czech Hydrometeorological Institute and adapted to planned coal consumption ("actual" emissions). For the 2016–2020 period, the emission ceilings set in the Transitional National Plan of the Czech Republic [41] were used if the "actual" emissions were higher. In the same vein, the upper limit values from the BREF Draft 2 version [42] were attributed for the post-2020 period.

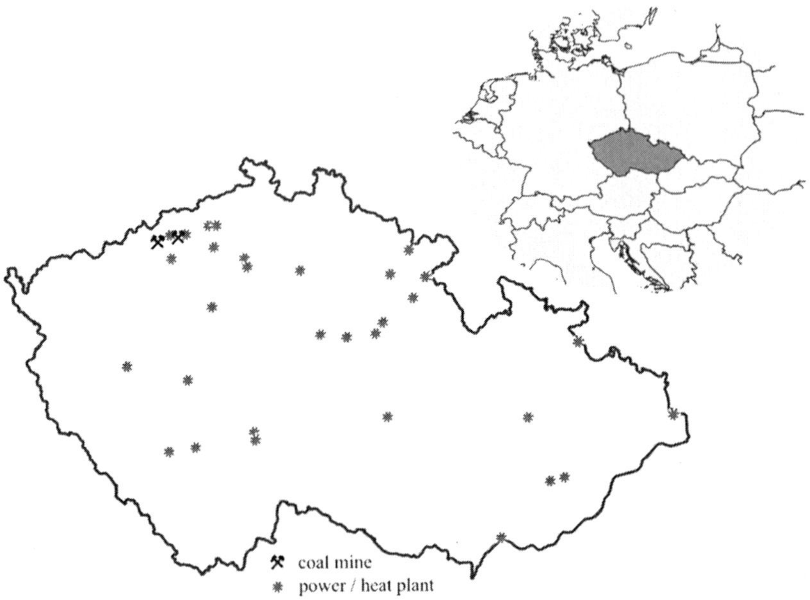


**Figure 3.** Location of the two coal mines and 33 power and heating plants.

These emission characteristics refer to (or close to) the full load operation of these LCPs, but the proportional allocation of coal from Bilina and CSA mines—particularly in the variant regarding maintained mining limits—results in substantial shortages of coal from the two mines for our set of LCPs. To avoid the need to address the series of resulting pitfalls (unrealistic operation conditions leading to higher emissions, unrealistically low flue gas volumes spread to lower troposphere layers affecting dispersion modelling, *etc.*), a full load of LCPs was modelled and only the share of emissions proportional to the volume of coal originating from Bilina and/or CSA was then used for a subsequent calculation of the health impacts. The additional coal was assumed to possess the average parameters of the remaining brown coal mined in the Czech Republic. A sketch of total estimated emissions from selected LCPs for the analysed period 2015–2050 is depicted in Figure 4.

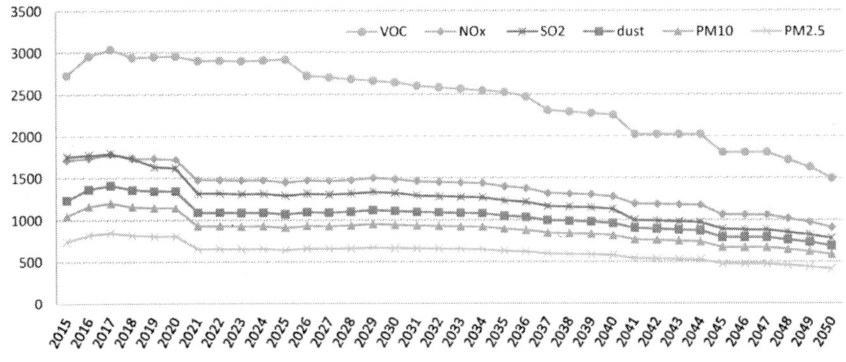


**Figure 4.** Modelled annual emissions from 33 large combustion plants in full load operation (in tonnes, except for $SO_2$ and $NO_x$ in tonnes/10).

# 5. RESULTS

## 5.1. Health Impacts from Coal Mining

The highest annual average concentrations of $PM_{10}$ attributable to coal mining at Bilina can be as high as 30 μg/m$^3$ locally around overburden and coal transfers, but decrease rapidly with distance. In the most exposed inhabited area (parts of 4 municipalities closest to the mine's borders) the annual contributions to $PM_{10}$ concentration levels are at most about 1–2 μg/m$^3$ and about 0.25–1.0 μg/m$^3$ in adjacent settlements of a further 4 municipalities. Annual concentrations of suspended $PM_{2.5}$ are estimated at considerably lower levels, *i.e.*, peaking at about 1.5 μg/m$^3$ at the mine's northern edge and decreasing rapidly with distance. The increases in adjacent settlements are relatively small, around 0.1–0.4 μg/m$^3$ in the four closest municipalities and below 0.1 μg/m$^3$ in more remote municipalities.

Modelled annual concentrations of $PM_{10}$ and $PM_{2.5}$ attributable to coal mining at the CSA mine are generally somewhat lower compared to the Bilina mine, the highest annual $PM_{10}$ concentrations in inhabited areas are at most 1.6 μg/m$^3$ in 2015 and 1.5 μg/m$^3$ in 2030 and 2050, and the highest annual $PM_{2.5}$ concentrations in inhabited areas are (mostly irrespective of variant and year) below 0.4 μg/m$^3$.

Using concentration-response functions defined for $PM_{10}$ and $PM_{2.5}$ exposures and the population exposed to respective concentrations, attributable cases of respective health effects were estimated for the "snapshot" years. These estimates were then interpolated over the whole 2015–2050 period (effectively until 2037 in the variant where mining limits are kept in place at Bilina, and until 2024 in the variants with the mining limits kept in place at CSA or until 2034 in the event of the partial limit abolition at the CSA mine) while taking account of the forecast volume of coal extraction (*i.e.*, assuming a linear correlation between coal and overburden extraction and related emissions) and population resettlement at the CSA mine in Variants 3 and 4.

Table 2 details the estimated health effects from the mining of coal for both variants at the Bilina mine and for the three variants considered for the CSA mine up to 2050. In short, were the mining limits to be repealed at Bilina the health impacts will more than double, *i.e.*, an increase from 121 to 272 attributable asthma episodes in children or from 2400 to 5600 attributable restricted activity days. This on the other hand more or less corresponds to an almost doubling of total coal extraction (from 135 million tonnes within the limits to 258 million tonnes, including the coal beyond the limits).

In the event of the partial abolition of the mining limits at the CSA mine, the estimated health impacts will roughly double compared to maintaining the mining limits. In the event of the total abolition of mining limits the health impacts will be approximately 5.5 times higher compared to the situation where limits would remain in place. Again, this roughly corresponds to an increase in volume of coal extraction (from 31 million tonnes within the limits to a total of 75 million tonnes in the event of the partial revision of mining limits to a total of 177 million tonnes until 2050 in the event of the total abolition of the mining limits).

**Table 2.** Health effects from mining of coal at Bilina and CSA mines in 2015–2050 period.

| Health Outcome | Unit | Bilina Mine | | CSA Mine | | |
|---|---|---|---|---|---|---|
| | | Within Limits | Limits Abolished | Within Limits | Partial Abolition | Total Abolition |
| Infant mortality | Cases | 0.003 | 0.007 | 0.0003 | 0.0006 | 0.0017 |
| Chronic bronchitis in adults | New cases | 4.38 | 10.4 | 0.4 | 0.9 | 2.6 |
| Children asthma symptoms | Asthma episodes | 121.1 | 271.5 | 12 | 25 | 68 |
| Bronchitis in children | New cases | 14 | 30. 9 | 1 | 3 | 8 |
| Adult mortality | YOLLs | 27.5 | 65.2 | 3 | 6 | 16 |
| Cardiovascular hospital admissions | Cases | 1.1 | 2.58 | 0.1 | 0.2 | 0.6 |
| Respiratory hospital admissions | Cases | 0.1 | 0.23 | 0.01 | 0.02 | 0.06 |
| Work days lost | Days | 1031 | 2327 | 105 | 216 | 582 |
| Restricted activity days | Days | 2396 | 5605 | 246 | 511 | 1389 |

Note: YOLLs stands for Years of Life Lost.

On a per tonne (of extracted coal) basis the health impacts of mining at the Bilina mine are more than twice as high as health impacts of mining at the CSA mine. This is due to the denser population in the settlements adjacent to the Bilina mine and a planned relocation of inhabitants from Horni Jiretin in the event of the abolition of the coal mine limits at the CSA mine.

Table 3 summarizes the estimated health impacts of all four mining limit revision variants put forward by the Ministry of Industry and Trade.

**Table 3.** Estimated health impacts of mining limit revision variants in the 2015–2050 period.

| Health Outcome | Unit | Variant 1 | Variant 2 | Variant 3 | Variant 4 |
|---|---|---|---|---|---|
| | | Within Limits | Limit Lifted at BILINA | Limits Lifted at Bilina and CSA Partially | Both Limits Lifted |
| Infant mortality | Cases | 0.0033 | 0.0072 | 0.0075 | 0.0086 |
| Chronic bronchitis in adults | New cases | 4.8 | 10.8 | 11.3 | 13.0 |
| Children asthma symptoms | Asthma episodes | 133 | 284 | 297 | 339 |
| Bronchitis in children | Cases | 15 | 32 | 34 | 39 |
| Adult mortality | YOLLs | 30 | 68 | 71 | 81 |
| Cardiovascular hospital admissions | Cases | 1.2 | 2.7 | 2.8 | 3.2 |
| Respiratory hospital admissions | Cases | 0.11 | 0.24 | 0.25 | 0.29 |
| Work days lost | Days | 1136 | 2431 | 2543 | 2908 |
| Restricted activity days | Days | 2642 | 5851 | 6116 | 6994 |

Note: YOLLs stands for Years of Life Lost.

## 5.2. Monetized Impacts from Coal Mining

To establish monetized health impacts from coal mining the estimated physical health impacts are multiplied by unit costs. The latter are adjusted at the Czech level to EU GDP per capita (in purchasing parity power) and predicted GDP growth in the 2015–2050 period as all the impacts are incurred in the Czech territory. The estimated health damages are presented in Table 4 for the respective mines, and in Table 5 for the respective revised mining limit variant. Table 4 clearly confirms elevated impacts at the Bilina mine compared to the CSA mine.

**Table 4.** Monetized impacts from future mining variants at the Bilina and CSA mines in 2015–2050 period (thousands of euros).

| Health Outcome | Bilina Mine | | CSA Mine | | |
|---|---|---|---|---|---|
| | Within Limits | Limits Abolished | Within Limits | Partial Abolition | Full Abolition |
| Infant mortality | 9.2 | 25.1 | 0.8 | 2.0 | 7.0 |
| Chronic bronchitis in adults | 291.6 | 842.6 | 26.9 | 64.3 | 228.6 |
| Children asthma symptoms | 6.2 | 16.9 | 0.6 | 1.3 | 4.7 |
| Bronchitis in children | 10.1 | 26.9 | 0.9 | 2.2 | 7.6 |
| Adult mortality | 1972 | 5687 | 185 | 439 | 1552 |
| Cardiovascular hospital admissions | 3.0 | 8.6 | 0.3 | 0.7 | 2.4 |
| Respiratory hospital admissions | 0.3 | 0.8 | 0.0 | 0.1 | 0.2 |
| Work days lost | 165.8 | 452.4 | 15.4 | 36.3 | 126.3 |
| Restricted activity days | 273.9 | 778.5 | 25.6 | 60.7 | 213.7 |
| Total (limited set of impacts) | 1976 | 5696 | 185 | 440 | 1555 |
| Total (extended set of impacts) | 2732 | 7839 | 255 | 607 | 2143 |

**Table 5.** Monetized impacts by revised mining limit variants in the 2015–2050 period (thousands of euros).

| Health Outcome | Variant 1 | Variant 2 | Variant 3 | Variant 4 |
|---|---|---|---|---|
| Infant mortality | 10.0 | 26.0 | 27.1 | 32.1 |
| Chronic bronchitis in adults | 318.5 | 869.5 | 906.8 | 1071.2 |
| Children asthma symptoms | 6.8 | 17.4 | 18.2 | 21.6 |
| Bronchitis in children | 11.0 | 27.8 | 29.1 | 34.5 |
| Adult mortality | 2157 | 5871 | 6126 | 7239 |
| Cardiovascular hospital admissions | 3.3 | 8.9 | 9.3 | 11.0 |
| Respiratory hospital admissions | 0.3 | 0.8 | 0.8 | 1.0 |
| Work days lost | 181.2 | 467.8 | 488.6 | 578.7 |
| Restricted activity days | 299.5 | 804.1 | 839.2 | 992.3 |
| Total (limited set of impacts) | 2161 | 5881 | 6137 | 7251 |
| Total (extended set of impacts) | 2988 | 8094 | 8446 | 9982 |

Damage is reported both for a limited set of impacts and for an extended set of impacts. The vast majority of impacts is represented by adult (chronic) mortality, making over 99% of monetized impacts quantified in the limited set and over 72% of impacts in the extended set of impacts.

### *5.3. Health Impacts from Coal Use*

Projected emissions of pollutants per facility were plugged into EcoSenseWeb model. The resulting health impacts were recalculated to reflect the subset of additive concentration-response functions suggested by the HRAPIE project. No direct impact of $NO_2$ emissions were estimated, however, but secondary inorganic aerosols (including nitrates) are evaluated in the same manner as primary particulate matter.

Total health impacts from the use of coal from the Bilina and CSA mines by revised mining limit variant are shown inTable 6. Overall, the estimated attributable health impacts are substantial, including tens of thousands years of life lost both from chronic and acute exposure to air pollution, several thousands of new cases of chronic bronchitis in adults, tens of thousands asthma symptoms in asthmatic children and millions of milder health outcomes such as restricted activity days and days of work loss. The assessment accounts not only for impact of primary emissions released from large combustion sources, but source-receptor matrices also provide estimates of the contribution of released emissions (mainly $NO_x$, $SO_2$and VOCs) to secondary pollutants (ozone, inorganic aerosols/particles) and their health impacts. These secondary particles are the main culprits of estimated health impacts, responsible for almost 95% of the total impact from particulate mass.

**Table 6.** Health effects from the use of coal from Bilina and CSA by revised mining limit variant in the 2015–2050 period.

| Health Outcome | Unit | Variant 1 | Variant 2 | Variant 3 | Variant 4 |
|---|---|---|---|---|---|
| Chronic mortality | YOLLs | 40,797 | 68,465 | 80,136 | 106,930 |
| Post-neonatal infant mortality | Cases | 6 | 10 | 12 | 16 |
| Chronic bronchitis | New cases | 3062 | 5142 | 6022 | 8048 |
| Bronchitis in children | Cases | 9996 | 16,784 | 19,657 | 26,263 |
| Acute mortality | Yolls | 304 | 514 | 604 | 820 |
| Asthma symptoms in asthmatic children | New cases | 109,958 | 184,787 | 216,598 | 289,990 |
| Cardiovascular hospital admissions | Cases | 3308 | 5567 | 6524 | 8754 |
| Respiratory hospital admissions | Cases | 490 | 825 | 967 | 1301 |
| Minor restricted activity days | Days | 1,285,065 | 2,177,167 | 2,556,027 | 3,470,902 |
| Restricted activity days | Days | 5,639,809 | 9,464,720 | 11,079,845 | 14,786,501 |
| Work loss days | Days | 2,266,459 | 3,811,767 | 4,470,263 | 5,996,024 |

Note: YOLLs stands for Years of Life Lost.

In order to illustrate the temporal distribution of health impacts by the respective variants the following Figure 5 depicts mortality impacts from chronic exposure to $PM_{2.5}$ (both primary and secondary particles) in terms of life years lost.

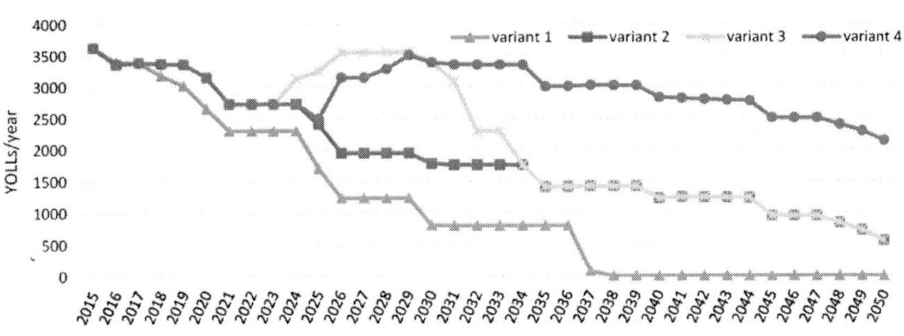


**Figure 5.** Chronic mortality impacts from exposure to fine particulates by variant (YOLLs per year).

## 5.4. Monetized Impacts from Coal Use

To arrive at monetized health impacts from coal use we multiply the estimated physical health impacts by unit costs that were localized to country specific values and adjusted for regionally specific predicted GDP growth, *i.e.,* differentiating spatial and temporal differences in the monetary valuation of impacts.

The total monetized health impacts from coal use in large (heating and) power plants are shown in Table 7. The estimates are shown for the four variants and two alternative sets of impacts considered, *i.e.,* either limited set impacts only or extended set impacts (see Table 1 for endpoints contained in the limited set). The limited set of impacts gives estimated monetary damages ranging from 2.7 billion euros in Variant 1 to 7.8 billion euros in Variant 4. Damage from Variants 2 and 3 lies within this range with 4.8 billion euros in Variant 2 and 5.6 billion euros in Variant 3. Over 90% of these monetized impacts are due to chronic mortality from exposure to secondary particles. Using the extended set these impacts are estimated at 3.9 (Variant 1), 6.9 (Variant 2), 8 (Variant 3) and 11.1 (Variant 4) billion euros for the whole 2015–2050 period. Irrespective of the variant assessed, around 65% of these impacts are due to chronic mortality. Additional impacts in the extended set make about 30% of total estimated damages.

**Table 7.** Total monetized health impacts from coal use in 2015–2050 period (in million euros).

| Health Impacts by Compounds | Variant 1 | Variant 2 | Variant 3 | Variant 4 | Variant 1 | Variant 2 | Variant 3 | Variant 4 |
|---|---|---|---|---|---|---|---|---|
| | Limited Set | | | | Extended Set | | | |
| **Mortality** | | | | | | | | |
| Primary particles | 143 | 256 | 300 | 418 | 143 | 256 | 300 | 418 |
| Secondary particles | 2510 | 4472 | 5253 | 7281 | 2510 | 4472 | 5253 | 7281 |
| Ozone | 19 | 34 | 40 | 56 | 19 | 34 | 40 | 56 |
| **Morbidity** | | | | | | | | |
| Primary particles | 0.4 | 0.6 | 0.7 | 1.0 | 62 | 107 | 125 | 172 |
| Secondary particles | 6 | 11 | 13 | 18 | 1079 | 1875 | 2200 | 3005 |
| Ozone | 3 | 6 | 7 | 9 | 63 | 109 | 128 | 177 |
| **Total** | 2682 | 4779 | 5613 | 7783 | 3875 | 6852 | 8047 | 11,109 |

The emissions released from the modelled large Czech power plants contribute to transboundary pollution as they are emitted high above the ground and thus the impacts are exported well beyond Czech borders. The regional distribution of monetized impacts is shown in Figure 6. These estimates suggest that only slightly over 10% of total damage is incurred by the Czech population, and that its two larger neighbouring countries, Germany and Poland, both bear a higher share of the damage, 31% and 13%, respectively. The remainder of the EU countries bears a further 35% of monetized impacts and the last 10% of monetized impacts is borne by populations in all non-EU European, five North African, five Middle Eastern and two Asian ex-Soviet countries.

## 5.5. Total Monetized Impacts from Coal Mining and Use

The final step in this assessment lies in combining the estimated health impacts from coal mining and coal use. This summation is provided in Table 8, but the results do not differ from the tables on the impacts of coal use. The overwhelming majority (>99%) of quantified health impacts originates from coal use; only between 0.07% and 0.12% of the total sum for respective health impacts is attributed to coal mining.

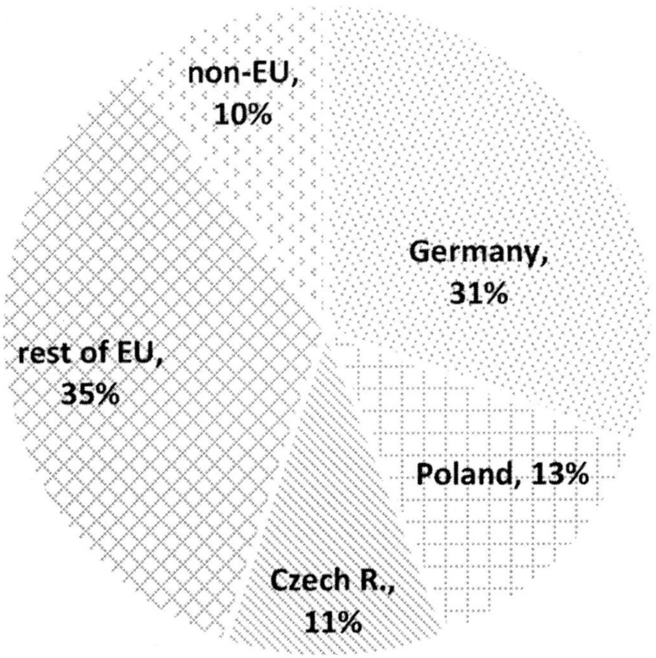


**Figure 6.** Regional distribution of monetized health impacts. Notes: "rest of EU countries" encompasses the remaining 25 EU member countries and "other countries" comprises all remaining European non-EU countries, North African and Middle East countries.

Finally, to estimate the net consequences of mining limit revision the results should be related to Variant 1 taken as the status quo. The revision of coal mining limits in Variant 2 (*i.e.*, abolishing mining limits at the Bilina coal mine only) increases the estimated health impacts by about 2–3 billion euro or 77% (virtually irrespective to whether the limited or extended set of impacts is used). If the third variant is pursued (*i.e.*, limits revised at Bilina and partially at the CSA mine), the monetized health impacts will be higher by 3–4 billion euro, or in relative terms more than twice as high (+108%). Finally, if the limits are abolished at both the Bilina and CSA mines the health impacts will reach 5–7 billion euro or almost triple the price (+187%) compared to the status quo.

**Table 8.** Health impacts from both coal mining and use for energy generation over 2015–2050 period (in million euros).

| Health Impacts by Phase | Variant 1 | Variant 2 | Variant 3 | Variant 4 |
|---|---|---|---|---|
| | | Mining | | |
| limited set of impacts | 2 | 6 | 6 | 7 |
| extended set of impacts | 3 | 8 | 8 | 10 |
| | | Use | | |
| limited set of impacts | 2682 | 4779 | 5613 | 7783 |
| extended set of impacts | 3875 | 6852 | 8047 | 11,109 |
| | | Total | | |
| limited set of impacts | 2684 | 4785 | 5619 | 7790 |
| extended set of impacts | 3878 | 6860 | 8055 | 11,119 |

# 6. DISCUSSION AND CONCLUSIONS

Over the last decade energy policies in most EU countries have faced several substantial challenges, from climate change targets for limiting $CO_2$ emissions and stabilizing its atmospheric concentration, to energy security, most frequently triggered by interrupted gas deliveries from the Russian Federation, to an increased uptake of renewable energy sources, raising the fears about the stability of energy systems. Among those many issues and the discussion started by the process of updating the National Energy Policy revealed an apparent conflict over the coal mining limits in the Northern Bohemia Coal Basin. To enrich such a discussion, this study makes use of the impact-pathway approach to estimate the health impacts of coal extraction and use for electricity and heat generation in the Czech Republic. Unlike previous studies, a detailed modelling exercise was conducted to estimate impacts from dust originating from coal extraction activities, along with a comprehensive estimation of the damage to health from electricity (and heat) generation in large combustion plants.

We find that lifting of the mining limits is likely to lead to damage worth several billions of euros over the 2015–2050 period. If the limits are lifted at the Bilina mine only, the related damage to health from coal extraction and use will be in the range of 2–3 billion euros. If the limits are revised fully at the Bilina mine and partially at the CSA mine, this will lead to damage of about 3–4 billion euros. Finally, if both mining limits are lifted the related damages from extraction and use will more than double to 5–7 billion euros. The major part of the damage (~55%) will be borne by the German, Polish and Czech population. This last finding, *i.e.*, that a substantial share of the impact is "exported" well beyond Czech borders, is somewhat startling, but a similar result is reported by Brandt and colleagues [43], who estimated that total health-related external costs from all Danish emissions in Europe account for 4.9 billion euros per year while in Denmark for only 817 million euros per year, *i.e.*, about 17% of the total.

From the perspective of international environmental policy, one should ask how this aligns with the fact that the Czech Republic is a contractual party to both the Convention on Long-Range Transboundary Air Pollution ("CLRTAP"), as well as the Convention on Environmental Impact Assessment in Transboundary Context ("Espoo Convention") that aim to limit transboundary pollution and provide the means for participating in impact assessments of projects capable of affecting the environment beyond borders. In short, neither of the two treaties will empower neighbouring countries to voice their concerns about those potential impacts on their populations if mining beyond the current limits takes place. Perhaps the only exception would be if a new power plant were planned (e.g., a new plant in Pocerady as envisioned in our Variant 4) then a neighbouring country can take part in an environmental impact assessment as mandated by the Espoo Convention.

Another finding is that airborne pollution impacts from electricity and heat generation vastly outnumber impacts from dust emitted during coal mining. This is roughly in line with previous studies that considered the damage to health from airborne emissions from the coal cycle, including the mining stage [11,19], although the level of detail largely differs. While it is possible to compare impacts from mining and electricity generation directly, as we use dispersion models (although accommodated to a spatial range of dispersion), and the same CR functions and monetary values, one should be aware that the much higher impacts from power generation take place over a much larger space. Coal mining analysis focuses on short range effects only because (based *i.e.*, on EIA documentation) dust is by and large a dominant emission from mining activities. These emissions are typically emitted just above ground level when leaving the mining pit. Hence dust concentrations due to mining activities are significantly elevated in a restricted area within and closely adjacent to the mine pit only, *i.e.*, more than 1 μg/m$^3$ increase in annual $PM_{10}$ concentration affects no more than 1000 residents there. In this respect, we did not account for the possible negative health effects of unfavourable meteorological conditions that may lead to temporarily elevated dust concentrations possibly affecting a greater population for a shorter period. In addition, it should be noted that the impact of mining may not be fully captured as a dominant constituent of dust emissions from mining activities is coarse fraction ($PM_{10}$ contribution is roughly 20 times higher than $PM_{2.5}$), but health effects that usually dominate in the quantification of impacts are linked to $PM_{2.5}$ (adult mortality, work days lost, restricted activity days).

The picture is different in the case of power generation where emissions are released from high stacks usually at about 100+ m above the ground. The stack height is not the only reason for dealing with emissions from power generation on a regional scale however. An even more important role is played by $NO_x$ and $SO_2$ emissions acting as precursors of secondary particles and ozone, as these transformations take place in the atmosphere on a larger scale than usually occurs with the dispersion of primary particles. This means that impacts from exposure not only take place over much larger area, but also in different forms—not only as exposure to primary pollutants, but also secondary pollutants—ozone, sulphates and nitrates—originating from chemical transformations in the atmosphere. And in fact these latter ones, sulphates and nitrates, are those which account for about 95% of total health impacts. This finding also projects a note of uncertainty into the calculation, as the current scientific evidence considers particulate matter components at the respective fraction level (*i.e.,* components of $PM_{10}$ or $PM_{2.5}$) to be equally harmful, but this evidence is relatively disperse and may be revised with more epidemiological knowledge to come.

Apart from these explicit limitations in our study (stemming from the disregarding of other than airborne pollution, and other coal cycle phases than coal mining and power generation) a huge legacy of environmental burden lies in Northern Bohemia that profoundly affects the quality of life of people living in the region. This encompasses not only the well documented long-term impacts on health [44], but also other dimensions of wellbeing that the damage function approach can barely capture. As anecdotal evidence of a compromised liveability we note that this region hosts the highest number of socially excluded localities and has the lowest prices of residential housing among all regions of the Czech Republic. These latter effects indicate a much broader range of—often interlinked—social and environmental burden imposed by coal mining and related activities on the region that existing costing studies are usually not able to encompass. Indeed, several studies already have pointed out to the wider social and psychological effects of mining (and post-mining) associated with environmental and health inequalities in Appalachia [45], Australia [46,47] and in Canada [48]. This is definitely an interesting topic for future research on environmental/social justice, as well as the long-term perspective for the region and people in the post-carbon future when the mine will close.

The policy lesson from this external cost quantification exercise (and environmental concerns in general) is rather mixed. In spite of the health impacts documented here, and even more importantly in facing climate change mitigation imperatives, the Czech government decided in late 2015 on revising the mining limits at the Bilina mine, *i.e.*, pursuing Variant 2. The timing of this decision paradoxically coincides with negotiation of COP21's Paris Agreement, where the Czech Republic as a part of EU committed itself to reduce greenhouse gas emissions by at least 40% by 2030. The key argument for such a decision was the need to secure the coal for the heating sector, but at the same time the national energy utility CEZ J.S.C. (operating the Bilina mine through its subsidiary) is about to set in operation a new supercritical power plant in Ledvice in the vicinity of the mine. In addition, the Ministry of Industry and Trade was instructed to analyse the need for brown coal as a part of periodical review of NEP in 2020, and in the event of substantial failures in achieving the goals of NEP2015 (*i.e.*, an increase in renewables, nuclear and energy savings) the possibility looms that the mining limits at the CSA mine may be revised as well.

## ACKNOWLEDGMENTS

The analysis reported in this article was supported by the Technology Agency of the Czech Republic, project No. TD020183. Scenarios and respective data were collected and developed under a service contract for the Ministry of Industry and Trade of the Czech Republic. The collaboration of the consultancy ATEM Ltd. on the development of scenarios, emission balances and dispersion modelling of dust emissions from coal mining within the service contract is gratefully acknowledged. Responsibility for errors and omissions remains with the authors.

## AUTHOR CONTRIBUTIONS

Vojtěch Máca contributed to the study design and data acquisition, developed the impact and damage assessment of coal mining, and drafted the manuscript. Jan Melichar contributed to the study design and data acquisition, developed the impact and damage assessment of coal use, and revised the manuscript.

## CONFLICTS OF INTEREST

The authors declare no conflict of interest.

## REFERENCES

1. National Energy Policy of the Czech Republic; Ministry of Industry and Trade of the Czech Republic: Prague, Czech Republic, 2015.
2. Government Resolution of 30 October 1991 No. 444 on the Report on Territorial Environmental Limits for Brown Coal Mining and Energy Generation in the North Bohemian Brown Coal Basin; Government of the Czech Republic: Prague, Czech Republic, 1991. (In Czech)

3. Ministry of Industry and Trade of the Czech Republic. Analysis of the Supply Needs of Brown Coal for Heating with Respect to the Proposed Options of Territorial Environmental Limits Revision; Ministry of Industry and Trade of the Czech Republic: Prague, Czech Republic, 2015. (In Czech)

4. Communication from the Commission—A Framework Strategy for a Resilient Energy Union with a Forward-Looking Climate Change Policy, COM (2015) 80 Final; European Commission: Brussels, Belgium, 2015.

5. Gerbaulet, C.; Egerer, J.; Oei, P.-Y.; Paeper, J.; Hirschhausen, C. Die Zukunft der Braunkohle in Deutschland im Rahmen der Energiewende; Deutsches Institut für Wirtschaftsforschung: Berlin, Germany, 2012.

6. Burtraw, D.; Krupnick, A.; Sampson, G.; Isaac, W.; Chu, J.; Beasley, B. The True Cost of Electric Power: An Inventory of Methodologies to Support Future Decisionmaking in Comparing the Cost and Competitiveness of Electricity Generation Technologies; Resources for the Future: Washington, DC, USA, 2012.

7. Rowe, R.D.; Lang, C.M.; Chestnut, L.G. Critical factors in computing externalities for electricity resources. Resour. Energy Econ. 1996, 18, 363–394.

8. Estimating Externalities of Coal Fuel Cycles. Report No. 3 on the External Costs and Benefits of Fuel Cycles: A Study by the US Department of Energy and the Commission of the European Communities; McGraw-Hill/Utility Data Institute: Washington, DC, USA, 1995.

9. National Research Council. Hidden Costs of Energy: Unpriced Consequences of Energy Production and Use; National Academies: Washington, DC, USA, 2009.

10. ExternE: Externalities of Energy. Methodology 2005 Update; Bickel, P., Friedrich, R., Eds.; Office for Official Publications of the European Communities: Luxembourg, Luxembourg, 2004.

11. ExternE: Externalities of Energy. Vol. 10: National Implementation; Aróstegui, M., Leal, J., Linares, P., Sáez, R., Varela, M., Eds.; Office for Official Publications of the European Communities: Luxembourg, Luxembourg, 1999.

12. Hendryx, M.; Ahern, M.M.; Nurkiewicz, T.R. Hospitalization patterns associated with Appalachian coal mining. J. Toxicol. Environ. Health A 2007, 70, 2064–2070.

13. Esch, L.; Hendryx, M. Chronic cardiovascular disease mortality in mountaintop mining areas of central Appalachian states. J. Rural Health 2011, 27, 350–357.

14. Hendryx, M.; Zullig, K.J. Higher coronary heart disease and heart attack morbidity in Appalachian coal mining regions. Prev. Med. 2009, 49, 355–359.

15. Ahern, M.; Hendryx, M. Cancer mortality rates in appalachian mountaintop coal mining areas. J. Environ. Occup. Sci.2012, 1, 63–70.

16. Hendryx, M.; O'Donnell, K.; Horn, K. Lung cancer mortality is elevated in coal-mining areas of Appalachia. Lung Cancer 2008, 62, 1–7.

17. Ahern, M.M.; Hendryx, M.; Conley, J.; Fedorko, E.; Ducatman, A.; Zullig, K.J. The association between mountaintop mining and birth defects among live births in central Appalachia, 1996–2003. Environ. Res. 2011, 111, 838–846.

18. Fernández-Navarro, P.; García-Pérez, J.; Ramis, R.; Boldo, E.; López-Abente, G. Proximity to mining industry and cancer mortality. Sci. Total Environ. 2012, 435–436, 66–73.

19. Sevenster, M.; Croezen, H.; van Valkengoed, M.; Markowska, A.; Doenszelmann, E. External Costs of Coal. Global Estimate; CE Delft: Delft, The Netherlands, 2008.

20. Bjureby, E.; Britten, M.; Cheng, I.; Kazmierska, M.; Mezak, E.; Munnik, V.; Nandi, J.; Pennington, S.; Rochon, E.; Schulz, N.; et al. The True Cost of Coal: How People and the Planet Are Paying the Price for the World's Dirtiest Fuel; Greenpeace International: Amsterdam, The Netherlands, 2008.

21. Huscher, J.; Smith, D. The Unpaid Health Bill: How Coal Power Plants Make Us Sick; Health and Environment Alliance: Brussels, Belgium, 2013.

22. Epstein, P.R.; Buonocore, J.J.; Eckerle, K.; Hendryx, M.; Stout, B.M.; Heinberg, R.; Clapp, R.W.; May, B.; Reinhart, N.L.; Ahern, M.M.; et al. Full cost accounting for the life cycle of coal. Ann. N. Y. Acad. Sci. 2011, 1219, 73–98.

23. Mahapatra, D.; Shukla, P.; Dhar, S. External cost of coal based electricity generation: A tale of Ahmedabad city. Energy Policy 2012, 49, 253–265.

24. Nkambule, N.; Blignaut, J. The external costs of coal mining: The case of collieries supplying Kusile power station. J. Energy South. Africa 2012, 23, 85–93.

25. Inglesi-Lotz, R.; Blignaut, J. Estimating the opportunity cost of water for the Kusile and Medupi coal-fired electricity power plants in South Africa. J. Energy South. Africa 2012, 23, 76–84.

26. Wang, L.; Watanabe, T.; Xu, Z. Monetization of external costs using lifecycle analysis—A comparative case study of coal-fired and biomass power plants in Northeast China. Energies 2015, 8, 1440–1467.

27. Schleisner, L. Comparison of methodologies for externality assessment. Energy Policy 2000, 28, 1127–1136.

28. HEI NPACT Review Panel HEI's National Particle Component Toxicity (NPACT) Initiative. Executive Summary; HEI Research Reports 177 & 178; Health Effects Institute: Boston, MA, USA, 2013; pp. 177–178.

29. Review of Evidence on Health Aspects of Air Pollution—REVIHAAP Project; World Health Organization: Copenhagen, Denmark, 2013.

30. Committee on the Medical Effects of Air Pollutants. Statement on the Evidence for Differential Health Effects of Particulate Matter According to Source or Components; Public Health England: London, UK, 2015.

31. Preiss, P.; Klotz, V. EcoSenseWeb V1.3: User's Manual & Description of Updated and Extended Draft Tools for the Detailed Site-Dependent Assessment of External Costs; Institute for Rational Use of Energy, University of Stuttgart: Stuttgart, Germany, 2008.

32. Holland, M. Implementation of the HRAPIE Recommendations for European Air Pollution CBA Work 2014. Available online: http://ec.europa.eu/environment/air/pdf/CBA HRAPIE implement.pdf (accessed on 20 November 2015).

33. Holland, M. Cost-Benefit Analysis of Final Policy Scenarios for the EU Clean Air Package 2014. Available online: http://ec.europa.eu/environment/air/pdf/TSAP%20CBA.pdf (accessed on 20 November 2015).

34. Desaigues, B.; Ami, D.; Bartczak, A.; Braun-Kohlová, M.; Chilton, S.; Czajkowski, M.; Farreras, V.; Hunt, A.; Hutchison, M.; Jeanrenaud, C.; et al. Economic valuation of air pollution mortality: A 9-country contingent valuation survey of value of a life year (VOLY). Ecol. Indic. 2011, 11, 902–910.

35. Ščasný, M.; Massetti, E.; Melichar, J.; Carrara, S. Quantifying the ancillary benefits of the representative concentration pathways on air quality in Europe. Environ. Resour. Econ. 2015, 62, 383–415.

36. Massetti, E.; Bosello, F.; Carrara, S.; Enei, R.; Leimbach, M.; Parrado, R.; Stevanovic, M.; Havlík, P.; Piontek, F.; Popp, A. Scenarios of Global

Challenges with Full Adaptation; GLOBAL-IQ Deliverable 5.1; Fondazione Eni Enrico Mattei: Venice, Italy, 2014.

37. Ludwig, L.; Neumann, J. Updating Income Elasticity Estimates in EPA's BenMAP Air Pollution Benefits Estimation System. 2012. Available online: http://www3.epa.gov/ttnecas1/regdata/Benefits/IncomeElasticityUpdate_Recommendationswithappendices.pdf (accessed on 20 November 2015).

38. U.S. Environmental Protection Agency. Emissions Factors & AP 42, Compilation of Air Pollutant Emission Factors; U.S. Environmental Protection Agency: Washington, DC, USA, 2011.

39. Brown Coal Reserach Institute. Summary of Existing Knowledge and the Proposal for Calculation of Dust Emissions from Surface Mine; Brown Coal Reserach Institute: Most, Czech Republic, 2014. (In Czech)

40. ATEM Ltd. Quantification of Environmental Impacts (from Air Pollution and Noise) of Brown Coal Surface Mining in the North Bohemian Brown Coal Basin at BILINA and CSA Opencast Mines and Utilization of Extracted Coal in Combustion Processes for the Production of Electricity and Heat in the Czech Republic; Ministry of Industry and Trade of the Czech Republic: Prague, Czech Republic, 2015. (In Czech)

41. European Commission. Decision C (2015) 2298 on the Notification by the Czech Republic of a Transitional National Plan Referred to in Article 32 of Directive 2010/75/EU of the European Parliament and of the Council on Industrial Emissions; European Union: Brussels, Belgium, 2015.

42. LCP BREF Technical Working Group. Draft 2 of LCP BREF Review; European Commission, Joint Research Centre: Seville, Spain, 2015.

43. Brandt, J.; Silver, J.D.; Christensen, J.H.; Andersen, M.S.; Bønløkke, J.H.; Sigsgaard, T.; Geels, C.; Gross, A.; Hansen, A.B.; Hansen, K.M.; et al. Contribution from the ten major emission sectors in Europe and Denmark to the health-cost externalities of air pollution using the EVA model system—An integrated modelling approach. Atmos. Chem. Phys.2013, 13, 7725–7746.

44. Šrám, R.J.; Beneš, I.; Binková, B.; Dejmek, J.; Horstman, D.; Kotĕsovec, F.; Otto, D.; Perreault, S.D.; Rubeš, J.; Selevan, S.G.; et al. Teplice program—The impact of air pollution on human health. Environ. Health Perspect. 1996, 104 (Suppl. 4), 699–714.

45. Cordial, P.; Riding-Malon, R.; Lips, H. The effects of mountaintop removal coal mining on mental health, well-being, and community health in Central Appalachia. Ecopsychology 2012, 4, 201–208.

46. Higginbotham, N.; Freeman, S.; Connor, L.; Albrecht, G. Environmental injustice and air pollution in coal affected communities, Hunter Valley, Australia. Health Place 2010, 16, 259–266.

47. Morrice, E.; Colagiuri, R. Coal mining, social injustice and health: A universal conflict of power and priorities. Health Place 2013, 19, 74–79.

48. Shandro, J.A.; Veiga, M.M.; Shoveller, J.; Scoble, M.; Koehoorn, M. Perspectives on community health issues and the mining boom-bust cycle. Resour. Policy 2011, 36, 178–186.

# Chapter 7

# Progress in Developments of Dry Coal Beneficiation

**Yuemin Zhao • Xuliang Yang • Zhenfu Luo • Chenlong Duan • Shulei Song**

*School of Chemical Engineering & Technology, China University of Mining & Technology, Xuzhou 221116, China*

## ABSTRACT

China's energy supply heavily relies on coal and China's coal resource and water resource has a reverse distribution. The problem of water shortages restricts the applications of wet coal beneficiation technologies in drought regions. The present situation highlights the significance and urgency of developing dry beneficiation technologies of coal. Besides, other countries that produce large amounts of coal also encounter serious problem of lack of water for coal beneficiation, such as American, Australia, Canada, South Africa, Turkey and India. Thus, dry coal beneficiation becomes the research hot-points in the field of coal cleaning worldwide in recent years. This paper systematically reviewed the promising research efforts on dry coal beneficiation reported in literature in last 5 years and discussed the progress in developments of dry coal beneficiation worldwide. Finally, we also elaborated the prospects and the challenges of the development of dry coal beneficiation.

**Keywords:** Dry coal beneficiation Air dense medium fluidized bed Density segregation Vibrated fluidized bed

# 1 INTRODUCTION

China's energy supply is heavily reliant on coal and this situation will last for decades to come. Now, China is the largest coal producer and consumer in the world. In 2012, China's coal production is up to 3.66 billion tons and coal consumption accounts for 68.4 % of its energy consumption. Thus, in order to improve energy efficiency and ensure the security of energy supply, China must increase the beneficiation ratio of run-of-mine coal. In 2013, the Chinese government released its toughest plan so far to combat air pollution, *Air Pollution Prevention Plan of Action*, in an effort to ease mounting public concern over air quality. In this plan, it is clearly pointed out that the beneficiation ratio of run-of-mine coal will be improved to more than 70 % till 2017 and apparently, a lot of continued efforts must be made to achieve this goal.

Meanwhile, more than 70 % China's coal reserves in regions of Northwest China and North China and unfortunately, these regions are almost dry and have prolonged coal weather each year, which puts many obstacles to the deployment of wet beneficiation technologies for coal cleaning. Thus, it is imperative to develop efficient dry coal beneficiation technologies. Besides, other countries producing large amounts of coal also encounter serious problem of lack of water for coal beneficiation, such as American, Australia, Canada, South Africa, Turkey and India. Thus, in recent years, dry coal beneficiation technologies have progressively become the research hot-points in the field of coal cleaning worldwide and a lot of promising research efforts have been reported in literature.

Overall, in the section of dry coal beneficiation, the most significant properties of coal that facilitate the separation process are density, shape, friction, electricity, and magnetite. According the different beneficiating mechanisms, dry coal beneficiation reported in recent literature are mainly classified into the following five categories: (I) air dense medium fluidized bed separation with/without external force field, (II) fluidized bed separation based on the difference of settling velocity, (III) compound dry separation, (IV) triboelectrostatic separation and (V) magnetic separation. These five categories of technologies have their own advantages respectively in processing certain coal or yielding clean coal product with certain quality. Generally speaking, technologies belong to the categories (I), (IV) and (V) usually have high separation efficiency but high operational cost, which are suitable for producing high-quality clean coal. In contrast, technologies in categories (II) and (III) don't need additional dense medium or power and usually have larger capacities and low processing cost, but low separation efficiency due to the original limitation of separation mechanism. These technologies are suitable for producing steam coal. Besides, the electrostatic separation technologies and the magnetic separation technologies have high requirements for coal properties and certain degree of dissociation, thus, the handling capacities are limited. Considering these limitation, these two types of beneficiation technologies are only used in very special purpose. In the following sections, the representative research works in terms of the aforementioned technologies in the last five years are reviewed in detail and finally, we discuss the prospects and the challenges of the development of dry coal beneficiation.

# 2 DRY BENEFICIATION WITH FLUIDIZED BED

Dry beneficiation of coal with an air dense-medium fluidized bed (ADMFB) uses a pseudofluid system of the mix of dense medium (such as magnetite powder) and fine coal powder as the separating medium and, within it, the feed coal conducts the sink-float processes based on Archimedes' principle. The light and heavy particles separate from each other by the separating density with light particles floating and heavy particles sinking (Chen and Yang 2003; Luo and Chen 2001; Luo et al. 2002a, 2003, 2007). The ADMFB separation differs in principle from pneumatic separating devices (using air as separating medium) such as air-tables and has comparatively high *E* values (Luo and Chen 2001).

## 2.1 Separation with air dense medium fluidized bed

China University of Mining and Technology (CUMT) has carried out numerous research works on ADMFB separation in the last about 30 years and developed a series of dry beneficiation techniques for coal cleaning including the bubbling fluidized bed (Luo and Chen 2001; Luo et al.2002a; Zhao et al. 2011a, 2011b), the vibrated fluidized bed (Luo et al. 2008; Yang et al. 2013a), and the magnetically fluidized bed (Fan et al. 2001, 2002, 2003; Luo et al. 2002b). Zhao et al. (2010) carried out systematic studies experimentally and numerically on fluidization characteristics of air dense medium fluidized bed with fine magnetite powder and pointed out that the increase of superficial air velocity will significantly improve the bed activity, but meanwhile, deteriorate the uniformity and stability of fluidization. Therefore, the superficial air velocity no more than 2.0 $u_{mf}$ (minimum fluidization velocity) is suggested for coal beneficiation. In addition, a method of numerical simulation of the fluidization of ADMFB was proposed to study the bubbling characteristics and the particles motions and the simulation results were consistent with the experimental results, as shown in Fig. 1.

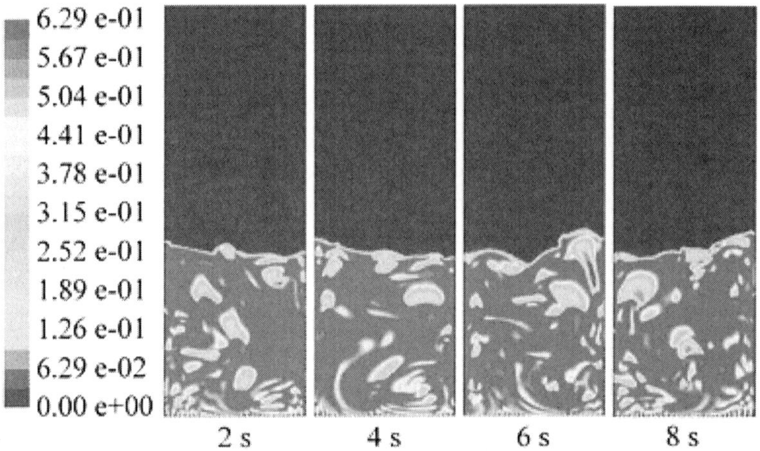


**Figure 1.** Bubbling and particles motions observed by numerical simulation of ADMFB (Zhao et al.2010)

Furthermore, Zhao et al. (2011) established a modularized industrial-scale ADMFB separation system with a capacity of 40–60 t/h, as show in Fig. 2. This system uses the steel structure instead of the recent reinforced concrete structure, leading to a reduction of the construction coast, the area and the number of workers by 60 %, 75 % and 80 %, respectively. The separation results show that this modularized system can effectively separate 50–6 mm coal with an *E*value in the range of 0.05–0.07.

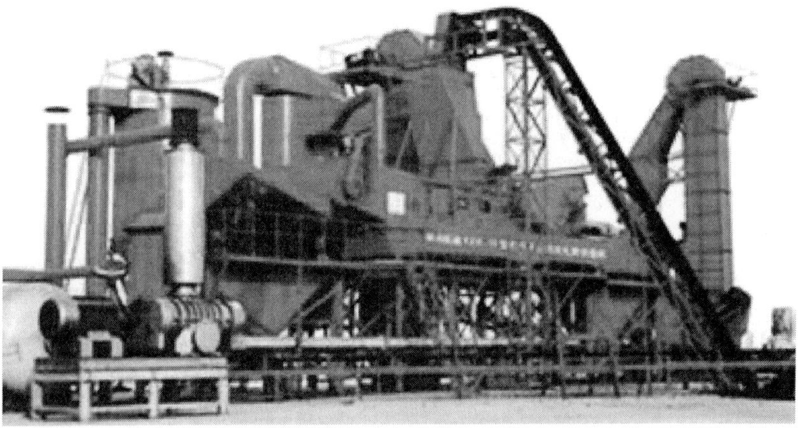

**Figure 2.** Modularized industrial-scale ADMFB separator

Luo et al. (2013) studied the effect of a secondary gas-distribution layer on the fluidization characteristics of an ADMFB for dry coal beneficiation and the experimental results show that the secondary layer with an optimal depth of 30 mm can significantly reduce the variance in both the bed pressure drop and the bed density, leading to an improvement in the fluidization quality, as shown in Fig. 3. It is also pointed out that the secondary layer can divide large bubbles passing through the region into small bubbles and can increase the pressure drop of the gas distributor. This work will provide a foundation for the design of the discharge structure of the bed and for calculating the capacity of the bed.

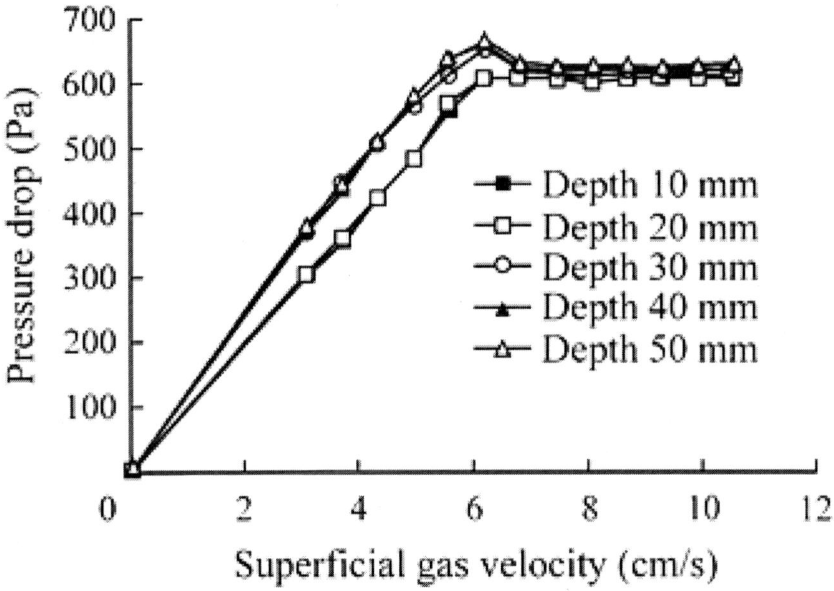


**Figure 3.** Fluidization curves of an ADMFB with different secondary layer depth (Luo et al. 2013)

In similarity with China, India is heavily dependent on coal for meeting its energy requirements in economic development (Sahu et al. 2011). In these years, many research works on using the ADMFB separation for Indian coal cleaning have been done by Indian scholars. Sahu et al. (2009, 2011, 2013) used an ADMFB separator to beneficiate India high ash coal with a size range of −25 + 6 mm and studied the stability of fluidization to make an expansion bed with a nanobubbling condition. It was pointed out that the stability of the fluidized bed had a significant effect on sharp separation between clean coal and gangue. A continuous ADMFB separator with a capacity of 600 kg/h was established, as shown in Fig. 4. The separation results show that the ash content is reduced from 40 % in feed coal to around 32 %–35.5 % in clean coal product with a 60 %–72 % yield and the separation efficiency *E* value is 0.12.

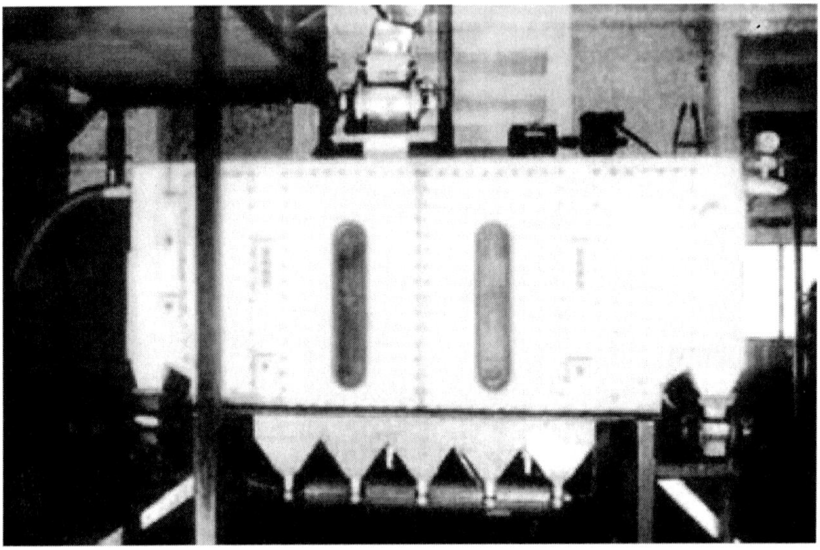

**Figure 4.** Continous ADMFB separator for beneficiating Indian high ash coal (Sahu et al. 2011)

Mohanta et al. (2011, 2012, 2013a, b) had made many efforts to optimize the operational parameters and the feed coal properties in order to achieving an optimum beneficiation performance of an ADMFB separator. It was pointed out that when the feed coal size is below 15 mm, the size effect on sharpness in separation becomes significant and the *E* values decrease faster. The experimental results indicate that for processing finer coal of size less than 15 mm, the ADMFB separator does not offer any real performance advantages better than the traditional process like heavy-medium cyclone and water-only cyclone. They also carried out a detailed investigation to examine the interdependencies among these parameters and their interactional effect on the separation performance of an ADMFB separator. The optimization results show that the optimum conditions were: superficial air velocity from 18.94 to 20.42 cm/s, bed height from 25.94 to 29.36, and coal to magnetite weight ratio of 0.02. A correlation for the theoretical prediction of minimum fluidization velocity was proposed in the following:

$$u_{\mathrm{mf}} = \frac{\mu}{d_{\mathrm{p}}\rho_{\mathrm{f}}}\left(\sqrt{(41.96)^2 + 0.049\mathrm{Ar}} - 41.96\right)$$

where $u_{mf}$ is the minimum fluidization velocity; $\mu$, $d_p$ and $\rho_f$ are the air viscosity, the particle diameter and the air density, respectively; Ar is the Archimedes number. The predictive adequacy and reliability was evaluated by adopting a statistical analysis approach on the data available in the literature and the results indicate that this new correlation is useful and accurate for predicting the minimum fluidization velocity and designing an ADMFB.

Researchers in University of Alberta in Canada (Prashant et al. 2010; Azimi et al. 2013a, b) have also done many works on ADMFB separation. Prashant et al. (2010) studied the effect of operating parameters such as the type of media, fluidizing velocity and separating time on beneficiation performance investigated under both batch and continuous ADMFB separators which are demonstrated in Figs. 5 and 6 respectively. The separation results show that the ash content of −6 + 2 mm feed coal is reduced from 25 % to 10 % with a yield of 80 %.

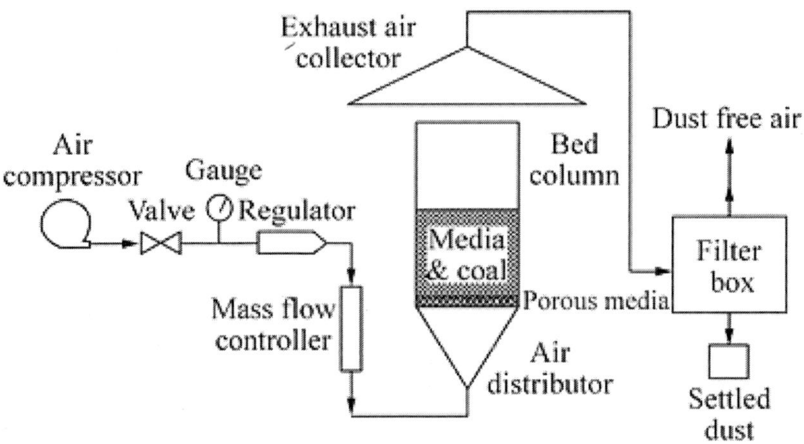


**Figure 5.** Schematics of a laboratory batch ADMFB separator (Prashant et al. 2010)

Azimi et al. (2013a, b) used an ADMFB to separate low-rank coals in Canada and carried out a detail study of the factors including superficial air velocity, residence time, and bed height affecting the beneficiation performance of a low-ash lignite coal. The experimental results show that the optimum operating condition is superficial air velocity of 15 cm/s, residence time of 90 s and bed height of 15 cm and in this condition, the beneficiation results revealed that higher ash removal (23 %) and recoveries (86 %) are obtainable with a clean coal ash content, recovery, and separation efficiency of 10.6 %, 95.63 %, and 15.29 %, respectively. In addition, it was also pointed out that feeding more coal to ADMFB resulted in higher organic material recovery and lower ash content of the product and system separation efficiency.

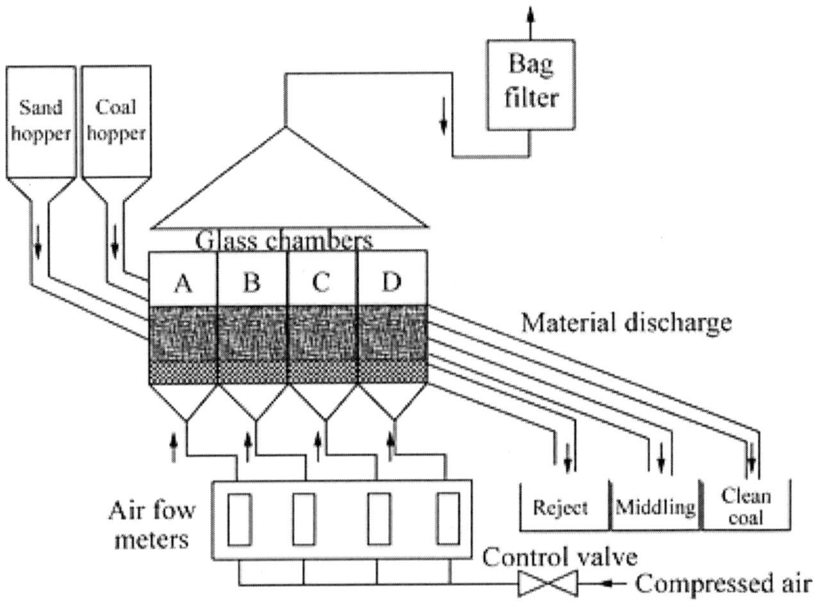


**Figure 6.** Schematics of a laboratory continuous ADMFB separator (Prashant et al. 2010)

## 2.2 Separation with vibrated fluidized bed

The conventional ADMFB separation is not available recently to separate fine coal smaller than 6 mm in size because of low separation efficiency and difficult in dense medium recovery and product purification. Luo et al. (2008) introduced the vibration energy into conventional ADMFB for separating dry fine coal particles and systemically studied the vibrational energy transmission, the interaction between vibration and air and the separation performance of vibrated air dense medium fluidized bed (VADMFB). The results show that the bubble formation in a VADMFB is efficiently restricted to small bubbles due to the cutting effect derived from the horizontal vibration component and the extruding effect from the vertical vibration component. An empirical correlation of the critical vibration frequency above which the bubble can be restrained and broken was proposed:

$$f > \left(\frac{6Q}{\pi}\right)^{-1/5} g^{3/5}$$

where *f*, *q* and *g* are vibration frequency, air flow rate and gravitational acceleration, respectively. The synergy between vibration and air make the fine coal bed can be fluidized with both micro-bubbles and a uniform bed density. The separation results show that the VADMFB has a good separation performance for −6 mm fine coal under optimal operating conditions with an *E* value of 0.07.

Macpherson and Galvin (2010) and Macpherson et al. 2010, 2011) in the University of Newcastle in Australia introduced the Reflux Classifier, whose water-based version had been successfully employed in industry for gravity separation of −2 + 0.25 mm coal, into the field of dry coal beneficiation. This new Reflux Classifier uses sand (−335 + 125 micron) as a dense-medium and uses vibration at two distinct levels to improve fluidization stability, as shown in Fig. 7. There are two parts: a vibrated fluidized bed in the lower section and a device consisting of parallel inclined channels in the upper section. The addition of an incline above the fluidized bed provides a more stable system allowing for grater separation efficiency and minimizing the effect of changing conditions. The density cut-point can be varied from 1,418 to 2,130 g/cm$^3$ by varying the underflow rate and the *E* value was within the range of 0.06–0.46 depending on particle size and gas rate.

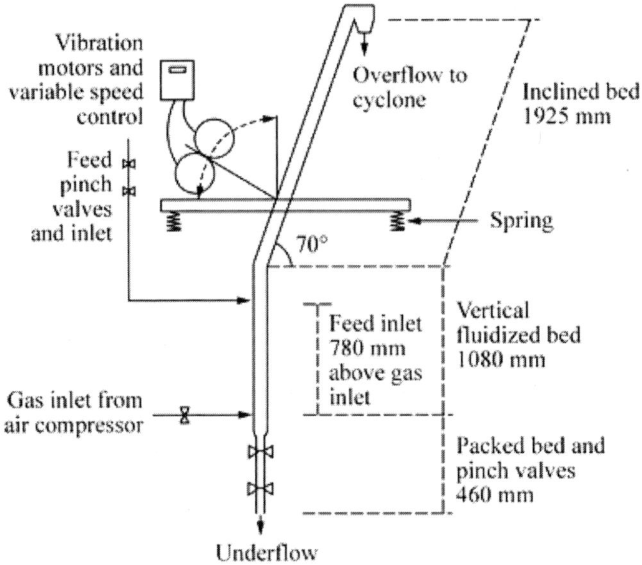


**Figure 7.** Schematic diagram of the reflux classifier using air-sand dense-medium and vibration (Macpherson et al. 2011)

## 2.3 Separation with magnetically stabilized air dense medium fluidized bed

Song et al. (2012a, b) in China University of Mining & Technology studied the continuous separation of −6 + 0.5 mm fine coal by using a crossflow magnetically stabilized air dense medium fluidized bed (MSADMFB) with the 0.074–0.045 mm magnetite beads as dense medium, as shown in Fig. 8. The fluidization results show that the range of steadily operational air velocity in MSADMFB is broader than that in a conventional ADMFB when they are at stable fluidization. The external magnetic field compels the magnetic grains to form parallel magnetic chains following the magnetic induction lines, which enlarge the bed voidage and form uniform air channels. Air bubbles cannot be produced when the air flows through the channels. Thus, a MSADMFB comparatively has a more stable bed density and smaller pressure fluctuation. The separation results show that the cross-flow MSADMFB can achieve successfully the separation of fine coal of −6 + 0.5 mm with a *E* value in the range of 0.068–0.095. It is also pointed out that the separation efficiency turns worse gradually with the decrease of the size of the fine raw coal.

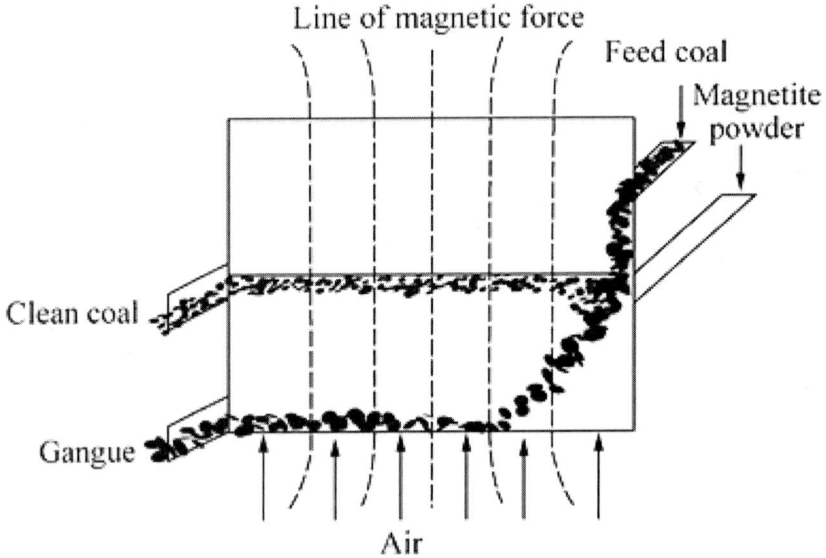


**Figure 8.** Schematic diagram of the crossflow magnetically stabilized air dense medium fluidized bed (Song et al. 2012b)

# 3 FLUIDIZATION BENEFICIATION WITHOUT DENSE MEDIUM

For fine coal dry beneficiation, the fluidization separation using dense medium has several problem need to be solved, including the efficient recovery of fine dense medium and the purification of product. Meanwhile, the complex process and the relatively high operational costs due to the recovery and loss of dense medium also present great obstacle on the industrial applications of the fluidization separation with dense medium. Thus, some recent studies on fluidization beneficiation without artificial dense medium have been carried out in order to provide an efficient and economical solution for fine coal cleaning.

## 3.1 Vibro-fluidization beneficiation based on density segregation

Yang et al. (2013a, b) introduced the density segregation phenomenon in the field of gas–solid fluidization into the research on fine coal dry beneficiation and adopted a vibrated fluidized bed to foster the formation of fluidization environment that intensifies density segregation within the bed of fine coal, leading to an effective fine coal beneficiation performance. Figure 9demonstrates the schematic diagram of the experimental apparatus and Fig. 10 depicts the separation mechanism. Particles in the region of a bubble having considerable lower solid volume fraction than the surrounding bulk phase conduct sink-float processes and particles with higher density tend to sink preferentially over the lighter particles, which leads to local density segregation. Thus, after the function of periodic bubbling, the local density segregation evolves the density segregation of total bed, leading to stratification of the particulate bed with the layers of clean coal, middling and gangue distribute along the bed height from top to bottom. The experimental results show that the operational parameters including superficial air velocity, vibration intensity, bed height and fluidizing time have significant influences on the segregation performance. The separation results show that the probable error *E* values of −6 + 3 and −3 + 1 mm fine coal separated in a continuous separation system using a vibrated fluidized bed are 0.19–0.225 and 0.175–0.195, respectively, indicating that the fine coal separation in a vibrated gas-fluidized bed system is useful to and more effective for fine coal cleaning.

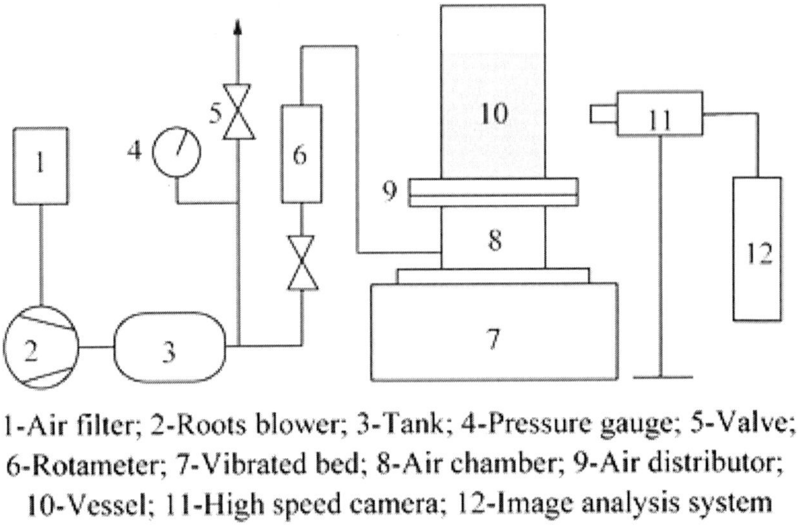


**Figure 9.** Schematic diagram of the experimental apparatus (Yang et al. 2013b)

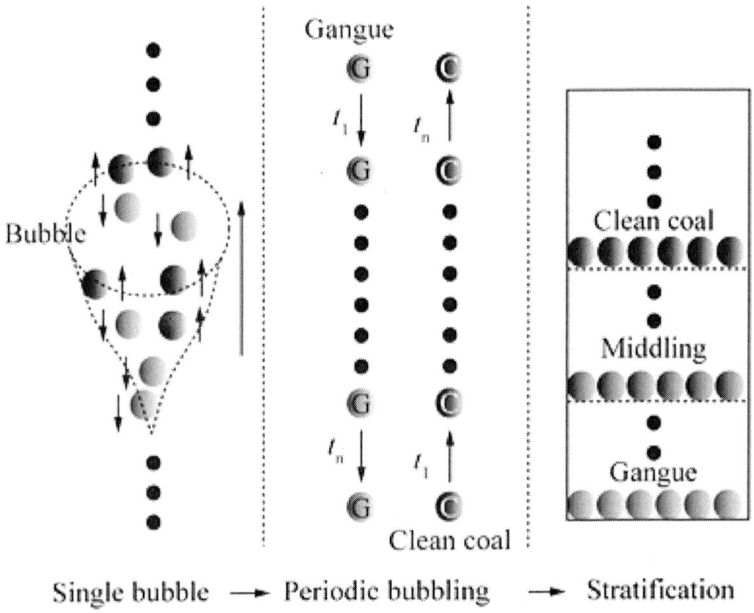


**Figure 10.** Separation mechanism of vibro-fluidization beneficiation based on density segregation (Yang et al. 2013a)

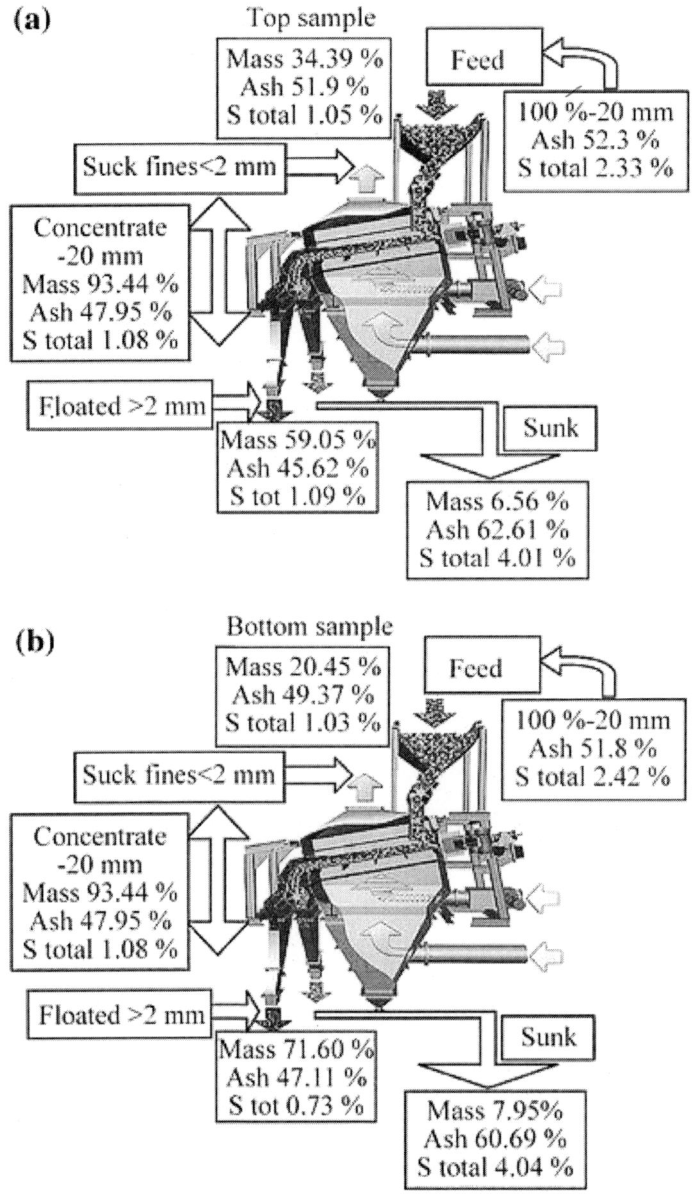


**Figure 11.** Detailed separation results of air jig studied by Sampaio et al. (2008)

### 3.2 Dry jigging

The air jig is a deep-bed separator that deploys the difference in hindered settling velocity of particles with different density, which is analogous to the proved wet jig. Air is supplied into the jig in two forms: a continuous flow and a superimposed pulsated airflow that provides the impetus for stratification and consolidation trickling. Sampaio et al. (2008) employed dry jigging to beneficiate Candiota coal in Brazil. This coal is low rank and can't be treated by any wet beneficiation technologies. The separation results show that the sulfur content reduces from 2.33 % in feed coal to 1.08 % in clean coal, providing a cheaper way than washing combustion gases. The detailed separation results are given in Fig. 11. Charan et al. (2011) used air jig manufactured by Allmineral Company in Germen to beneficiate Indian high-ash non-coking coals which contain high amounts of mineral matter. The first commercial air jig with a capacity of 50 t/h was installed and commissioned to separate −40 + 5 mm high-ash coals with an ash content of 40 %. The separation results show that a clean coal product with an ash content of 33 % was produced.

## 4 COMPOUND DRY BENEFICIATION

Recently, researchers have studied and developed some innovative dry coal beneficiation technologies depending on not only the density difference, but the difference of other properties including coefficient of friction and shape. This compound dry beneficiation enhances the stratification process of coal and gangue in many aspects and leads to a stable and efficient separation performance.

### 4.1 FGX dry separator

The FGX dry separator is firstly developed by China's researchers and already has several hundred commercial installations. It consists of a perforated separating bed, a vibrating mechanism, and a hanging support mechanism, shown as in Fig. 12. The deck vibration frequency, longitudinal deck angle, feeder frequency, and baffle plate height all have significant effects on the separation performance. Coal particles conduct the spiral flip motions under the synergy of vibration and air flow. The lighter particles rise to the top of the particulate layer and are collected in the front section of the separating bed as the clean coal product. Meanwhile, the heavy particles stay in the bottom of the particulate layer and keep contact with the bed. Thus, with the function of vibration and riffles fitted on the bed, these heavy particles move forward to the narrow section of the bed and finally are discharged as gangue. Particles with intermediate density are discharged as middling. The

FGX dry separator finally generates three products: clean coal product, middling, and gangue. Two dust collection systems are employed to clean the recycled air and to remove the dust from air before being emitted into the atmosphere.

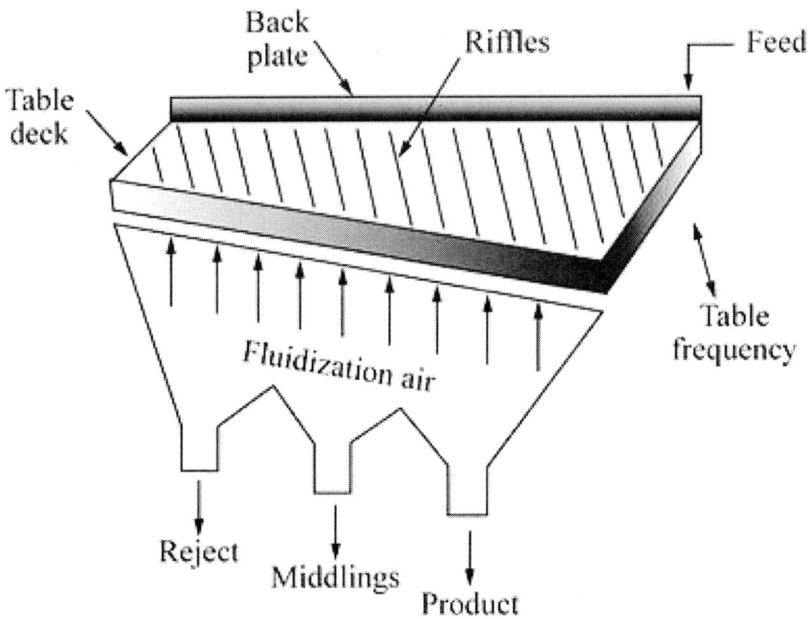


**Figure 12.** Schematic diagram of the FGX dry separator and its processing system (Honaker et al.2008)

Zhang et al. (2011) used a FGX dry separator with a capacity of 10 t/h to clean raw coals extracted from Illinois mines in America. The separation performance of the FGX dry separator was evaluated by separating the −63.5 + 4.75 mm coal and the results show that the specific gravity of separation and the probable error *E* values are 1.98 g/cm3 and 0.17, respectively. A modified log-logistic partition model was established using experimental data reported in literature and in this study to predict the FGX dry separator coal-cleaning performance, given in the following:

$$PN = 100 * \frac{1}{1 + \exp^{a*\ln\frac{x}{b}}}$$

$$X = D_m/D_{50}$$

where *a* and *b* are fitting constants; $D_m$ is the mean density and $D_{50}$ is the separation density.

Honaker et al. (2008) deployed a 5 t/h pilot-scale FGX dry separator to produce clean coal having qualities that meet contract specifications and maximize the amount of high-density rock rejected prior to transportation and processing. The separation results clearly indicate that the FGX dry separator is able to reject more than 70 % of the high-density rock in a run-of-mine coal at high separation density values of around 1.8–2.2 g/cm$^3$ with an *E* valued 0.25.

## 4.2 Air table

The air table has a flat deck with the uniformly distributed apertures and riffles. Ambient air after filtering enters the deck and fluidizes the feed coal. The feed coal stratifies depending on the difference in the terminal velocity of the particles. Particles with smaller density move to the top of the particulate layer and then travel down the slope towards the discharge open. Particles with larger density settle to the bottom of the particulate layer travel in the direction of the deck's vibration along the riffles. The schematic diagram of this separation process is shown in Fig. 13.

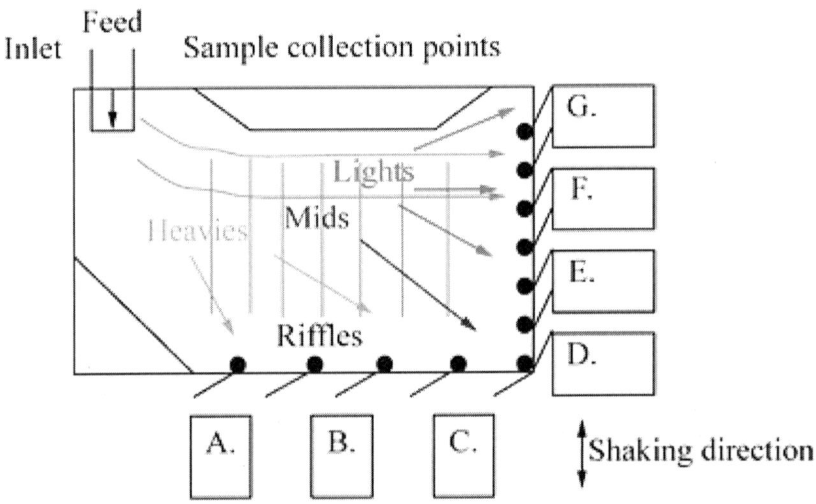


**Figure 13.** Detailed separation results of air jig studied by Sampaio et al. (2008)

Patil and Parekh (2011) used a dry air table for processing of −6.3 + 1.4 mm coal from a mine located in Western Kentucky. The separation results show that the ash content is reduced from 27 % to 10 % with a clean coal yield of 75 %–80 % and the combustible recovery is 95 % with the ash rejection of

77 %–80 %. In addition, the pyritic sulfur is reduced by about 33 % and the heat content increases from 23,997 to 29,595 kJ/kg, indicating excellent separation efficiency.

Çicek (2008) developed a modified air table to beneficiate Turkish coal by a dry cleaning method and the separation results show that the coal samples having three size fraction of 8–5, 5–3 and 3–1 mm can be efficiently beneficiated by this modified air table with *E* values of 0.21, 0.14 and 0.09, respectively, indicating a satisfactory separation performance.

## 5 TRIBOELECTROSTATIC SEPARATION

The triboelectrostatic beneficiation is an advanced dry fine coal cleaning technology and can effectively process fine coal of less than 300 μm (Dwari and Hanumantha Rao 2008; Zhang et al. 2009). During the process of triboelectrostatic separation, coal particles are charged by contact or friction with other particles or with a third material including the walls of a container or pipe and then conduct free-fall process through an electric field that deflects the particles according to the magnitude and sign of their charge. The mechanism of triboelectrostatic separation determines that the feed coal must achieve a certain degree of dissociation and the coal particles and the gangue particles mainly exist in the form of monomer. Therefore, this technology has a comparative small handling capacity and is usually used for producing high value-added clean coal product.

Zhang et al. (2009) deployed the triboelectrostatic separation of mineral matters from clean coal with density of < 1.35 g/cm$^3$ and the samples of feed coal with a size smaller than 75 μm was separated and analyzed with XRF, sulphur and ash analyzer. Figure 14 depicted the principle of triboelectrostatic separator and the sampling rule. The separation results showed that a quantity of quartz of 69.31 %–71.27 %, kaolin of 75.66 %–81.93 % and pyrite of 86.74 %–90.52 % could be removed and also indicated that coal would be charged positively and quartz, kaolin, pyrite and calcite would be charged negatively, leading to efficient separation of coal and these mineral matters.

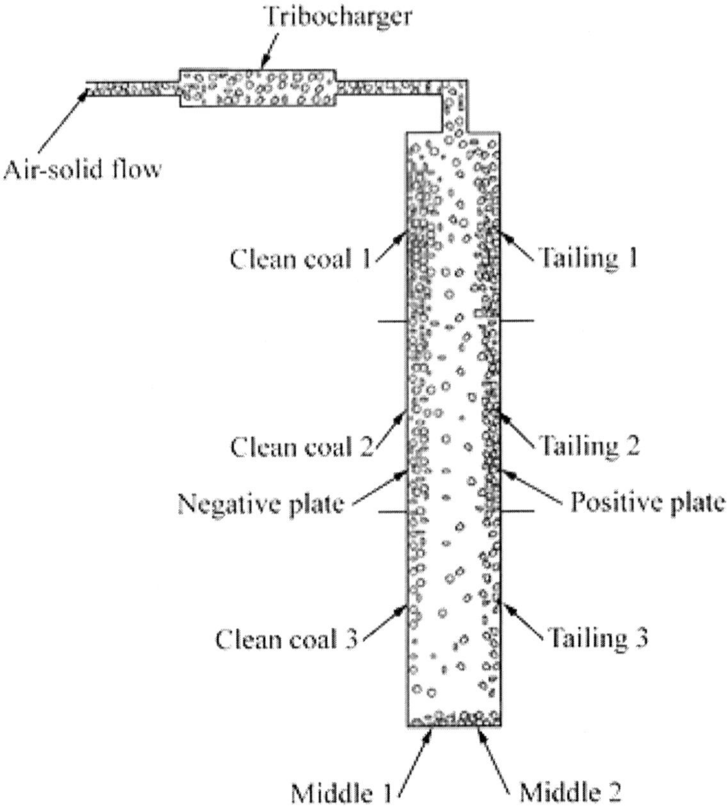


**Figure 14.** Principle of triboelectrostatic separator and sampling rule (Zhang et al. 2009)

Dwari and Hanumantha Rao (2008, 2009) used a new laboratory fluidized bed triboelectrostatic separator to beneficiate −300 μm Indian thermal non-coking coal from Ramagundam coal mines, shown as in Fig. 15. The tribocharger consisted of the internal baffles made up of copper metal and the coal and mineral particles charged with positive and negative polarities respectively. It was pointed out that the magnitude of particles charge is relevant with the efficiency of contact electrification in fluidized bed tribocharger. The separation results showed that the ash content can be reduced to 18 % and 33 % from 43 % in feed coal with an yield of about 30 % and 67 %, respectively.

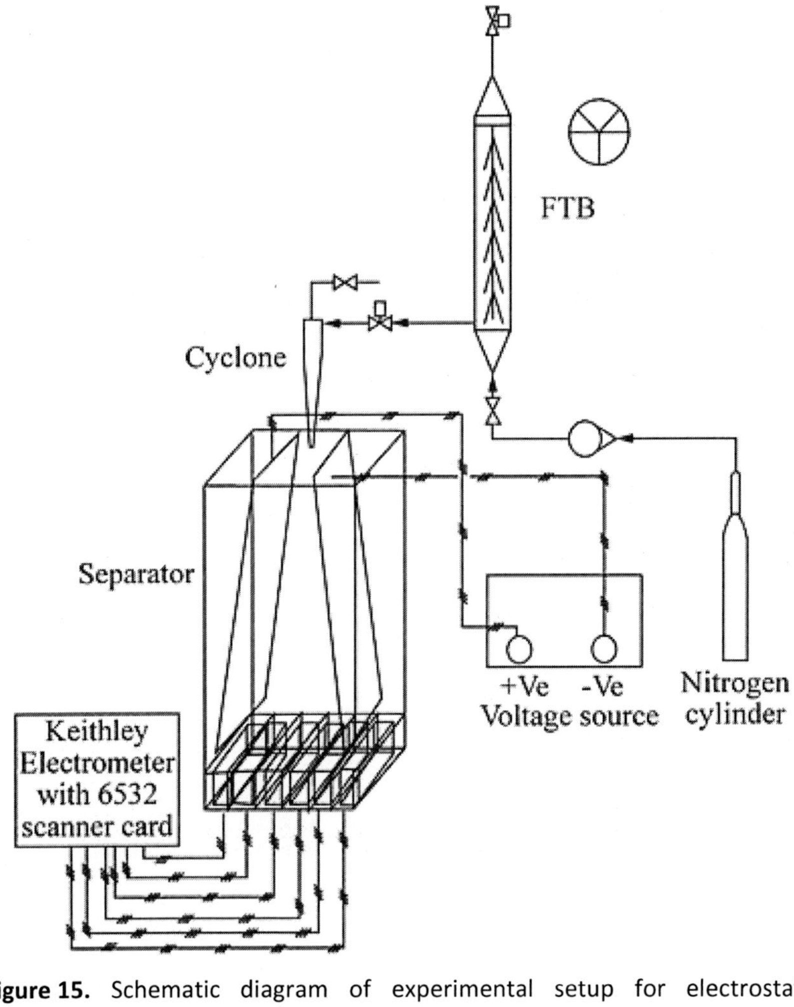


**Figure 15.** Schematic diagram of experimental setup for electrostatic separation (Dwari and Hanumantha Rao 2009)

# 6 DRY MAGNETIC SEPARATION

Dry magnetic separation technology beneficiates coal powder depending on the different magnetic susceptibilities of coal and mineral materials under high gradient magnetic field. In similarity to triboelectrostatic separation technology, dry magnetic separation technology also requires that the feed coal has high degree of dissociation in order to facilitate the separating process of coal and gangue depending on magnetic susceptibilities difference. Meanwhile, dry magnetic separation technology also has comparative small handing capacity.

Jiao et al. (2009) used dry magnetic separation to improve desulphurization and deash efficiency of fine coal and investigated the relation between magnetic susceptibility and density, size as well as magnetic field intensity. The results showed that there is a linear correlation between magnetic susceptibility and density, as shown in Fig. 16. It was also pointed out that the magnetism of high density coal and low density coal was opposite at the cut density of 1.6 g/cm$^3$. Furthermore, the diamagnetism property of low density coal weakened and the paramagnetism of high density coal enhanced along with the size reduction of fine coal. The separation results showed that the desulphurization and deash rates achieved 55.52 % and 64.41 %, respectively.

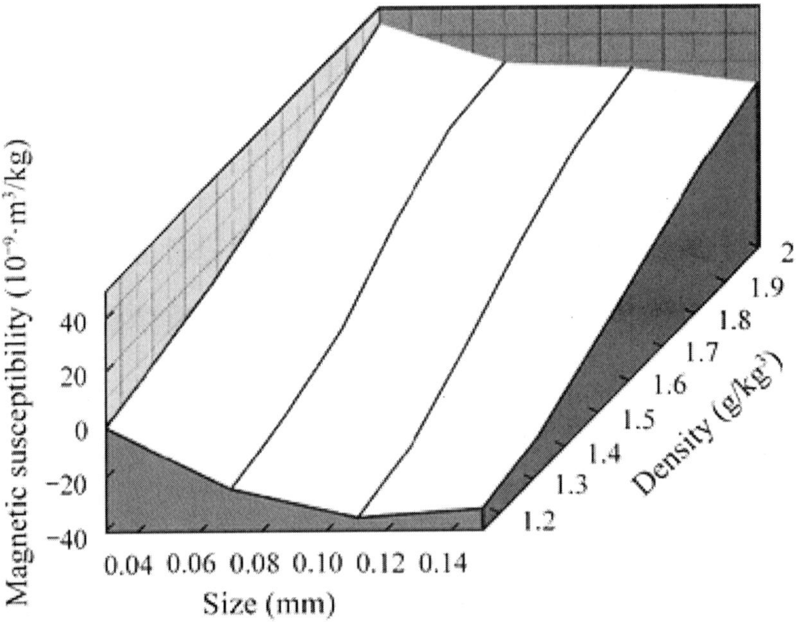


**Figure 16.** The correlation between magnetic susceptibility and densiy and size (Jiao et al. 2009)

## 7 PROSPECTS AND CHALLENGES

Dry coal beneficiation has an inherent advantage since it uses no process water and reduces the costs that are associated with process water, fines dewatering and slurry confinement. In particular, dry coal beneficiation is more suitable for coal cleaning in dry regions that lack available processing water. Meanwhile, the low-rank coal easily conducts the process of argillation when using wet coal beneficiation, yielding the difficulties in slurry treatment and product dewatering. Therefore, dry coal beneficiation is comparatively more suitable for low-rank coal cleaning and upgrading. Countries that heavily relay on coal for energy supply all progressively exploit and utilize low-rank coal to meet the increasing required energy consumption and protect the hard coal resource. Thus, it is imperative to develop high-efficiency dry coal beneficiation to support the utilization of low-rank coal.

However, there are a lot of works need to be done in order to form a reliable and stable solution that consists of several dry coal beneficiation technologies. Especially the separation stability and the separation efficiency of dry coal beneficiation technologies should be further improved in future. Furthermore, some demonstrational industrial dry coal beneficiation systems should be established for engineering verification and academic studies, providing an advanced research platform to carry out sufficient industry-university joint investigations. The significance of developing dry coal beneficiation should be paid sufficient attentions and the policy support and adequate financial support are required to facilitate the considerable progress in coal dry cleaning.

## ACKNOWLEDGMENTS

The study is supported by the National Key Basic Research Program of China (2012CB214904), the National Natural Science Foundation of China (51221462; 51134022; 51174203), the Research Fund for the Doctoral Program of Higher Education (20120095130001) and the Natural Science Foundation of Jiangsu Province (BK20140209).

## REFERENCES

1. Azimi E, Karimipour S, Rahman M, Szymanski J, Gupta R (2013a) Evaluation of the performance of air dense medium fluidized bed (ADMFB) for low-ash coal beneficiation. Part 1: effect of operating conditions. Energy Fuels 27(10):5595–5606
2. Azimi E, Karimipour S, Rahman M, Szymanski J, Gupta R (2013b) Evaluation of the performance of air dense medium fluidized bed (ADMFB) for low-ash coal beneficiation. Part 2: characteristics of the beneficiated coal. Energy Fuels 27(10):5607–5616
3. Charan GT, Chattopadhyay US, Singh KMP, Kabiraj SK, Haldar DD (2011) Beneficiaron of high-ash, Indian non-coking coal by dry jigging. Miner Metall Process 28(1):21–23
4. Chen QR, Yang YF (2003) Development of dry beneficiation of coal in China. Coal Prep 23(1–2):3–12

5. Çicek T (2008) Dry Cleaning of Turkish Coal. Energy Sources Part A 30(7):593–605

6. Dwari RK, Hanumantha Rao K (2008) Non-coking coal preparation by novel tribo-electrostatic method. Fuel 87(17–18):3562–3571

7. Dwari RK, Hanumantha Rao K (2009) Fine coal preparation using novel tribo-electrostatic separator. Miner Eng 22(2):119–127

8. Fan MM, Chen QR, Zhao YM, Luo ZF (2001) Fine coal (6-1 mm) separation in magnetically stabilized fluidized beds. Int J Miner Process 63(4):225–232

9. Fan MM, Chen QR, Zhao YM, Guan YP, Li B (2002) Magnetically stabilized fluidized beds for fine coal separation. Powder Technol 123(2–3):208–211

10. Fan MM, Chen QR, Zhao YM, Luo ZF, Guan YP (2003) Fundamentals of a magnetically stabilized fluidized bed for coal separation. Int J Coal Prep Utili 23(1):47–55

11. Honaker RQ, Saracoglu M, Thompson E, Bratton R, Luttrell GH, Richardson V (2008) Upgrading coal using a pneumatic density-based separator. Int J Coal Prep Utili 28(1):51–67

12. Jiao HG, Cui JY, Liu P, Chen QR, Tie ZX (2009) Experimental study of magnetic property and dry magnetic separation of fine coal. J China Univ Min Technol 38(1): 131–134, 148

13. Luo ZF, Chen QR (2001) Dry beneficiation technology of coal with an air dense-medium fluidized bed. Int J Miner Process 63(3):167–175

14. Luo ZF, Chen QR, Zhao YM (2002a) Dry beneficiation of coarse coal using an air dense medium fluidized bed (ADMFB). Coal Prep 22(1):57–64

15. Luo ZF, Zhao YM, Chen QR, Fan MM, Tao XX (2002b) Separation characteristics for fine coal of the magnetically fluidized bed. Fuel Process Technol 79(1):63–69

16. Luo ZF, Zhao YM, Tao XX, Fan MM, Chen QR, Wei LB (2003) Progress in dry coal cleaning using air-dense medium fluidized beds. Coal Prep 23(1–2):13–20

17. Luo ZF, Zhu JF, Fan MM, Zhao YM, Tao XX (2007) Low density dry coal beneficiation using an air dense medium fluidized bed. J China Univ Min Technol 17(3):306–309

18. Luo ZF, Fan MM, Zhao YM, Tao XX, Chen QR, Chen Z (2008) Density-dependent separation of dry fine coal in a vibrated fluidized bed. Powder Technol 187(2):119–123

19. Luo ZF, Tang LG, Dai NN, Zhao YM (2013) The effect of a secondary gas-distribution layer on the fluidization characteristics of a fluidized bed used for dry coal beneficiation. Int J Miner Process 118:28–33

20. Macpherson SA, Galvin KP (2010) The effect of vibration on dry coal beneficiation in the reflux classifier. Int J Coal Prep Utili 30(6):283–294

21. Macpherson SA, Iveson SM, Galvin KP (2010) Density based separations in the reflux classifier with an air–sand dense–medium and vibration. Miner Eng 23(2):74–82

22. Macpherson SA, Iveson SM, Galvin KP (2011) Density-based separation in a vibrated Reflux Classifier with an air-sand dense-medium: tracer studies with simultaneous underflow and overflow removal. Miner Eng 24(10):1046–1052

23. Mohanta S, Chakraborty S, Meikap BC (2011) Influence of coal feed size on the performance of air dense medium fluidized bed separator used for coal beneficiation. Ind Eng Chem Res 50(18):10865–10871

24. Mohanta S, Daram AB, Chakraborty S, Meikap BC (2012) Characteristics of minimum fluidization velocity for magnetite powder used in an air dense medium fluidized bed for coal beneficiation. Part Part Syst Charact 29(4):228–237

25. Mohanta S, Chakraborty S, Meikap BC (2013a) Optimization process of an air dense medium fluidized bed separator for treating high-ash non-coking indian coal. Miner Process Extr Metall Rev 34(4):240–248

26. Mohanta S, Rao CS, Daram AB, Chakraborty S, Meikap BC (2013b) Air dense medium fluidized bed for dry beneficiation of coal: technological challenges for future. Part Sci Technol 31(1):16–27

27. Patil DP, Parekh BK (2011) Beneficiation of fine coal using the air table. Int J Coal Prep Utili 31(3–4):203–222

28. Prashant D, Xu ZH, Szymanski J, Gupta R, Boddez J (2010) Dry cleaning of coal by a laboratory continuous air dense medium fluidized bed separator. In: Honaker RQ (ed) Processding of the international coal preparation congress 2010. SME, Lexington, pp 608–616

29. Sahu AK, Biswal SK, Parida A (2009) Development of air dense medium fluidized bed technology for dry beneficiation of coal_A review. Int J Coal Prep Utili 29(4):216–241

30. Sahu AK, Tripathy A, Biswal SK, Parida A (2011) Stability Study of an air dense medium fluidized bed separator for beneficiation of high-ash Indian coal. Int J Coal Prep Utili 31(3–4):127–148

31. Sahu AK, Tripathy A, Biswal SK (2013) Study on particle dynamics in different cross sectional shapes of air dense medium fluidized bed separator. Fuel 111:472–477

32. Sampaio CH, Aliaga W, Pacheco ET, Petter E, Wotruba H (2008) Coal beneficiation of Candiota mine by dry jigging. Fuel Process Technol 89(2):198–202

33. Song SL, Zhao YM, Luo ZF, Tang LG (2012a) Motion behavior of particles in air-solid magnetically stabilized fluidized beds for separation. Int J Min Sci Technol 22(5):725–729

34. Song SL, Zhao YM, Luo ZF, Tang LG, Yang XL (2012b) Fine coal particles separation by air-solid magnetic fluidization. Meitan Xuebao/J China Coal Soc 37(9):1586–1590

35. Yang XL, Zhao YM, Luo ZF, Chen ZQ, Song SL, Duan CL (2013a) Energy transfer mechanism of vibro-fludization and its separation for fine coal. Zhongguo Kuangye Daxue Xuebao/J China Univ Min Technol 42(2):266–270

36. Yang XL, Zhao YM, Luo ZF, Song SL, Duan CL, Dong L (2013b) Fine coal dry cleaning using a vibrated gas-fluidized bed. Fuel Process Technol 106:338–343

37. Zhang XX, Duan DY, Tian B, Wang JS, Deng F, Li HS, Ma RX (2009) Research on the triboelectrostatic separation of minerals from coal. Procedia Earth and Planet Sci 1(1):845–850

38. Zhang B, Akbari H, Yang F, Mohanty MK, Hirschi J (2011) Performance optimization of the fgx dry separator for cleaning high-sulfur coal. Int J Coal Prep Utili 31(3–4):161–186

39. Zhao YM, Luo ZF, Chen ZQ, Tang LG, Wang HF, Xing HB (2010a) The effect of feed-coal particle size on the separating characteristics of a gas-solid fluidized bed. J S Afr Inst Min Metall 110(5):219–224

40. Zhao YM, Tang LG, Luo ZF, Liang CC, Xing HB, Wu WC, Duan CL (2010b) Experimental and numerical simulation studies of the fluidization characteristics of a separating gas-solid fluidized bed. Fuel Process Technol 91(2):1819–1825

41. Zhao YM, Li GM, Luo ZF, Liang CC, Tang LG, Chen ZQ, Xing HB (2011a) Modularized dry coal beneficiation technique based on gas-solid fluidized bed. J Cent South Univ Technol 18(2):374–380

42. Zhao YM, Liu XJ, Liu KL, Luo ZF, Wu WC, Song SL, Tang LG (2011b) Fluidization characteristics of a gas-paigeite-powder bed to be utilized for dry coal beneficiation. Int J Coal Prep Utili 31(3–4):149–160

# Chapter 8

# Research on Effectiveness of Coal Mine Safety Supervision System Reform on Three Types of Collieries in China

**Quanlong Liu • Xinchun Li • Fuyuan Guan**

*School of Management, China University of Mining and Technology, Xuzhou 221116, China*

## ABSTRACT

Coal mine safety supervision system plays an important role in the coal mine safety management in China. However, the current supervision system is established on the basis of learning the advanced experience from other developed countries. It needs to be further improved according to national conditions. Therefore, the effectiveness of coal mine safety supervision system reform on three types of collieries are assessed by using time series analysis method based on comparative analysis of the supervision system before and after the reform in this paper. The regression results show that the structural reform is not conductive to the improvement of coal mine safety situation in the short term, but conductive significantly in the long term. Specifically, the effects in township coal mines are more significant than state-owned key coal mines in the long run, but negative effects also exist in the short term. The negative effects in state-owned key coal mines are non-significant compared with township coal mines. Moreover, the regression results are analyzed from the aspects of the closure policy of illegal small township coal mines at the end of 1998 and shortage of the new supervision system. Finally, the suggestions on improving the new supervision system are put forward based on the above analysis.

**Keywords:** Coal mine safety supervision Time series analysis Structural reform Death rate per million tonnes Effectiveness of supervision

## 1 INTRODUCTION

Coal accounts for more than 70 % of China's energy. The coal-dominated energy structure is unlikely to be changed for a long period because China is rich in coal, poor in oil and gas (Wang2006). In recent years, frequent coal mine accidents not only caused huge losses of life and property, but also had a negative influence on the society. Although the data of total accidents, death toll and death rate per million tonnes from *China Coal Industry Statistical Yearbook*have decreased year after year (Table 1), the coal mine safety situation is still very grim compared with some developed countries. Therefore, coal mine safety remains one of the most significant outstanding problems in China (Liu et al. 2011; Li 2012). The complex mining geological condition, backward technology and equipment, insufficient skills of miners, and weak safety foundation are the fact that does not dispute for the bad coal mine safety situation in China. But coal mine safety supervision system plays a dominant role in regulating collieries and bear great responsibility for China's bad coal mine safety situation. Consequently, China began to reform fundamentally the coal mine safety management system at the end of 1999 and established a new coal mine safety supervision system which is "State Supervision, Local Regulation and Enterprise Responsibility", namely the State Administration of Coal Mine Safety and the local coal mine safety regulation department share the task of administrative enforcement on coal mine safety production (Liu and Li 2013). But how was the effectiveness of the coal mine safety supervision system reform?

Many scholars at home and abroad studied the current problems of China's coal mine supervision system from different aspects to explain the high occurrence of coal mine accidents. Wright (2004) have analyzed the regulation of China's township and village collieries, they pointed out that the current regulatory policy can't solve the problem fundamentally and a targeted regulation system should be set up. A number of studies have quantitatively analyzed the effectiveness of coal mine safety supervisions (Viscusi 1979, 1986; Lewis-Back and Alford1980; Gray and Jones 1991), and the results showed that there exist significant correlation between coal mine accidents rate and the intensity of government supervision. Chinese scholar Xiao (2009, 2010) have empirically studied the effectiveness of China's coal mine safety regulation based on VAR model, and he drew the conclusion that

China's coal mine safety regulation was effective in the long run. However, there is less research on quantitative study of China's coal mine safety supervision, especially on quantitative study of the three types of collieries, and most research to date has focused on qualitative analysis. Therefore, in this paper, the effectiveness of coal mine safety supervision system reform on the three types of collieries (state-owned key coal mines, local state-owned coal mines and township coal mines) are studied by using time series analysis method.

**Table 1.** Safety situation after the coal mine safety supervision system reform in China

| Time | State-owned key coal mines | | | Local state-owned coal mines | | | Township coal mines | | |
|---|---|---|---|---|---|---|---|---|---|
| | Output (million tonnes) | Death toll | Death rate per million tonnes (%) | Output (million tonnes) | Death toll | Death rate per million tones (%) | Output (million tonnes) | Death toll | Death rate per million tones (%) |
| 1998 | 503.49 | 542 | 1.02 | 242.02 | 910 | 3.76 | 531.98 | 4,575 | 8.60 |
| 1999 | 512.71 | 572 | 0.92 | 253.89 | 947 | 3.73 | 360.31 | 4,666 | 12.95 |
| 2000 | 535.74 | 765 | 1.44 | 201.22 | 827 | 4.11 | 269.20 | 3,933 | 14.61 |
| 2001 | 618.57 | 781 | 1.27 | 254.63 | 1,044 | 4.10 | 245.95 | 3,645 | 14.82 |
| 2002 | 714.58 | 904 | 1.27 | 267.10 | 1,023 | 3.83 | 433.53 | 5,068 | 11.69 |
| 2003 | 814.05 | 892 | 1.07 | 293.67 | 881 | 3.00 | 612.48 | 4,661 | 7.61 |
| 2004 | 938.79 | 854 | 0.93 | 301.11 | 816 | 2.71 | 742.25 | 4,357 | 5.87 |
| 2005 | 1,024.21 | 984 | 0.93 | 279.41 | 570 | 2.04 | 792.77 | 4,384 | 5.53 |
| 2006 | 1,119.56 | 704 | 0.63 | 319.90 | 611 | 1.91 | 882.01 | 3,431 | 3.89 |
| 2007 | 1,214.91 | 475 | 0.38 | 318.60 | 411 | 1.29 | 960.26 | 2,900 | 3.02 |
| 2008 | 1,377.81 | 454 | 0.33 | 246.01 | 401 | 1.63 | 995.78 | 2,360 | 2.37 |
| 2009 | 1,526.34 | 580 | 0.38 | 394.25 | 294 | 0.75 | 1,091.92 | 1,757 | 1.61 |
| 2010 | 1,624.16 | 478 | 0.29 | 519.73 | 255 | 0.49 | 1,199.72 | 1,700 | 1.42 |
| 2011 | 1,689.11 | 351 | 0.21 | 549.16 | 231 | 0.42 | 1,259.96 | 1,391 | 1.10 |

# 2 MATERIALS AND METHODS

## 2.1 Comparative analysis of the supervision system before and after the reform

China's coal administrative supervision system and coal industry production system had been repeatedly changed with the characteristics of frequently separating and integrating in turn after long intervals (Yan 2009). Premier Zhou firstly put forward the policy of "safety first" in the first national coal conference in 1949 and then the Ministry of Fuel Industry was established which managed coal, electricity and oil industry. In 1953, the Technical Supervision Bureau was established which was subordinate to the Ministry of Fuel Industry, it marked the initial formation of coal mine safety management system, "administrative management, trade union supervision and labor department inspection". In July 1955, the Ministry of Coal Industry and its subordinate Safety Supervision Bureau were established by withdrawing the Ministry of Fuel Industry in the second session of the first National People's

Congress. But coal mine safety supervision had not been paid enough attention in the actual coal production, especially in the period of "Great Leap Forward" and "Cultural Revolution", which was interrupted (Wang 2004). In short, the management system was the "almighty management mode" in this period.

After the Third Plenary Session of the 11th Central Committee, China's coal mine safety management entered a new stage of recovery and development, and gradually institutionalized, it showed a change from the "almighty management mode" to "supervision management mode". In 1983, the Ministry of Coal Industry promulgated the *Regulations of Coal Mine Safety Supervision*. In 1993, the State Council proposed the coal mine safety management system which is "enterprise responsibility, state supervision, sectional management and public surveillance" according to the development of the reform of market system and state-owned coal mining enterprises. In 1998, the organ of the State Council reformed, and the Ministry of Coal Industry was canceled and its coal mine safety work was allocated to the Safety Production Bureau of State Economic and Trade Commission.

China began to reform fundamentally the coal mine safety management system at the end of 1999. On December 30 1999, the General Office of the State Council of the People's Republic of China promulgated the "Circular on Printing and Distributing the Implementation Plan on the Reform of Coal Mine Safety Management System" and drafted the new *Regulations of Coal Mine Safety Supervision*, and began to establish a new coal mine safety supervision system which was vertical management (Zhang 2001). In 2001, the new coal mine safety supervision system was composed of 19 provincial administration of coal mine safety bureaus and 68 sub-administration of coal mine safety offices, which was three-level and vertical supervision system included the state, province and region levels. In March 2003, the State Administration of Work Safety (the State Administration of Coal Mine Safety) became the institutions directly under the State Council and was responsible for the comprehensive management of national safety production and coal mine safety supervision. In 2005, the State Administration of Work Safety was upgraded to a ministry-level agency, and the State Administration of Coal Mine Safety was set up separately and upgraded to a vice-ministerial level agency under the State Administration of Work Safety. In 2006, the general office of the State Council promulgated "Views on the Relevant Issues about Strengthening the Coal Industry Management" and transferred the functions related to coal mine safety from the State Development and Reform Commission to the State Administration of Coal Mine Safety. Since then, China's coal mine safety supervision was dual leadership of the State Administration of Coal Mine Safety and the local government, and mainly by the State Administration of Coal Mine Safety (Wang 2010), namely the State

Administration of Coal Mine Safety and the local coal mine safety regulation departments share the task of administrative enforcement on coal mine safety production, as shown in Fig. 1.

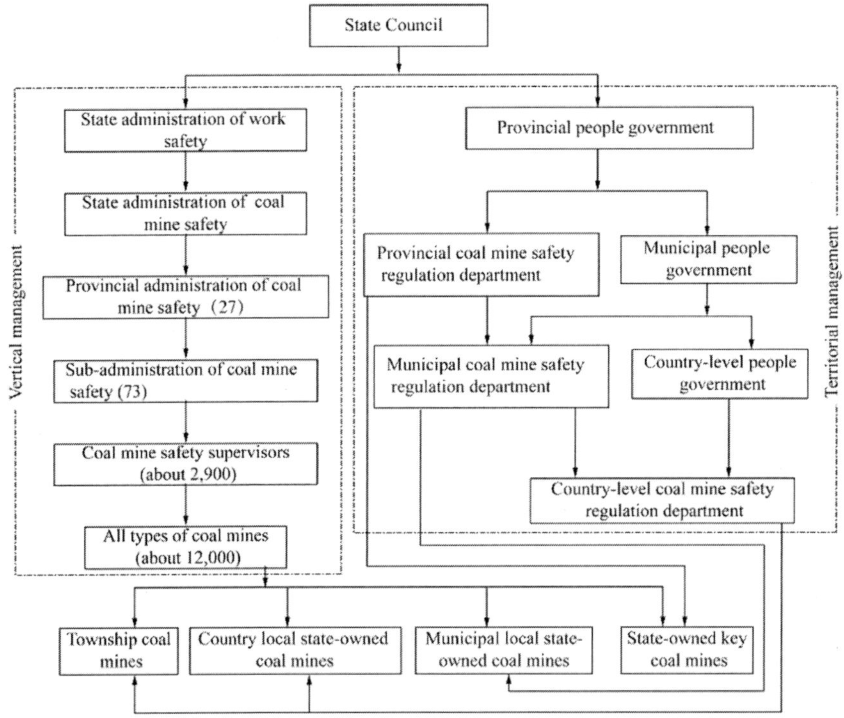


**Figure 1.** Structure of coal mine safety supervisions system in China

## 2.2 Model design and data

The time series analysis method was used in assessing the effectiveness of many policies by many scholars, and it has improved continuously and has been proved to have strong explanatory power on assessing the effectiveness of structural reform (Zheng and Cui 2011). The basic idea of this method is that select a continuous period data which can reflect the safety situation and design the econometric model. Firstly, the econometric model was designed as follows according to the above comparative analysis of supervision system before and after the reform.

$$Y_t = \beta_0 + \beta_1 X_{1t} + \beta_2 D_{1t} + \beta_3 D_{2t} + e_t$$

where $Y_t$ is the variable used to represent the annual safety situation of coal mines; $X_{1t}$ is the time variable, also called the trend variable and used to assess the time, value from 1 to N; $D_{1t}$ is the dummy variable, and given the value 0 before 2,000 and 1 after 2,000; $D_{2t}$ is the dummy variable that assess the time, and given the value 0 before 2,000 and 1, 2, 3, ... after 2,000; $\beta_0$,$\beta_1$, $\beta_2$ and $\beta_3$ are the regression coefficient; and $e_t$ is the residuals.

In the above model, $\beta_0$ and $\beta_1$ represent the safety level of coal mine and variation trend respectively, namely the intercept and slope of linear regression. And $\beta_2$ and $\beta_3$ represent the effects after the structural reform in 2000. Specifically, $\beta_2$ represents level effects, namely short-term effects; and $\beta_3$ represents trend effects, namely long-term effects. Therefore, the effectiveness of the structural reform can be obtained from assessing whether $\beta_0$ and $\beta_1$ are affected or not, namely detecting the statistical significance of $\beta_2$ and $\beta_3$. If $\beta_2$ is significantly different from 0, then the supervision system reform has a short-term effects on the improvement of coal mine safety, and vice versa. And if $\beta_3$ is significantly different from 0, then the supervision system reform has a long-term effects on the improvement of coal mine safety, and vice versa. Finally, the effectiveness of the supervision system reform on state-owned key coal mines, local state-owned coal mines and township coal mines can be obtained by using the above econometric model.

In the econometric model, the value of $X_{1t}$, $D_{1t}$ and $D_{2t}$ have been given except $Y_t$. There are many indicators which can represent the annual safety situation of coal mines, such as the data of annual total accidents, death, et al. However, in this paper, we selected the death rate per million tonnes as the assessment indicator for the following considerations. Firstly, death is the most serious accident consequences in coal mine production. Secondly, the death rate per million tonnes has a high correlativity with other data and can reflect other data indirectly. Thirdly, it is more generic and not be affected by other factors, such as output of coal, death toll, et al.

The data of death rate per million tonnes in state-owned key coal mines, local state-owned coal mines and township coal mines are collected from *China Coal Industry Statistical Yearbook*and the website of State Administration of Coal Mine Safety, and the sample interval is 1989–2011. The value of $X_{1t}$, $D_{1t}$, $D_{2t}$, and $Y_t$ are shown in the following Table 2 based on the above analysis.

## 2.3 Empirical results

The regression coefficients of the econometric model are obtained by using the econometric analysis software EViews (Zheng and Cui 2011), and they are tested with F-test, *t* test, Heteroskedasticity test and Autocorrelation test. Furthermore, the model is modified continually until it passed all the tests at the significance level of 5 %. Finally, the regression results of the model are sort out in Table 3.

**Table 2.** Data of $Y_t$, $X_{1t}$, $D_{1t}$, and $D_{2t}$ in 1989–2011

| Time | $Y_t$ | | | $X_{1t}$ | $D_{1t}$ | $D_{2t}$ |
|---|---|---|---|---|---|---|
| | State-owned key coal mines | Local state-owned coal mines | Township coal mines | | | |
| 1989 | 1.74 | 6.30 | 13.00 | 1 | 0 | 0 |
| 1990 | 1.43 | 5.00 | 12.79 | 2 | 0 | 0 |
| 1991 | 1.06 | 6.20 | 10.10 | 3 | 0 | 0 |
| 1992 | 1.01 | 4.50 | 9.20 | 4 | 0 | 0 |
| 1993 | 1.12 | 4.90 | 8.50 | 5 | 0 | 0 |
| 1994 | 1.19 | 4.82 | 8.32 | 6 | 0 | 0 |
| 1995 | 1.16 | 4.90 | 8.13 | 7 | 0 | 0 |
| 1996 | 1.17 | 4.02 | 7.70 | 8 | 0 | 0 |
| 1997 | 1.45 | 4.13 | 8.44 | 9 | 0 | 0 |
| 1998 | 1.02 | 3.76 | 8.60 | 10 | 0 | 0 |
| 1999 | 0.92 | 3.73 | 12.95 | 11 | 0 | 0 |
| 2000 | 1.44 | 4.11 | 14.61 | 12 | 1 | 1 |
| 2001 | 1.27 | 4.10 | 14.82 | 13 | 1 | 2 |
| 2002 | 1.27 | 3.83 | 11.69 | 14 | 1 | 3 |
| 2003 | 1.07 | 3.00 | 7.61 | 15 | 1 | 4 |
| 2004 | 0.93 | 2.71 | 5.87 | 16 | 1 | 5 |
| 2005 | 0.93 | 2.04 | 5.53 | 17 | 1 | 6 |
| 2006 | 0.63 | 1.91 | 3.89 | 18 | 1 | 7 |
| 2007 | 0.38 | 1.29 | 3.02 | 19 | 1 | 8 |
| 2008 | 0.33 | 1.63 | 2.37 | 20 | 1 | 9 |
| 2009 | 0.38 | 0.75 | 1.61 | 21 | 1 | 10 |
| 2010 | 0.29 | 0.49 | 1.42 | 22 | 1 | 11 |
| 2011 | 0.21 | 0.42 | 1.10 | 23 | 1 | 12 |

**Table 3.** Regression results

| Explanatory variables | State-owned key coal mines | | | Local state-owned coal mines | | | Township coal mines | | |
|---|---|---|---|---|---|---|---|---|---|
| | Coefficient | *t*-stat | *P*-stat | Coefficient | *t*-stat | *P*-stat | Coefficient | *t*-stat | *P*-stat |
| $C$ ($\beta_0$) | 1.436 | 13.236 | 0.0000 | 6.113 | 25.280 | 0.0000 | 11.177 | 9.109 | 0.0000 |
| $X_{1t}$ | −0.038 | −2.393 | 0.0278 | −0.227 | −6.369 | 0.0000 | −0.231 | −1.274 | 0.0218 |
| $D_{1t}$ | 0.549 | 3.815 | 0.0013 | 1.044 | 3.253 | 0.0044 | 6.037 | 3.811 | 0.0012 |
| $D_{2t}$ | −0.087 | −3.858 | 0.0012 | −0.157 | −3.126 | 0.0058 | −1.085 | −4.508 | 0.0002 |
| $R^2$ | 0.845 | | | 0.955 | | | 0.828 | | |
| *F*-stat | 32.63 | | | 127.84 | | | 30.58 | | |
| *D*–*W* test | 1.91 | | | 2.14 | | | 1.82 | | |

The following results can be drawn from the Table 3.

(1)The structural reform has had a big influence on the safety situation of coal mines and its work is effective on the whole. Specifically, the regression coefficients of $C$,$X_{1t}$, $D_{1t}$ and $D_{2t}$ are all significant under the significance level of 5 %, and their symbols of t-stat are positive, negative, positive and negative respectively. And the results show that there are different degrees of improvement trend of safety situation in state-owned key coal mines, local state-owned coal mines and township coal mines.

(2)Coal mine safety situation in state-owned key coal mines is better than local state-owned coal mines, and local state-owned coal mines is better than township coal mines before the structural reform according to $\beta_0$ (state-owned key coal mines) >$\beta_0$(local state-owned coal mines) >$\beta_0$ (township coal mines). This is correspond to actual situation that the state-owned key coal mines mostly have large production scale and high equipment and technology level while the township coal mines mostly have small production scale, less investment and backward equipment and technology.

(3)In the short term, the structural reform is not conductive to the improvement of coal mine safety situation, and negative effects are different in the three types of collieries. Specifically, the negative effects in state-owned key coal mines are non-significant compared with township coal mines.

(4)In the long term, the structural reform is conductive significantly to the improvement of coal mine safety situation, and positive effects are also different in the three types of collieries. Specifically, the effects of the new supervision system in township coal mines are more significant than the effects in state-owned key coal mines. Therefore, the township coal mines have much room for improvement compared with the state-owned coal mines.

# 3 RESULTS ANALYSES

The regression results are mainly analyzed from the aspects of the closure policy of illegal small township coal mines at the end of 1998 and shortage of the new supervision system.

## 3.1 The closure policy of illegal small township coal mines at the end of 1998

The structural reform is not conductive to the improvement of coal mine safety situation in the short term, and this result can also be shown in Table 1, which the death rate per million tonnes fluctuated greatly in 1998–2002, especially in the township coal mines. This result is much more related with the closure policy of illegal small township coal mines at the end of 1998.

The closure policy has mainly brought two aspects of negative influence. Firstly, the closure of small coal mines was carried out in batches, so when a number of small coal mines was closed, other small coal mines would have a sense of crisis and then they would produce hastily and didn't pay attention to safety issues more before they were shut down, which lead to the increase of accidents. Secondly, the supply of coal decreased greatly and may even in short supply owning to closing many small coal mines, which would lead to high coal prices and profits and then many other coal mines would be possible to increase their outputs and ignore the safety issues. Many illegal small township coal mines couldn't be completely shut down. Some of them still recovered production behind closed doors, and they produced hastily and didn't pay attention to safety issues more for compensating the considerable loss in their rectification period. In short, the negative effects from the closure period and recovery period greatly lead to the safety record worsened in the short term.

## 3.2 The shortage of the new coal mine safety supervision system

The regression results show that the structural reform is conductive significantly to the improvement of China's coal mine safety situation in the long run and its effect is significant at the significance level of 5 %, but the goodness of fit of the data are not very good. From the aspect of the shortages of the new coal mine safety supervision system, the reasons are as follows.

(1)The vertical supervision system has caused unclear rights and responsibilities between the State Administration of Coal Mine Safety and the local coal mine regulation departments. Because of lacking effective coordination mechanisms, the two kinds of department act of their own free will for their interests, and even some central supervision departments and local regulation departments are the one department in some areas and they undertake the function of supervision and management at the same time (Zhen 2009).

(2)The Administration of Coal Mine Safety is short of independence and authority. In the process of law enforcement, they have no independent power of penalty and compulsory right to execution on local regulation departments' illegal enforcement or coal mines' illegal production (Xiao 2010).

(3)The local coal mine safety regulation departments are of serious malpractice on regulating their territorial mines. The local government has great law enforcements in the coal mine safety supervision and regulation work, but in order to develop its local economy, it often ignore national interests and long-term interests and cause the prevalence of local protectionism.

In short, the above shortages of the new coal mine safety supervision system have weakened its supervision effects, and this also increased the probability of accidents to a large extent.

# 4 CONCLUSIONS AND SUGGESTIONS

In this paper, we studied the effectiveness of coal mine safety supervision system reform on state-owned key coal mines, local state-owned coal mines and township coal mines by using time series analysis method. The regression results show that the structural reform has had a big influence on the safety situation of coal mines and its work is effective on the whole. In the short term, the structural reform is not conductive to the improvement of coal mine safety situation, and negative effects are different in the three types of coal mines. Specifically, the negative effects in state-owned key coal mines are non-significant compared with township coal mines. In the long term, the structural reform is conductive significantly to the improvement of coal mine safety situation, and positive effects are also different in the three types of coal mines. Specifically, the effects of the new supervision system in township coal mines are more significant than the effects in state-owned key coal mines. Therefore, the Administration of Coal Mine Safety should take measures to perfect its supervision system on the basis of the above conclusions and analysis. (1) Ensure the independence and authority of the Administration of Coal Mine Safety, and establish effective supervision system to avoid its abuse of power at the same time; (2) avoid frequent changes of supervision organization and coordinate its relationship with the legislation departments, administration departments and justice department;

(3) stabilize the policy on the township coal mines and encourage long-term legal business, and also periodically inspect the township coal mines which have passed the security acceptance; (4) weaken the beneficial relations between local government and township coal mines. The tax from the township coal mines can be mostly submitted to central government and then return to local government according to their different demands, and the rest can be used as safety fund for granting appropriate subsidies to the legitimate township coal mines.

## ACKNOWLEDGMENTS

This work was supported by the National Natural Science Foundation Projects of China under Grant 71271206; and Innovation Project of Graduate Education for Jiangsu Province under Grant KYZZ_0377.

## REFERENCES

1. Gray WB, Jones CA (1991) Are OASA health inspections effective? a longitudinal study in the manufacturing sector. Rev Econ Stat 73(3):504–508
2. Lewis-Back MS, Alford JR (1980) Can government regulate safety? The coal mine example. Am Polit Sci Rev 74(3):745–756
3. Li JK (2012) China strategic coal stockpile and its supervision mechanism. Economy & Management Publishing House, Beijing
4. Liu QL, Li XC (2013) Study on the efficiency of the structural reform of coal mine safety supervision system in China. China Popul Resour Environ 23(11):161–167
5. Liu QL, Li XC, Zhang QC (2011) Study on the risk measurement and the coupling analysis of multi hazard source in coal gas accident. J Saf Coal Mines 42(7):189–192
6. Viscusi WK (1979) The impact of occupational safety and health supervision. Bell J Econ 10(1):117–140
7. Viscusi WK (1986) The impact of occupational safety and health supervision in 1973–1983. Rand J Econ 17(4):567–580
8. Wang SG (2004) The regulation of coal mine safety production: the transformation of China's governance mode. Comp Stud 13:79–110
9. Wang MZ (2006) Innovate the safety supervision and constructing the harmonious society. Mod Occup Saf 12:62–64

10. Wang BJ (2010) Safety management of modern coal mine production in China. China Sci Technol Rev 06:190-190

11. Wright T (2004) The political economy of coal mine disasters in China: your rice bowl or your life. China Q 179:629–646

12. Xiao XZ (2009) The economic analysis of coal mine safety supervision in China. Capital University of Economics and Business Press, Beijing

13. Xiao XZ (2010) Theory and practice of coal mine safety supervision in China. Science press, Beijing

14. Yan Y (2009) The changes in China's coal mine safety supervision system. Contemp China Hist Stud 16:42–51

15. Zhang YJ (2001) Analysis of the township coal mine safety supervision system. China Coal 27(10):48–50

16. Zhen Y (2009) Reflection on China's coal mine safety production supervision. J Shandong Inst Bus Technol 23(04):31–34

17. Zheng FT, Cui HX (2011) Economic analysis of safety supervision. Huazhong University of Science and Technology Press, Wuhan

# Index